Neurotrauma

Evidence-Based Answers to Common Questions

Thieme

Neurotrauma

Evidence-Based Answers to Common Questions

Alex B. Valadka, M.D., F.A.C.S.

Associate Professor of Neurosurgery
Baylor College of Medicine
Chief of Neurosurgery
Ben Taub General Hospital
Houston, Texas

Brian T. Andrews, M.D., F.A.C.S.

Chairman, Division of Neurosurgery
Vice Chairman, Department of Neurosciences, California Pacific Medical Center
Attending Neurosurgeon
Department of Neurological Surgery
University of California–San Francisco
San Francisco, California

Foreword by
Donald P. Becker, M.D.

Thieme
New York • Stuttgart

Thieme Medical Publishers, Inc.
333 Seventh Ave.
New York, NY 10001

Assistant Editor: Jennifer Berger
Editor: Timothy Hiscock
Vice President, Production and Electronic Publishing: Anne T. Vinnicombe
Production Editor: Print Matters, Inc.
Marketing Director: Phyllis Gold
Sales Director: Ross Lumpkin
Chief Financial Officer: Peter van Woerden
President: Brian D. Scanlan
Compositor: Techset Composition Limited
Printer: Maple-Vail Book Manufacturing Group

Library of Congress Cataloging-in-Publication Data

Valadka, Alex B.
Neurotrauma: evidence-based answers to common questions/[edited by] Alex B. Valadka,
Brian T. Andrews; foreword by Donald P. Becker.
p.; cm.
Includes bibliographical references and index.
ISBN 1-58890-266-8 (HC : TMP) – ISBN 3-13-130781-1 (HC : GTV)
1. Nervous system–Wounds and injuries. 2. Brain–Wounds and injuries.
3. Head–Wounds and injuries. 4. Spinal cord–Wounds and injuries.
5. Evidence-based medicine. I. Andrew, Brian T. II. Title.
[DNLM: 1. Craniocerebral Trauma–therapy. 2. Evidence-Based Medicine.
3. Spinal Cord Injuries–therapy. WL 354 N49449 2005]
RD593.V354 2005
617.4'81044–dc22

Important note: Medical knowledge is ever-changing. As new research and clinical experience broaden our knowledge, changes in treatment and drug therapy may be required. The authors and editors of the material herein have consulted sources believed to be reliable in their efforts to provide information that is complete and in accord with the standards accepted at the time of publication. However, in view of the possibility of human error by the authors, editors, or publisher of the work herein or changes in medical knowledge, neither the authors, editors, or publisher, nor any other party who has been involved in the preparation of this work, warrants that the information contained herein is in every respect accurate or complete, and they are not responsible for any errors or omissions or for the results obtained from use of such information. Readers are encouraged to confirm the information contained herein with other sources. For example, readers are advised to check the product information sheet included in the package of each drug they plan to administer to be certain that the information contained in this publication is accurate and that changes have not been made in the recommended dose or in the contraindications for administration. This recommendation is of particular importance in connection with new or infrequently used drugs.

Printed in the United States of America

5 4 3 2

TMP ISBN 1-58890-266-8
GTV ISBN 3 13 130781 1

To my children, Patrick and Jaclyn, for their long-suffering and often inconvenient indulgence of their father's work in neurotrauma and critical care.

Alex B. Valadka

To my wife Linda for being there always. And to the members of the AANS/CNS Section on Neurotrauma and Critical Care for their devotion to our field.

Brian T. Andrews

Contents

IV. Spinal Cord Injury

V. Postacute Care

VI. Sports Medicine

VII. Trauma Systems

Foreword

The modern effort to use sound scientific principles in the management of traumatically brain injured patients followed the introduction of intracranial pressure monitoring. Other technologies, including the application of controlled ventilation, cerebral blood flow monitoring, computed tomographic brain scanning, and sophisticated brain electrophysiological monitoring, enhanced methodologies for earlier diagnosis and continuous evaluation of a brain-injured patient's intracranial pathobiological condition. Dependable neurological evaluation scales (e.g., the Glasgow Coma Scale) contributed a critical method for defining and comparing patients according to their level of coma. In 1977, a published report in the *Journal of Neurosurgery* from the brain injury group at the Medical College of Virginia demonstrated an astounding 30% reduction in mortality rate for those with severe brain injuries after application of early diagnosis and treatment of mass lesions coupled with modern organized intensive care management.

The mortality reduction translated directly into an increase in good outcomes. The percentage of poor functioning survivors (severely disabled or vegetative individuals) did not increase. That report has subsequently been confirmed in multiple studies utilizing various designs. The management principles initially promulgated in that publication, which were based on scientific knowledge and expert opinion, are today widely applied, and the outcome data are generally accepted as accurate.

The knowledge that traumatic brain injury management could be defined according to scientific principles provided the stimulus for this area to be the first identified by organized neurosurgery for the development of "guidelines." This resulted in the 1995 creation by the Brain Trauma Foundation of *Guidelines for the Management of Severe Head Injury*.

These guidelines, although useful and widely referenced, have limitations, primarily because the pathobiology of traumatic brain injury is complex and because the physiological, chemical, and anatomic status of the injured brain will often change from hour to hour and day to day. Controlled, randomized, and blinded studies in brain trauma are notoriously difficult to construct, in large part because patients vary in degree, extent, and location of pathobiological cellular and subcellular injury. Thus brain trauma guidelines demanding a full and rigorous scientific basis presently have major limitations.

Alex B. Valadka and Brian T. Andrews, the editors of this book, make a remarkably useful contribution by enhancing the guidelines concept with the addition of expert opinion. The result is a readable, workable, interesting, and up-to-date book, which provides authoritative information that will no doubt be applied to and improve patient management. Their selection of authors to provide expert opinion is especially outstanding, and I enjoyed reading the individual chapters because of the practical and accurate presentations. Patients with severe traumatic brain injury and individuals caring for them will benefit from this timely and carefully developed contribution.

Donald P. Becker, M.D.
Los Angeles, CA 2004

Preface

The introduction and widespread acceptance of the guidelines process has had a noticeable impact on the care of neurotrauma patients. Guidelines serve to remind us of what we should be doing all the time: treating our patients based on the best available evidence. However, the downside of a rigorous guidelines process is that it does not allow the formulation of meaningful recommendations on a topic for which well-conducted clinical trials have not been carried out and reported. In certain quarters, this problem has led to some backlash against guidelines and to a sense of disillusionment with how little they often tell us.

This book is intended to combine clinical evidence with the wisdom and experience of experts in order to give answers to specific questions. The questions themselves were chosen in no particular order. Instead, they arose on daily rounds and during everyday conversations with colleagues and trainees. For the purposes of this book, these questions were organized into sections on resuscitation and initial assessment, general critical care, brain injury, spinal cord injury, recovery, sports medicine, and trauma systems. Undoubtedly, many other questions could have been asked, and new questions will continue to arise. Such topics can easily form the basis of future books, monographs, and review articles.

The target audience for this book is anyone who needs information about these questions. Certainly, students and residents fit this category, but physicians who are unfamiliar with this material, who may not have had to use it for a long time, or who would like an update or simple verification that they are treating patients in an acceptable manner could also benefit from this book. In addition to neurosurgeons, interested specialists might include intensivists, trauma surgeons, emergency physicians, neurologists, anesthesiologists, pediatricians, and virtually anyone else who comes into contact with these patients. Allied health practitioners who might be interested in these questions include nurses, physician assistants, certified registered nurse anesthetists, paramedics, speech therapists, respiratory therapists, and a host of others.

This book would not have been possible without the efforts of a great many people. The authors of the individual chapters tolerated our insistence that they adhere to a strict format for their chapters. They also put up with numerous edits, revisions, and rewrites with a minimum of complaining. At Thieme, Brian Scanlan was always optimistic that this book would be completed, even when such optimism did not seem warranted. Finally, Sylvia Melendez spent countless hours finding references, verifying the accuracy of citations, organizing mountains of correspondence and hundreds of e-mails, proofreading each version of each chapter several times, and shepherding this project along to its completion.

We hope that the readers find this book to be interesting and informative. Most of all, we hope that the material contained in these pages may help at least a few neurotrauma patients achieve better outcomes.

Alex B. Valadka, M.D., F.A.C.S.
Houston, Texas
Brian T. Andrews, M.D., F.A.C.S.
San Francisco, California

Contributors

Brian T. Andrews, M.D., F.A.C.S.
Chairman, Division of Neurosurgery
Vice Chairman, Department of Neurosciences,
California Pacific Medical Center
Attending Neurosurgeon
Department of Neurological Surgery
University of California–San Francisco
San Francisco, CA

John L.D. Atkinson, M.D.
Associate Professor
Department of Neurosurgery
Mayo Clinic
Rochester, MN

Julian E. Bailes, M.D.
Chairman
Department of Neurosurgery
West Virginia University School of Medicine
Morgantown, WV

Donald P. Becker, M.D.
Professor
Division of Neurosurgery
University of California–Los Angeles
Director
UCLA Brain Tumor Program
Director
Neurosurgery Skull Base Lab at UCLA
Los Angeles, CA

Christopher M. Bono, M.D.
Assistant Professor
Department of Orthopaedic Surgery
Boston University Medical Center
Boston, MA

Mark G. Burnett, M.D.
Department of Neurosurgery
University of Pennsylvania
Philadelphia, PA

Robert C. Cantu, M.D.
Chief of Neurosurgery
Director
Service of Sports Medicine
Emerson Hospital
Concord, MA

Jeff W. Chen, M.D., Ph.D., F.A.C.S.
Director of Neurotrauma
Department of Neurological Surgery
Legacy Emanuel Hospital
Portland, OR

Guy L. Clifton, M.D.
Professor and Chairman
Department of Neurosurgery
Director, Vivian L. Smith Center for Neurological
Research
University of Texas Medical School at Houston
Houston, TX

Pejman Cohan, M.D.
Assistant Professor
Department of Medicine
Division of Endocrinology and Metabolism
University of California–Los Angeles
Los Angeles, CA

Shon W. Cook, M.D.
Division of Neurosurgery
University of California–Los Angeles
Los Angeles, CA

William M. Coplin, M.D.
Associate Professor
Departments of Neurology and
Neurological Surgery
Wayne State University
Medical Director, Neurotrauma and
Critical Care
Chief of Neurology
Detroit Receiving Hospital
Detroit, MI

Manuela Cormio, M.D.
Department of Anestesia e Rianimazione
Universita Milano-Bicocca
Hospitale S. Gerardo Monza
Monza, Italy

Harel Deutsch, M.D.
Assistant Professor
Department of Neurosurgery
Rush Medical College
Rush University Medical Center
Chicago, IL

Ann-Christine Duhaime, M.D.
Professor
Department of Neurosurgery
Dartmouth Medical School
Lebanon, NH

J. Paul Elliott, M.D.
Rocky Mountain Neurological Associates
Englewood, CO

Christopher N. Faber, M.D.
Division of Respiratory Diseases and Critical Care Medicine
Allegheny General Hospital
Pittsburgh, PA

Azadeh Farin, B.S.
Department of Neurosurgery
University of California–San Diego
San Diego, CA

Michael G. Fehlings, M.D., Ph.D., F.R.S.C.
Professor
Krembil Chair in Neural Repair and Regeneration
Department of Surgery
University of Toronto
Krembil Neuroscience Center
Toronto Western Hospital
Toronto, ON

Henry Feuer, M.D.
Indianapolis Neurosurgical Group
Indianapolis, IN

Fred H. Geisler, M.D., Ph.D.
Illinois Neuro-Spine Center
Rush-Copley Medical Center
Aurora, IL

Jamshid Ghajar, M.D., Ph.D.
Brain Trauma Foundation
New York, NY

Jonas J. Gopez, M.D.
Department of Neurosurgery
Temple University
Philadelphia, PA

Roger Hartl, M.D.
Assistant Professor
Department of Neurosurgery
Weill-Medical College of Cornell University
New York, NY

Robert F. Heary, M.D.
Associate Professor
Director, The Spine Center of New Jersey
Department of Neurosurgery
UMDNJ–Robert Wood Johnson Medical School
Newark, NJ

Roman Hlatky, M.D.
Department of Neurosurgery
Baylor College of Medicine
Ben Taub General Hospital
Houston, TX

Colonel John B. Holcomb, M.D.
Commander, United States Army Institute of Surgical Research
Fort Sam Houston, TX

Matthias Jaeger, M.D.
Department of Neurosurgery
University of Leipzig
Leipzig, Germany

Daniel F. Kelly, M.D.
Associate Professor
Division of Neurosurgery
University of California–Los Angeles
Los Angeles, CA

Karl L. Kiening, M.D.
Professor
Department of Neurosurgery
University Hospital Heidelberg
Heidelberg, Germany

J. Kraus, M.D., Ph.D.
Department of Neurology
Wayne State University
Detroit, MI

Peter B. Letarte, M.D.
Department of Neurosurgery
Loyola University Medical Center
Maywood, IL

Jeffrey M. Lobosky, M.D.
Associate Clinical Professor
Department of Neurological Surgery
University of California–San Francisco
San Francisco, CA

John A. Lopez, M.D.
Department of Neurosurgery
University of Colorado
Denver, CO

John M. Luce, M.D.
Professor of Medicine and Anaesthesia
University of California-San Francisco
Director, Medical-Surgical Intensive Care Unit
San Francisco General Hospital
San Francisco, CA

R. Loch Macdonald, M.D., Ph.D.
Professor
Department of Neurosurgery
University of Chicago Medical Center
Chicago, IL

Donald W. Marion, M.D., M.Sc.
Senior Research Fellow
The Brain Trauma Foundation
New York, NY

Lawrence F. Marshall, M.D.
Professor and Chief
Division of Neurosurgery
Acting Director of Neurotrauma, Children's Hospital
University of California at San Diego
San Diego, CA

Richard J. Meagher, M.D.
Department of Neurosurgery
Temple University
Philadelphia, PA

Jürgen Meixensberger, M.D.
Professor
Department of Neurosurgery
University of Leipzig
Leipzig, Germany

Christopher Mendello, M.D.
Division of Pulmonology/Critical Care and Sleep Medicine
Wayne State University
Detroit, MI

José A. Menéndez, M.D.
Department of Neurological Surgery
Washington University
St. Louis, MO

Daniel B. Michael, M.D., Ph.D.
Adjunct Assistant Professor
Departments of Anatomy and Cell Biology and Neurosurgery
Wayne State University
Detroit, MI

Vincent J. Miele, M.D.
Department of Neurosurgery
West Virginia University School of Medicine
Morgantown, WV

J. Paul Muizelaar, M.D., Ph.D.
Professor and Chairman
Department of Neurological Surgery
University of California at Davis
Sacramento, CA

Raj K. Narayan, M.D.
Professor and Chairman
Department of Neurological Surgery
University of Cincinnati College of Medicine
Mayfield Clinic
Cincinnati, OH

David W. Newell, M.D.
Professor
Department of Neurological Surgery
University of Washington
Seattle, WA

Nelson M. Oyesiku, M.D., Ph.D.
Associate Professor
Department of Neurosurgery
Emory University School of Medicine
Atlanta, GA

Justin Pik, M.B., F.R.A.C.S.
Clinical Fellow
Division of Neurosurgery and Spinal Program
University of Toronto
Krembil Neuroscience Center
Toronto Western Hospital
Toronto, ON

Donald S. Prough, M.D.
Professor and Chairman
Department of Anesthesiology
University of Texas Medical Branch
Galveston, TX

Daniel K. Resnick, M.D., M.S.
Associate Professor
Department of Neurosurgery
University of Wisconsin
Madison, WI

Claudia S. Robertson, M.D.
Professor
Department of Neurosurgery
Baylor College of Medicine
Houston, TX

Juan Sahuquillo, M.D., Ph.D.
Professor
Department of Neurosurgery
Vall d'Hebron University Hospital
Autonomous University of Barcelona
Barcelona, Spain

Asita S. Sarrafzadeh, M.D.
Clinic of Neurosurgery
Charité Campus
Virchow Medical Center
Humboldt University
Berlin, Germany

Thomas M. Scalea, M.D.
Physician-in-Chief
R. Adams Cowley Shock Trauma Center
University of Maryland Medical Center
Baltimore, MD

Rudolph J. Schrot, M.D.
Department of Neurosurgery
University of California–Davis
Sacramento, CA

Lali H.S. Sekhon, M.B.B.S., Ph.D., F.R.A.C.S.
Clinical Fellow
Division of Neurosurgery
University of Toronto
Krembil Neuroscience Center
Toronto Western Hospital
Toronto, ON

Sherman C. Stein, M.D.
Clinical Professor
Department of Neurosurgery
University of Pennsylvania
Philadelphia, PA

Nino Stocchetti, M.D.
Istituto Anestesia e Rianimazione
Universita di Milano
Milan, Italy

John F. Stover, M.D., Ph.D.
Division of Surgical Intensive Care Medicine
University Hospital Zurich
Zurich, Switzerland

Charles H. Tator, M.D., Ph.D.
Professor
Department of Surgery
University of Toronto
Toronto Western Hospital
Toronto, ON

Nancy R. Temkin, Ph.D.
Professor
Departments of Neurological Surgery and Biostatistics
University of Washington
Seattle, WA

Shelly D. Timmons, M.D., Ph.D.
Semmes-Murphey Neurologic and Spine Institute
University of Tennessee Health Science Center
Memphis, TN

Donald D. Trunkey, M.D.
Professor
Department of Surgery
Oregon Health and Science University
Portland, OR

Jamie S. Ullman, M.D., F.A.C.S.
Associate Professor
Department of Neurosurgery
Mount Sinai School of Medicine
New York, NY

Andreas W. Unterberg, M.D.
Professor
Department of Neurosurgery
University Hospital Heidelberg
Heidelberg, Germany

Alex B. Valadka, M.D., F.A.C.S.
Associate Professor of Neurosurgery
Baylor College of Medicine
Chief of Neurosurgery
Ben Taub General Hospital
Houston, TX

Paul M. Vespa, M.D.
Assistant Professor
Director of Neurocritical Care
Division of Neurosurgery
University of California Los Angeles
Los Angeles, CA

Sandra M. Wanek, M.D.
Critical Care Fellow
Department of Surgery
Oregon Health and Science University
Portland, OR

Jack E. Wilberger, M.D.
Professor and Chairman
Department of Neurosurgery
Allegheny General Hospital
Pittsburgh, PA

Antonios Zikos, D.O.
Assistant Professor
Department of Medicine
Division of Respiratory Diseases and Critical Care Medicine
Allegheny General Hospital
Pittsburgh, PA

Introduction

Why do we do the things we do? When it comes to taking care of our patients, common reasons include, "That's how I was told to do it as a resident," or "That's how we've always done it," or "I had a case once in which I didn't do that, and I regretted it."

Similarly, during neurosurgical training, residents observe that different attendings manage patients with the same problems in different ways. Of course, each of us thinks that our own way of doing things is the best, but what is our basis for that assumption? Such questions were the genesis of this book.

This book is a review of the literature that answers specific questions that frequently arise during the care of neurotrauma patients. The authors, who were chosen on the basis of their expertise in specific areas, were asked to sift through the data. Because the literature pertinent to most of these questions was expected to be rather weak, the authors were asked, when appropriate, to incorporate their expert opinions into their answers.

However, this book is not a collection of formal guidelines. Creation of formal guidelines is often a complex, collaborative, and multistep process. Instead, these chapters were written by an individual or by a small group of authors; a group process of evaluating the literature was not used.

All too often, rigorously constructed guidelines documents cannot make firm recommendations because no prospective, randomized, controlled, blinded trials have been (or can be) constructed to answer a specific question. In neurosurgery, perhaps the best example of this problem concerns the need for immediate evacuation of a large, rapidly expanding epidural hematoma in a previously awake patient whose neurologic condition abruptly deteriorates. No one would randomize half of such patients to the nonoperative arm of a clinical trial. Thus, "proof" of the benefit of immediate surgery can never be obtained, and therefore a standard of care that recommends immediate evacuation will never be promulgated if one adheres to a rigorous methodology that allows only strict interpretation of the published literature.

Instead, the authors of this book were encouraged to give their best advice, even if based more on experience than on evidence. After all, clinicians confronted with a sick patient or difficult clinical problem don't need laundry lists of therapeutic options that might be weakly supported by the literature. What might be more useful is a brief review of the relevant literature on a specific topic, followed, when appropriate, by some suggestions from an expert in the field. Readers who want to review the literature are encouraged to do so for themselves. Perhaps they might even conduct their own clinical studies to answer some of these questions!

Such an approach may sometimes cause these answers to deviate from the published literature. On the other hand, it also allows common sense and experience to play a role in the analysis of the available data. After all, the synthesis of published evidence with experience and common sense represents the optimal practice of "evidence-based" medicine.[1,2] Moreover, allowing authors to state their opinions explicitly acknowledges the biases and prejudices of individual reviewers. Such subjective sources of error often seem to be glossed over or even ignored in formal guidelines documents. This issue is quite important because the end product of a formal process of guidelines construction may be heavily influenced by the biases of the particular experts who participated in it.

The approach to literature review that is used in this book follows the common practice of classifying evidence as class I, class II, or class III (Table 1).[2] However, to avoid confusing the conclusions in these chapters with those reached by a formal guidelines process, a different format of weighting recommendations was used. This format classifies recommendations as level I, level II, or level III (Table 2).

The astute reader will notice that different authors may classify the same study differently. Sometimes these differences arise because the authors use the same article to answer different questions. For example, a particular study may do a very good job of investigating the effects of a treatment on intracranial pressure (class I data), but it may provide only very

Table 1 Strength of Evidence

Type of Evidence	Examples
Class I	Prospective, randomized, controlled, blinded clinical trials
Class II	Studies based on prospectively collected data and retrospective analyses of reliable data, e.g., observational and cohort studies
Class III	Studies based on retrospectively collected data, e.g., clinical series, registry-based reports, case reports, expert opinion

Table 2 Strength of Recommendations

Strength of Recommendation	Meaning
Level I	Accepted management strategies with a high degree of clinical certainty
Level II	Management strategies with moderate clinical certainty
Level III	Management strategies with unclear clinical certainty

Level I recommendations are generally based on class I evidence, level II recommendations on class II evidence, and level III recommendations on class III evidence. However, conflicting or flawed class I or class II evidence may support only level II or level III recommendations, respectively. On the other hand, a preponderance of class II or class III evidence may support level I or level II recommendations, respectively, especially for issues that are difficult or impossible to test in a randomized, prospective trial.

poor data about clinical outcome (class III data). At other times, however, authors may honestly disagree about the strength of a study. In such cases, we again encourage the reader to analyze the data and formulate his or her own answer.

Interest in evidence-based medicine is growing rapidly. The Internet contains many Web sites with considerable information about this topic. Among the more useful sites are *www.guidelines.gov*, the "Trauma Practice Guidelines" link on the Web site of the Eastern Association for the Surgery of Trauma (*www.east.org*), and the "Guidelines" link on the Web site of the Brain Trauma Foundation (*www2.braintrauma.org*).

References

1. Sackett DL, Straus SE, Richardson WS, et al. Introduction. In: Sackett DL, Straus SE, Richardson WS, et al. Evidence-Based Medicine: How to Practice and Teach EBM. Edinburgh: Churchill Livingstone, 2000:1–12.
2. Eastern Association for the Surgery of Trauma (EAST) Ad Hoc Committee on Practice Management Guideline Development. Utilizing evidence-based outcome measures to develop practice management guidelines: a primer. Website of the Eastern Association for the Surgery of Trauma, 2000. Available at: *http://www.east.org/tpg/primer.pdf.*

Neurotrauma

Evidence-Based Answers to Common Questions

◆ Part I ◆

Resuscitation and Initial Assessment

◆ 1 ◆

Does It Matter How Head-Injured Patients Are Resuscitated?

Thomas M. Scalea

Brief Answer

Although there are insufficient data to make specific level I recommendations about resuscitation, some general principles are well established. These include the prevention and prompt treatment of secondary insults such as hypoxia, hypotension, and cerebral edema and the initial transport of trauma patients to established trauma centers.

Background

Traumatic brain injury is the leading cause of injury-related death in the United States and the predominant cause of death in young people under the age of 44 years.[1–3] Although the exact magnitude of the problem of brain injury in the United States is unknown, data compiled by Rosenwasser et al[3] suggest that ~500,000 new cases of brain injury are seen in our nation's emergency departments (EDs) annually. Of these, 30 to 40% are moderate to severe, with a mortality and serious morbidity rate of nearly 10% each.[3]

Resuscitation of mild [Glasgow Coma Scale (GCS) score 13–15), moderate (GCS 9–12), and severe brain injuries (GCS ≤ 8) differs both in intensity and timing. During the last two decades, most research has focused on the pathophysiology and treatment of severe cerebral injury. Unfortunately, there is little consensus regarding the resuscitation of those patients sustaining a mild head injury. Certainly this subset of patients has a much lower risk of death or disability; however, as many as 1.4% of patients who are admitted awake and alert following a mild brain injury will deteriorate, and some will die.[4] Stein et al[4] retrospectively reviewed 1538 mild head injury patients and found that those presenting to the ED with an initial GCS score of 15 have a 13% risk of having positive computed tomography (CT) findings. This proportion increases to nearly 40% in those presenting with an initial GCS of 13 (class III data).[4] Shackford et al[5] demonstrated similar results (class III data). This is a compelling argument for expedient CT evaluation of these patients.[6]

Those who present with moderate to severe head injury are a much different subset of patients. Although there is some controversy surrounding the ideal resuscitation of patients with an initial GCS ≤ 12, it is well documented that any treatment modality employed in the care of these patients, beginning in the prehospital setting, must be aimed at preventing secondary brain injury.[1,7–10]

Brain injury can be categorized as either primary or secondary in nature. Primary injury is a direct result of the initial trauma. Impact to the skull results in displacement of the brain within its confines, often resulting in axonal shearing, contusion, or vascular disruption. Other than continued prevention campaigns, little can be done to ameliorate the effects of primary injury. Secondary insults are generally due to the evolution of the brain injury or to subsequent complications. Common causes of secondary brain injury include hypoxia, hypotension, cerebral ischemia, cerebral edema, alterations in cerebral blood flow, and intracranial hypertension. Aggressive resuscitation of head-injured patients can prevent secondary brain injury and improve morbidity and mortality.[1]

Literature Review

Emergency Medical Systems

Effective resuscitation of head-injured patients must begin upon activation of the Emergency Medical Services (EMS) system. It is imperative that providers of advanced life support are dispatched to the accident scene and that the patient is transported expeditiously to a hospital that can provide the requisite level of care. In 1990, Smith et al[11] demonstrated that patients treated in trauma centers had a significantly lower mortality rate than those treated in nontrauma settings (class III data). Meredith et al[12] suggested the use of the straightforward motor component of the GCS (GMR) as an accurate means for EMS dispatchers to immediately identify patients in need of high-level prehospital care and mobilization of trauma center resources (class III data). Presumably the GMR is simple enough for a witness at the scene to assess. A citizen activating the EMS system could provide the dispatcher with the information that the patient is able or unable to accomplish simple tasks. This knowledge may alter triage decisions.

Pearl

Some studies have found that patients treated in trauma centers have a significantly lower mortality rate than those treated in nontrauma settings.

Pearl

The motor component score on the GCS, and specifically whether or not a patient can obey simple one-step commands, may be an accurate means for EMS dispatchers to immediately identify patients in need of high-level prehospital care and mobilization of trauma center resources.

Airway

In the past 20 years, the importance of early recognition of brain injury and the effects that the prevention of secondary injury have on outcome have been elucidated.[10] As in the resuscitation of any trauma patient, securing a patent airway is primary. Most patients with severe brain injuries are unable to protect their airways and require intubation. Hypoxia is among the most common and lethal of all secondary insults.[9] Chesnut et al[10] furnished evidence that prehospital hypoxia is highly predictive of increased morbidity and mortality in these patients (class II data).

The role of EMS providers in airway control is controversial. The time required to accomplish field intubation may result in a delay in transport. In the particular subset of severely head-injured patients with a subdural hematoma, it has been "strongly contended" that the single controllable factor most affecting morbidity and mortality is the timing of surgical intervention (class III data).[13] In fact, Haselsberger et al[14] demonstrated that when the time from injury to definitive care exceeds 2 hours, the mortality rate nearly doubles (class III data). However, there is also strong evidence that prehospital endotracheal intubation is associated with significantly improved survival (class III data).[15] It seems reasonable that if intubation will not significantly delay transport or if transport time to definitive care is expected to be prolonged (as in many rural areas), airway control should be accomplished. In urban settings with short transport times, it may not be necessary, particularly with the realization that field intubation may compromise spinal immobilization. Certainly, any patient who is unresponsive, apneic, or at risk for aspiration must have some attempt at airway control.

Pearl

If intubation will not significantly delay transport, or if transport time to definitive care is expected to be prolonged (as in many rural areas), airway control should be accomplished.

Breathing

In the past, severely head-injured patients were thought to benefit from routine and aggressive hyperventilation. While hyperventilation does initially decrease intracranial pressure (ICP) by causing cerebral vasoconstriction, this vasoconstriction increases cerebral vascular resistance and reduces cerebral blood flow (CBF).[2] Marion et al[16] demonstrated that CBF often drops significantly in the 24 hours following head trauma. This is most pronounced in the first few hours (class II data). The additional decrease in CBF provided by hyperventilation places the patient at greater risk for cerebral ischemia.[2] Although there have not been any studies investigating the outcome of brain-injured patients following prehospital hyperventilation, the Brain Trauma Foundation's *Guidelines for Prehospital*

Management of Traumatic Brain Injury[17] suggest (at the level of an option) that ventilatory rates greater than 10 breaths per minute (for an adult) during patient transport should be used only as a temporizing measure for profoundly injured patients exhibiting signs of herniation (e.g., posturing, pupillary asymmetry, or fixed and dilated pupils). In the hospital setting, hyperventilation should be utilized only if increased ICP is refractory to other forms of treatment. If this intervention becomes necessary, ventilation should be guided by serial blood gases, with a target $PaCO_2$ between 30 and 35 mmHg.[18]

Pearl

In the prehospital setting, hyperventilation should be used only as a temporizing measure for profoundly injured patients exhibiting signs of herniation (e.g., posturing, pupillary asymmetry, or fixed and dilated pupils). In the hospital setting, hyperventilation should be utilized only if increased ICP is refractory to other forms of treatment.

Circulation

Once the patient's airway and breathing have been assessed and stabilized, circulation becomes the primary concern. Hypotension in the brain-injured patient is no less detrimental than hypoxia. Severe brain injury alters the permeability of the blood–brain barrier, impairs cerebral autoregulatory mechanisms, and increases the oxygen demands of the brain.[3] This decrease of CBF at a time when cerebral demands are highest and autoregulatory mechanisms are ineffective greatly affects prognosis. Brain-injured patients experiencing a single episode of prehospital hypotension [systolic blood pressure (SBP) <90 mmHg] have twice the mortality and significantly increased morbidity compared with those without hypotension (class III data).[19] In addition, the duration of hypotension almost certainly plays a critical role in determining outcome. As the duration of hypotension lengthens, the probability of favorable outcome decreases.[1] Blood pressure in the field should be monitored very closely, and any hypotension corrected immediately.

Until recently, aggressive volume resuscitation was thought to be contraindicated in victims of brain injury because of concerns about secondary cerebral edema and increased ICP. However, it is now generally recognized that hypovolemia reduces mean arterial pressure (MAP), which in turn lowers cerebral perfusion pressure (CPP). Thus, withholding fluids is potentially more harmful than aggressive fluid resuscitation.[2,10,19] Euvolemia seems to be ideal in these patients (class III data).[8] Although CPP is probably the best measure of the adequacy of cerebral resuscitation,[8,17,20] CPP cannot be calculated in the field. Unfortunately, the first sign of hypovolemia is often hypotension.

Pearl

Withholding fluids in head-injured patients is potentially more harmful than aggressive fluid resuscitation. Hypovolemia, particularly in the prehospital setting, may exacerbate secondary brain injury.

Many studies have attempted to identify the ideal resuscitation fluid for head-injured patients. In 1993, Vassar et al[21,22] published two prospective, randomized studies (class II) that included brain-injured patients resuscitated in the prehospital setting with hypertonic fluid instead of crystalloid solutions. The authors concluded that prehospital administration of 7.5% sodium chloride was associated with a significant increase in systolic blood pressure compared with infusion of Ringer's lactate. Additionally, Anderson et al[23] reported that early ICP was lower in animals resuscitated with hypertonic saline versus lactated Ringer's. Although there were no increases in complication rates from hypertonic resuscitation, neither study was able to demonstrate any improvement in outcome with the use of hypertonic solutions. Currently, the ideal fluid for use in head-injured patients is unknown. The American College of Surgeons' *Advanced Trauma Life Support Instructor's Manual* offers a general recommendation for rapid infusion of 2 L of isotonic crystalloid solution such as Ringer's lactate or normal saline as the initial bolus in adults with head trauma because underresuscitation, particularly in the prehospital setting, virtually ensures some degree of secondary brain injury.[24]

Mannitol has been used for decades as an osmotic diuretic. In the brain-injured patient, mannitol effectively improves ICP by providing intravascular volume expansion with a subsequently decreased hematocrit, reduced blood viscosity, improved cardiac index, and increased cerebral blood flow with improved oxygenation.[25] Miller and Leech[26] noted that each 1-mL reduction in cerebral blood volume after mannitol administration correlated with a decrease in ICP of 7 to 8 mm Hg under pathologic conditions (class III data). Within 5 minutes of intravenous administration, mannitol can reduce ICP by at least 26%.[2] Generally, mannitol is administered in a dose of 0.5 to 1 g/kg for traumatic brain injury. Some data suggest that repeat boluses may be more efficacious and may decrease the potential for "rebound" increases in ICP as compared with continuous infusion.[17] There has been some concern, however, that mannitol administration may cause hypotension secondary to its diuretic effect. There have been numerous studies attempting to determine the actual effect of mannitol on MAP.[25–28] However, the Brain Trauma Foundation has concluded that there is insufficient class I data to support the prehospital use of mannitol at this time.[17] Care should be taken to monitor for physiologic changes in blood pressure, urine output, serum osmolality, and sodium concentration.[20] ICP and MAP (and therefore CPP) monitoring is strongly recommended. CPP should guide diuretic therapy as well as fluid resuscitation. Maintaining a CPP at or above 70 mmHg is advised.[2,18,20]

Pearl

There are insufficient class I data to support the prehospital use of mannitol at this time.

Dextrose

EMS protocols often prescribe 50 mL of a 50% dextrose solution to all patients found to have a decreased level of consciousness. Some studies have shown that high serum glucose levels in patients with traumatic brain injury may worsen prognosis.[10,29] Serum glucose and lactate levels have been found to be elevated in patients with severe brain injuries.[30] This may well be the result of a stress response. Nonetheless, the anaerobic metabolism that accompanies severe head injury may cause glucose to be converted into large quantities of lactate, leading to intracellular acidosis.[20,29] Lam et al[29] examined the relationship between serum glucose levels and outcome in a study of 169 patients requiring surgical intervention for head injury. Their results indicated that peak 24-hour glucose levels >200 mg/dL were significantly associated with poor prognosis (class III data). Several authors have suggested the addition of a glucose measurement device to the prehospital armamentarium.[17] After a critical review of the literature, the Brain Trauma Foundation recommended that patients with altered mental status of undetermined etiology have a rapid glucose determination or be given glucose empirically.[17]

Intoxication

In addition to the patient's admission glucose level, prehospital providers and ED staff must consider the possible effects of alcohol intoxication and/or drug use in their trauma patients. Alcohol is often consumed by trauma patients prior to their injury, and its effects can tremendously complicate the neurologic exam. The GCS is frequently used to determine the extent of brain injury and has been shown to be a powerful independent predictor of outcome.[31] A study conducted by a group in Wales suggests that severe alcohol intoxication (greater than 240 mg/100 mL) reduces the GCS by two to three points in patients without head injuries (class III data).[32] This may alter the treatment protocol, particularly in patients with admission GCS scores of 6 to 10.

Recommendations (Level III)

The resuscitation of head-injured patients requires further investigation. The optimal type and volume of fluid to be administered, the preferred method of airway management, the role of mannitol, and the value and risks of empiric administration of dextrose in the prehospital environment remain topics of much controversy.

Although much remains unknown, it is possible to make general recommendations. Hypoxia should be prevented by the administration of supplemental oxygen. Endotracheal intubation should generally be considered unless transport times are exceptionally short. Prehospital hyperventilation should be avoided unless severely injured patients exhibit signs of herniation. Hypotension should be prevented by liberal use of crystalloids, with the goal of intravascular euvolemia; dehydrating head-injured patients is not recommended. Some studies suggest that hypertonic saline may be of benefit. Prehospital use of mannitol is generally not recommended.

References

1. Shackford SR. Effect of small-volume resuscitation on intracranial pressure and related cerebral variables. J Trauma 1997;42: S48–S53.
2. Silvestri S, Aronson S. Severe head injury: prehospital and emergency department management. Mt Sinai J Med 1997;64: 329–338.
3. Rosenwasser RH, Andrews DW, Jimenez DF. Penetrating craniocerebral trauma. Surg Clin North Am 1991;71:305–316.
4. Stein SC, Ross SE. Mild head injury: a plea for routine early CT scanning. J Trauma 1992;33:11–13.
5. Shackford SR, Wald SL, Ross SE, et al. The clinical utility of computed tomographic scanning and neurologic examination in the management of patients with minor head injuries. J Trauma 1992;33:385–394.
6. Jeret JS, Mandell M, Anziska B, et al. Clinical predictors of abnormality disclosed by computed tomography after mild head trauma. Neurosurgery 1993;32:9–16.
7. Lehr D, Baethmann A, Reulen HJ, et al. Management of patients with severe head injury in the preclinical phase: a prospective analysis. J Trauma 1997;42:S71–S75.
8. Wald SL. Advances in the early management of patients with head injury. Surg Clin North Am 1995;75:225–242.
9. Chandler CL, Cummins B. Initial assessment and management of the severely head-injured patient. Br J Hosp Med 1995;53: 102–108.

10. Chesnut RM, Marshall LF, Klauber MR, et al. The role of secondary brain injury in determining outcome from severe head injury. J Trauma 1993;34:216–222.
11. Smith JS Jr, Martin LF, Young WW, et al. Do trauma centers improve outcome over non-trauma centers: the evaluation of regional trauma care using discharge abstract data and patient management categories. J Trauma 1990;30:1533–1538.
12. Meredith W, Rutledge R, Hansen AR, et al. Field triage of trauma patients based on the ability to follow commands: a study in 29,573 injured patients. J Trauma 1995;38:129–135.
13. Wilberger JE Jr, Harris M, Diamond DL. Acute subdural hematoma: morbidity, mortality, and operative timing. J Neurosurg 1991;74:212–218.
14. Haselsberger K, Pucher R, Auer LM. Prognosis after acute subdural or epidural haemorrhage. Acta Neurochir (Wein) 1988;90: 111–116.
15. Winchell RJ, Hoyt DB. Endotracheal intubation in the field improves survival in patients with severe head injury. Trauma Research and Education Foundation of San Diego. Arch Surg 1997;132:592–597.
16. Marion DW, Darby J, Yonas H. Acute regional cerebral blood flow changes caused by severe head injuries. J Neurosurg 1991; 74:407–414.
17. Brain Trauma Foundation. Guidelines for prehospital management of traumatic brain injury. Available at: *www2.braintrauma.org/guidelines.php*.
18. Chesnut RM. Guidelines for the management of severe head injury: what we know and what we think we know. J Trauma 1997;42:S19–S22.
19. Wald SL, Shackford SR, Fenwick J. The effect of secondary insults on mortality and long-term disability after severe head injury in a rural region without a trauma system. J Trauma 1993;34:377–381.
20. Gruen P, Liu C. Current trends in the management of head injury. Emerg Med Clin North Am 1998;16:63–83.
21. Vassar MJ, Fischer RP, O'Brien PE, et al. A multicenter trial for resuscitation of injured patients with 7.5% sodium chloride. The effect of added Dextran 70. The Multicenter Group for the Study of Hypertonic Saline in Trauma Patients. Arch Surg 1993; 128:1003–1011.
22. Vassar MJ, Perry CA, Holcroft JW. Prehospital resuscitation of hypotensive trauma patients with 7.5% NaCl versus 7.5% NaCl with added dextran: a controlled trial. J Trauma 1993;34: 622–632.
23. Anderson JT, Wisner DH, Sullivan PE, et al. Initial small-volume hypertonic resuscitation of shock and brain injury: short- and long-term effects. J Trauma 1997;42:592–601.
24. American College of Surgeons Committee on Trauma. Advanced Trauma Life Support Instructor's Manual. Chicago: American College of Surgeons, 1996.
25. Israel RS, Marx JA, Moore EE, et al. Hemodynamic effect of mannitol in a canine model of concomitant increased intracranial pressure and hemorrhagic shock. Ann Emerg Med 1988;17:560–566.
26. Miller JD, Leech P. Effects of mannitol and steroid therapy on intracranial volume-pressure relationships in patients. J Neurosurg 1975;42:274–281.
27. Sayre MR, Daily SS, Stern SA, et al. Out-of-hospital administration of mannitol to head-injured patients does not change systolic blood pressure. Acad Emerg Med 1996;3:840–848.
28. Muizelaar JP, Wei EP, Kontos HA, et al. Mannitol causes compensatory cerebral vasoconstriction and vasodilation in response to blood viscosity changes. J Neurosurg 1983;59:822–828.
29. Lam AM, Winn HR, Cullen BF, et al. Hyperglycemia and neurological outcome in patients with head injury. J Neurosurg 1991;75:545–551.
30. De Salles AA, Muizelaar JP, Young HF. Hyperglycemia, cerebrospinal fluid lactic acidosis, and cerebral blood flow in severely head-injured patients. Neurosurgery 1987;21:45–50.
31. Marshall LF, Gautille T, Klauber MR, et al. The outcome of severe closed head injury. J Neurosurg 1991;75:S28–S36.
32. Brickley MR, Shepherd JP. The relationship between alcohol intoxication, injury severity and Glasgow Coma Score in assault patients. Injury 1995;26:311–314.

◆ 2 ◆

What Is the Best Way to Assess and Classify Head-Injured Patients?

Nelson M. Oyesiku

This type of question does not lend itself to the standard class I, II, or III method of reviewing the literature. Although such methodology is appropriate for evaluating many kinds of studies, investigations of grading schemes do not readily lend themselves to that type of analysis. For the sake of consistency, the studies discussed in this chapter can be considered to report class III data, but the limitations of using such a classification scheme for this topic should be remembered.

Brief Answer

It is recommended that clinicians be trained to use one of the currently available assessment tools for evaluation of both acute and long-term patients. The Glasgow Coma Scale (GCS) is the most extensive and rigorously evaluated tool for the acute assessment of brain-injured patients and is often considered to be the "gold standard," but other scales have also been demonstrated to be reliable. Likewise, the Glasgow Outcome Scale (GOS) (both the original version and the extended version) has been extensively evaluated as an outcome assessment tool for these patients, but again, other scales are available. Regardless of which scale is used, care must be taken that all assessments are performed and documented accurately.

Background

Traumatic brain injury (TBI) is a major public health problem, affecting more than 500,000 people in the United States each year. Its annual incidence is estimated to be 200 per 100,000 population. The neurologic condition of TBI patients on initial presentation is a key determinant for determining triage, therapy, and prognosis. Methods of clinically assessing the neurologic condition of TBI patients should be uniform, straightforward, and reliable. Advantages of effective assessment tools include reliability of documentation, ease of data access, consistency of evaluation methods, and accuracy of prognostication.

Various assessment systems have been developed for documenting a patient's status after TBI (Table 2-1). These include the GCS,[1] the Reaction Level Scale,[2,3] the Innsbruck Coma Scale,[4] the Edinburgh Coma Scale,[5–7] the Comprehensive Level of Consciousness Scale,[8] the Maryland Coma Scale,[9] the Glasgow-Liege Scale,[10,11] and the Head Injury Watch Sheet.[12] Some assessment tools undergo periodic refinement through serial iterations and remain in widespread use, whereas others have not become broadly disseminated.

One type of assessment scale is *disability-specific*. Scales of this type focus on neurologic deficits. They are generally based on the motor and sensory examination, with assignment of numerical values or letter grades. The second type of scale focuses on *functional*

Table 2-1 Selected Disability and Outcome Scales

First Author	Description of Study	Summary
Teasdale, 1974[1]	Description of the Glasgow Coma Scale	GCS is practical and useful
Jennett, 1975[46]	Description of the Glasgow Outcome Scale	GOS describes both duration and intensity of disability
Sugiura, 1977[7]	Discussion of the Edinburgh Coma Scale	This scale assesses the severity of traumatic brain injury (TBI) with more precision than the GCS
Yen, 1978[12]	Description of the Head Injury Watch Sheet	This sheet can help evaluate the efficacy of various modes of therapy
Artiola, 1980[27]	Description of the Oxford Coma Scale	This scale has good interobserver agreement and facilitates prompt detection of slight neurologic deterioration in patients
Salcman, 1981[9]	Description of the Maryland Coma Scale	A Maryland Coma Scale score of less than or equal to 35% on day 1 is associated with poor prognosis
Rappaport, 1982[54]	Description of the Disability Rating Scale for severe head trauma	DRS is easily learned, quickly completed, valid, predictive of outcome, and has a high interrater reliability; it is more sensitive than the GOS; it can identify patients most likely to benefit from intensive rehabilitation care
Stanczak, 1984[8]	Description of the Comprehensive Level of Consciousness Scale	This scale is probably too detailed for routine clinical use
Shores, 1986[29]	Preliminary validation of the Westmead Posttraumatic Amnesia Scale for measuring the duration of posttraumatic amnesia	The Westmead PTA Scale is a simple tool for routine use to enhance the accuracy of measuring the severity of head injury
Levin, 1987[41]	Investigation of the reliability and validity of the Neurobehavioral Rating Scale	The NRS reflects the severity and chronicity of TBI and has satisfactory interrater reliability
Born, 1988[11]	Description of the Glasgow-Liege Scale	Status of brainstem reflexes appears to be the factor with the best prognostic ability
Stalhammar, 1988[3]	Testing of the Reaction Level Scale (RLS 85) in neurosurgical patients	RLS 85 is easily learned and reliable
Crosby, 1989[26]	Development and testing of the Clinical Neurologic Assessment Tool	This tool is reliable, valid, convenient, and easily scored and can capture subtle changes in TBI patients
Gibson, 1989[24]	Description of the Leeds prognostic scale	Reliable predictive scale
Benzer, 1991[4]	Description of Innsbruck Coma Scale	This scale allows a highly accurate early prediction of nonsurvival
Stein, 1995[35]	Testing of the Head Injury Severity Scale	Adding a complication dimension to each severity category effectively divides patients into very different groups
Prasad, 1996[23]	Literature review to conduct a critical appraisal of the clinimetric properties of the GCS	The GCS has a good sensibility and reliability and well-established cross-sectional construct validity; when combined with age and brainstem reflexes, its predictive validity in traumatic coma is good; its validity as a predictive and evaluative instrument has not yet been studied adequately

outcome, such as the patient's ability to transfer, ambulate, or participate in activities of daily living. In general, the first type of scale is used for the acute assessment of patients with TBI, whereas both types are important for the assessment and description of patients who are past the acute stage of their injuries.

This chapter describes clinical assessment tools for TBI patients and discusses how to determine whether the available medical evidence supports the use of a particular assessment scale or scales. All studies report class III data.

Pearl

Disability-specific scales focus on neurologic deficits, whereas functional outcome scales focus on specific tasks. In general, the first type of scale is used for acute assessment of TBI patients, whereas both types of scales are used for longer-term assessments.

Literature Review

Disability Assessment

Glasgow Coma Scale

The most widely used and most extensively and rigorously evaluated tool for the acute classification and assessment of TBI patients is the GCS.[1] In its current form, it is based on eye opening (score of 1 to 4), verbal responsiveness (1 to 5), and motor responsiveness (1 to 6). The scale was originally designed as three separate subscales. Subsequently, the sum of the three scores was used as a measure of a patient's overall responsiveness. Common usage classifies patients with a GCS score of 3 to 8 as having severe injuries, those with a score of 9 to 12 as moderate injuries, and those with a score of 13 to 15 as mild injuries. The probability of a poor outcome increases with a decreasing GCS. It must be remembered, however, that different patients with the same total GCS score can have significantly different probabilities of death due to differences in the components making up that score.[13]

Pearl

The GCS is the most widely used and most extensively evaluated tool for the acute classification and assessment of TBI patients.

Observations in the early stages after injury define the depth and duration of coma. In combination with clinical features such as a patient's age and degree of brainstem function, these observations have been used to predict outcome.[14] However, to ensure reliability, the GCS should be measured in a standardized way and must be obtained through interaction with the patient. The assessment should be made only after pulmonary and hemodynamic resuscitation and only after pharmacologic sedation or paralytic agents have been metabolized.[15]

Studies of interobserver reliability of the GCS have documented overall consistency of assessment among medical, nursing, and paramedical personnel, but the distinction between "abnormal" and "normal" flexion movements has been reported to be a major source of disagreement.[16] Braakman et al[17] found a high interobserver agreement between experienced and nonexperienced observers in assessment of the motor response. In a study of intensive care unit nurses with varying degrees of experience in the use of the GCS, Ingersoll and Leyden[18] found that the rate of interobserver agreement in determination of the summed GCS score in TBI patients was 100% in straightforward cases, but this rate decreased when more complex patients (e.g., those with a tracheostomy) were assessed. Rowley and Fielding[19,20] found mean interobserver agreement rates of 88.5 to 98%. Although higher agreement rates were seen among trained and experienced practitioners, interobserver reliability coefficients were good within each group tested (groups were assigned based on experience). These results suggest that accuracy (or inaccuracy) of GCS determinations is more of a problem than consistency among different observers. The GCS is also useful and reliable in comparing patients from different countries.[21]

Jagger et al[22] found that the motor response score alone was a slightly better predictor of outcome than the GCS sum score. Prasad[23] assessed the utility of the GCS by reviewing published articles describing and using the scale. The GCS was found to have good sensibility and reliability (intraclass correlation coefficient of 0.8 to 1 for trained users). It also has a well-established cross-sectional construct validity. Its predictive validity in traumatic coma, when combined with age and brainstem reflexes, is good (sensitivity of 79 to 97%; specificity of 84 to 97%). This review concluded that, although the scale is an established discriminative instrument, its validity as a predictive and evaluative instrument has not yet been studied adequately.

Other Scales

The scale that later came to be known among Japanese researchers as the Edinburgh Coma Scale was described in the Japanese literature in 1973. The initial version (E1 CS) was modified in 1983 to become the E2 CS.[5–7] It has not gained widespread acceptance.

The Comprehensive Level of Consciousness Scale was proposed primarily as a research tool.[8] It consists of eight subscales: posture (scored 0–4), eye position at rest (0–6), spontaneous eye opening (0–4), general motor functioning (0–6), abnormal ocular movements (0–6), pupillary light reflexes (0–7), general responsiveness (0–8), and best communicative effort (0–7). This scale is said to be internally more consistent than the GCS. Although its interrater and test-retest reliability are similar to those of the GCS, it is not suitable for routine bedside use because of its detail.

The Head Injury Watch Sheet was described in 1978. It consists of assessment of consciousness and mental status (scored 0–12), motor response to pain (0–12), and pupillary reactivity (0–3 for each eye) for a maximum score of 30.[12] It has not seen widespread use.

The Reaction Level Scale (RLS85) is an eight-part scale for assessment of patient responsiveness. The RLS85 is easily learned and is based on the same concepts as the GCS, but the separate responses are directly weighted together in one scale that has eight categories. The RLS85 has good interobserver agreement[2,3]; in fact, one study found that the RLS85 had better interobserver agreement than the GCS sum score.[2]

The Innsbruck Coma Scale was introduced in 1981.[4] The scale scores eight items. A scale of 0 to 3 is used for reaction to acoustic stimuli, reaction to pain, body posture, eye opening, pupil size, pupil response to light, and position and movement of eyeballs; oral automatisms are scored on a 0 to 2 scale. This scale allows for highly accurate prediction of death in patients with scores of 0 or 1, even during the initial posttraumatic examination.

The Maryland Coma Scale was described in 1981.[9] Its components include eye opening; orientation; pupil, corneal, and caloric reflexes and grimace; type of stimulus required; verbal response; leg motor response; and arm motor response. It contains the three variables of the GCS, excludes responses that cannot be evaluated, and provides more information concerning the status of brainstem reflexes and motor lateralization.

In 1982, the Glasgow-Liege Scale, which combines the GCS with the quantified analysis of five brainstem reflexes, was developed.[10,11] Combining these two parameters in a single scale improves the precision of prognosis, especially for those TBI patients with initial and complete loss of consciousness (LOC).[10]

Gibson and Stephenson[24] devised the Leeds prognostic scale to identify severely injured patients whose death could be predicted with certainty within 12 hours of admission. They used several variables: age, unreactive pupils, intracranial pressure, systolic blood pressure, GCS score, presence of extracranial injuries, and presence of high-density lesions on computed tomography (CT) scan. They weighted each of these to reflect their influence on mortality. Scores ranged from 0 (best) to 24 (worst). None of the patients with a score higher than 11 survived. Based on these results and on calculated probabilities of survival, they proposed withdrawal of active treatment when a patient's score exceeded 13. However, when Feldman et al[25] tested the reliability of the Leeds scale in patients with TBI, they found that the scale failed to predict mortality with 100% accuracy. Their findings suggested that the Leeds prediction model is not infallible and that it should be applied cautiously when making decisions about the early termination of care in severely head-injured patients.

The Clinical Neurologic Assessment Tool is a 21-item instrument assessing response to verbal and tactile stimulation, ability to follow commands, muscle tone, body position, movement, chewing, and yawning in TBI patients.[26] This scale was developed to detect subtle changes in neurologic status. Its reliability has been shown to be high, and concurrent validity testing with the GCS has indicated a strong positive correlation. In one study, scores correctly classified 95.1% of patient observations into their respective GCS categories, leading the authors to conclude that this instrument is valid, convenient, and easily scored and that it captures subtle changes in the patient with TBI.

The Oxford scale, described in 1980, measures the duration of posttraumatic amnesia (PTA), which is defined as a failure of continuous memory.[27] This scale builds on the observations of Russell,[28] who proposed duration of LOC as a useful index of the severity of brain injury. The Oxford scale uses simple memory tests to categorize PTA by duration, from less than 10 minutes to more than 4 weeks. An extension of the Oxford scale is the Westmead PTA Scale.[29] Described in 1986, it is a more standardized measurement of the duration of PTA following TBI. It has a high degree of interrater reliability, takes about 3 minutes to administer, and requires a minimum of training.[30] As a predictor of neuropsychological outcome, duration of PTA as determined by the Westmead PTA Scale was reported to have predictive superiority over admission GCS score and duration of coma as determined by the GCS.[30]

Multiple classification systems have been devised to sort mild TBI by severity. In 1991, the American Congress of Rehabilitation Medicine defined mild TBI as an injury with at least one of the following: (1) any period of LOC lasting less than 30 minutes, with a GCS score of 13 to 15 after the period of LOC; (2) any loss of memory for events immediately before or after the accident, with duration of PTA of <24 hours; (3) any alteration in mental state at the time of the accident; (4) focal neurologic deficit that may or may not be transient.[31] In addition, various classification systems have been proposed to evaluate concussion in athletes after TBI. One of the better known is that proposed by Cantu: grade I, or mild, has no LOC and duration of PTA <30 minutes; grade II, or moderate, has LOC <5 minutes or PTA >30 minutes but <24 hours; and grade III, or severe, has LOC >5 minutes or PTA >24 hours.[32] A modification of this scheme adds a grade 0 for the athlete with only delayed onset of headache and difficulty concentrating (but without symptoms immediately after injury) and omits LOC from the definitions of grades I and II. Ommaya and Gennarelli[33] described syndromes of cerebral concussion based on experimental and clinical observation, with grades I to III involving no LOC and grades IV to VI associated with LOC. Gennarelli differentiates mild concussion with no LOC from a classic concussion with LOC. Mild concussion is divided into several levels of increasing severity of injury. Classic concussion is defined as an injury characterized by coma of up to 6 hours in duration.[34]

Pearl

A patient may sustain a concussion without ever losing consciousness.

Stein and Spettell[35] in 1995 introduced the Head Injury Severity Scale, a two-dimensional scale for rating the severity of closed head injury. This scheme begins with a five-interval severity classification (minimal through critical), determined primarily by the initial postresuscitation GCS score. The second dimension is predicated on the presence or absence of complications appropriate for each level of severity. They found that adding a complication dimension to each severity category had a significant effect on outcome and accurately divided patients into groups with very different risks, prognoses, and treatment requirements.

The Adelaide Coma Scale was designed for pediatric assessment. This scale takes the child's age and neurologic immaturity into account. However, the Adelaide scale by itself does not provide enough scope for assessment. Thus, if this scale is used, additional information must be considered, including specific pediatric indicators and an assessment of each child's behavior according to the main caregiver.[36]

Functional Outcome Scales

Rating scales are useful for longitudinal assessment of neuropsychological sequelae of TBI. Many different types of rating scales have been described. Many of these scales were not originally developed for patients with TBI. Instead, they have been modified and adapted as a result of validity studies. Methodologies for gathering data include (1) self-report, as in the Minnesota Multiphasic Personality Inventory[37]; (2) relative's or friend's report,[38] as in the Katz Adjustment Scale: Relative's Form[39]; (3) clinician's assessment, such as the Brief Psychiatric Rating Scale,[40] the Neurobehavioral Rating Scale,[41] and the European head injury evaluation chart[42]; and (4) multi-informant scales, such as the Neurobehavioral Functioning Inventory,[43] the Portland Adaptability Inventory,[44] and the European Brain Injury Questionnaire.[45] Most of these instruments are in the process of validation. In addition, the Wechsler Adult Intelligence Scale, the Halstead-Reitan Neuropsychological Battery, the GOS, and other tools have also been used to assess outcome. Each type of assessment tool contributes different kinds of information to the description of the neuropsychological sequelae and psychosocial consequences of TBI.

The most commonly used outcome measure is the GOS.[46] Originally, the GOS described outcomes as falling into one of five categories: death, persistent vegetative state, severe disability, moderate disability, and good recovery. *Vegetative state* refers to the inability to follow commands or communicate. *Severe disability* describes patients who are conscious but require assistance with basic needs like feeding, personal hygiene, grooming, and personal safety. *Moderately disabled* patients have some persistent neurologic or cognitive impairments, but they can take care of their basic physical and cognitive needs, can use public transportation, can work in a sheltered situation (but not in a nonsheltered setting), and can resume some social roles, although perhaps in a decreased capacity.

To increase sensitivity, the scale originally described in 1975 was expanded to an eight-point scale by subdividing the outcomes of severe disability, moderate disability, and good recovery into upper and lower categories.[47] Concerns have been expressed that gains in sensitivity from expansion of such classification schemes may be offset by decreased consistency of outcome classification, but others argue that consistency need not be sacrificed when such classification schemes are expanded.[48,49] Nevertheless, to counteract this potential problem, Teasdale and coworkers[47,50] proposed the use of a structured questionnaire to increase reliability. The extended GOS has been reported to provide an assessment of disability that is more complete than that given either by an alternative scale of functional disability (Disability Rating Scale, which is discussed below) or by an assessment of physical disability (Barthel Activities of Daily Living index).[51] Another attempt to improve upon the GOS is the Edinburgh Extended GOS, which was intended to retain the advantages of the existing GOS but also to allow comparison of patterns of recovery in behavioral, cognitive, and physical function.[52]

Pearl

The GOS is the most commonly used instrument to measure outcome from TBI. Using the extended GOS, which expands the original scale from five to eight categories, and administering it via a structured questionnaire may improve sensitivity and reliability.

The King's Outcome Scale for Childhood Head Injury is a specific pediatric adaptation of the adult GOS.[53] In an attempt to improve sensitivity, the King's scale expands the GOS categories associated with better outcomes; that is, severe disability, moderate disability, and good recovery. This instrument is quick and easy to use. Interrater reliability studies show that even with such an apparently simple scale, however, some training may be required.

The Disability Rating Scale (DRS) was developed by Rappaport et al.[54] It is a 30-point scale that rates eight dimensions of ability: eye opening; verbalization; motor responsiveness; cognitive skills for feeding, toileting, and grooming; overall level of functioning (in terms of physical and cognitive disability); and employability. Scoring is based on levels of function that range from normal to complete disability. The DRS is easily learned and can be completed quickly, with high interrater reliability.[54–56] It has been shown to be a valid predictor of outcome. The DRS has been reported to be more sensitive than the GOS in detecting and measuring clinical changes after severe TBI.[54,56]

The Coma Recovery Scale was developed for use during the acute phase of rehabilitation. It can detect subtle changes in neurobehavioral status and can help predict outcome in patients with severe alterations of consciousness. Acceptable levels of concurrent validity have been established with the DRS ($r = -0.93$) and with the GCS ($r = 0.90$). This scale also has adequate interrater reliability ($\kappa = 0.83$).[57]

Levin et al[41] utilized a more specific scale, the Brief Psychiatric Rating Scale (BPRS),[40] to assess behavioral changes following TBI. Although useful in quantifying information on behavioral sequelae, this scale was primarily designed for assessment of psychiatric disorders. Consequently, Levin et al developed the Neurobehavioral Rating Scale (NRS), which reflects both the severity and chronicity of closed head injury.[41] The interrater reliability and validity of the NRS are satisfactory.[41,58,59]

The Galveston Orientation and Amnesia Test (GOAT) was developed to evaluate cognition during the subacute stage of recovery from TBI.[60] This test measures orientation to person, place, and time, as well as memory for events that preceded and followed the injury. It may be used in the field, in the emergency room, or at the bedside. However, its method of scoring has been reported to cause some confusion; this problem is addressed by the Wolinsky Amnesia Information Test (WAIT).[61] In addition to the same questions as the GOAT, the WAIT asks for date of birth, additional details about the incident that caused the TBI, and current and immediate past presidents of the United States. The WAIT has satisfactory interrater reliability, and it compares favorably with the GCS and the GOAT in terms of concurrent validity. In terms of discriminative validity, the WAIT compares favorably to CT scan data.[61]

The Children's Orientation and Amnesia Test (COAT) was developed to assess cognition serially during early recovery from TBI in children and adolescents. COAT scores were a better predictor of verbal and nonverbal memory performance than the GCS score at 6 and 12 months after injury. The COAT has adequate reliability and validity as a measure of the duration of PTA in children and adolescents.[62]

The Glasgow Assessment Schedule is another measure of outcome from TBI. This scale provides for a comprehensive assessment. It distinguishes mildly and severely injured patients and rate of change over time. Interrater reliability and concurrent validity with a global rating scale are satisfactory. This instrument is mainly of use in longer-term management settings.[63]

Recommendations

Based on extensive class III evidence supplemented by widespread clinical experience, a level II recommendation may be made to use a currently available assessment tool to document both a patient's acute clinical condition and long-term outcome. The Glasgow Coma Scale and Glasgow Outcome Scale may be chosen for acute and long-term assessment, respectively, because of their widespread use and general clinical familiarity, but other scales may be used if desired. Care must be taken that all assessments are performed and documented accurately.

References

1. Teasdale G, Jennett B. Assessment of coma and impaired consciousness: a practical scale. Lancet 1974;2:81–84.
2. Starmark JE, Stalhammar D, Holmgren E, et al. A comparison of the Glasgow Coma Scale and the Reaction Level Scale (RLS85). J Neurosurg 1988;69:699–706.
3. Stalhammar D, Starmark JE, Holmgren E, et al. Assessment of responsiveness in acute cerebral disorders: a multicentre study on the reaction level scale (RLS85). Acta Neurochir (Wien) 1988;90:73–80.
4. Benzer A, Mitterschiffthaler G, Marosi M, et al. Prediction of non-survival after trauma: Innsbruck Coma Scale. Lancet 1991; 338:977–978.
5. Sugiura K, Muraoka K, Chishiki T, et al. The Edinburgh-2 coma scale: a new scale for assessing impaired consciousness. Neurosurgery 1983;12:411–415.
6. Sugiura K, Muraoka K, Kanazawa C, et al. A clinical study on a system of assessment of impaired consciousness (the second report). No To Shinkei 1978;30:1025–1029.
7. Sugiura K, Kanazawa C, Sato S, et al. A clinical study on a system of assessment of impaired consciousness (the first report). No To Shinkei 1977;29:879–883.
8. Stanczak DE, White JG III, Gouview WD, et al. Assessment of level of consciousness following severe neurological insult: a comparison of the psychometric qualities of the Glasgow Coma Scale and the Comprehensive Level of Consciousness Scale. J Neurosurg 1984;60:955–960.
9. Salcman M, Schepp RS, Ducker TB. Calculated recovery rates in severe head trauma. Neurosurgery 1981;8:301–308.
10. Born JD, Albert A, Hans P, et al. Relative prognostic value of best motor response and brain stem reflexes in patients with severe head injury. Neurosurgery 1985;16:595–601.
11. Born JD. The Glasgow-Liege Scale: prognostic value and evolution of motor response and brain stem reflexes after severe head injury. Acta Neurochir (Wien) 1988;91:1–11.
12. Yen JK, Bourke RS, Nelson LR, et al. Numerical grading of clinical neurological status after serious head injury. J Neurol Neurosurg Psychiatry 1978;41:1125–1130.
13. Teoh LS, Gowardman JR, Larsen PD, et al. Glasgow Coma Scale: variation in mortality among permutations of specific total scores. Intensive Care Med 2000;26:157–161.
14. Teasdale G, Jennett B. Assessment and prognosis of coma after head injury. Acta Neurochir (Wien) 1976;34:45–55.
15. The Brain Trauma Foundation. The American Association of Neurological Surgeons, The Joint Section on Neurotrauma and Critical Care. Management and prognosis of severe traumatic brain injury. Glasgow Coma Scale score. J Neurotrauma 2000; 17:563–571.
16. Teasdale G, Knill-Jones R, van der Sande J. Observer variability in assessing impaired consciousness and coma. J Neurol Neurosurg Psychiatry 1978;41:603–610.
17. Braakman R, Avezaat CJ, Maas AI, et al. Inter observer agreement in the assessment of the motor response of the Glasgow Coma Scale. Clin Neurol Neurosurg 1977;80:100–106.

18. Ingersoll GL, Leyden DB. The Glasgow Coma Scale for patients with head injuries. Crit Care Nurse 1987;7:26–32.
19. Rowley G, Fielding K. Reliability and accuracy of the Glasgow Coma Scale with experienced and inexperienced users. Lancet 1991;337:535–538.
20. Fielding K, Rowley G. Reliability of assessments by skilled observers using the Glasgow Coma Scale. Aust J Adv Nurs 1990;7:13–17.
21. Jennett B, Teasdale G, Galbraith S, et al. Severe head injuries in three countries. J Neurol Neurosurg Psychiatry 1977;40:291–298.
22. Jagger J, Jane JA, Rimel R. The Glasgow Coma Scale: to sum or not to sum? Lancet 1983;2:97.
23. Prasad K. The Glasgow Coma Scale: a critical appraisal of its clinimetric properties. J Clin Epidemiol 1996;49:755–763.
24. Gibson RM, Stephenson GC. Aggressive management of severe closed head trauma: time for reappraisal. Lancet 1989;2:369–371.
25. Feldman Z, Contant CF, Robertson CS, et al. Evaluation of the Leeds prognostic score for severe head injury. Lancet 1991;337:1451–1453.
26. Crosby L, Parsons LC. Clinical neurologic assessment tool: development and testing of an instrument to index neurologic status. Heart Lung 1989;18:121–129.
27. Artiola L, Fortuny I, Briggs M, et al. Measuring the duration of post traumatic amnesia. J Neurol Neurosurg Psychiatry 1980; 43:377–379.
28. Russell WR. Cerebral involvement in head injury. Brain 1932; 55:549–603.
29. Shores EA, Marosszeky JE, Sandanam J, et al. Preliminary validation of a clinical scale for measuring the duration of post-traumatic amnesia. Med J Aust 1986;144:569–572.
30. Shores EA. Comparison of the Westmead PTA Scale and the Glasgow Coma Scale as predictors of neuropsychological outcome following extremely severe blunt head injury. J Neurol Neurosurg Psychiatry 1989;52:126–127.
31. Esselman PC, Uomoto JM. Classification of the spectrum of mild traumatic brain injury. Brain Inj 1995;9:417–424.
32. Cantu RC. Guidelines for return to contact sports after a cerebral concussion. Phys Sportsmed 1986;14:75–83.
33. Ommaya AK, Gennarelli TA. Cerebral concussion and traumatic unconsciousness: correlation of experimental and clinical observations on blunt head injuries. Brain 1974;97:633–654.
34. Gennarelli TA. Mechanism and pathophysiology of cerebral concussion. J Head Trauma Rehabil 1986;1:23–29.
35. Stein SC, Spettell C. The Head Injury Severity Scale (HISS): a practical classification of closed-head injury. Brain Inj 1995;9: 437–444.
36. Westbrook A. The use of a paediatric coma scale for monitoring infants and young children with head injuries. Nurs Crit Care 1997;2:72–75.
37. Dahlstrom WG, Welsh GS, Dahlstrom LE. An MMPI handbook, Vol 1, Clinical Interpretation, revised ed. Minneapolis, MN: University of Minnesota, 1972.
38. Brooks N, Campsie L, Symington C, et al. The five year outcome of severe blunt head injury: a relative's view. J Neurol Neurosurg Psychiatry 1986;49:764–770.
39. Katz MM, Lyerly SB. Methods for measuring adjustment and social behavior in the community, I: Rationale, description, discriminative validity and scale development. Psychol Rep 1963; 13:503–535.
40. Overall JE, Gorham DR. The brief psychiatric rating scale. Psychol Rep 1962;10:799–812.
41. Levin HS, High WM, Goethe KE, et al. The neurobehavioral rating scale: assessment of the behavioral sequelae of head injury by the clinician. J Neurol Neurosurg Psychiatry 1987;50: 183–193.
42. Truelle JL, Brooks DN, Potagas C, et al. A European chart for evaluation of patients with traumatic brain injury. In: Christensen AL, Uzzell BP, eds. Brain Injury and Neuropsychological Rehabilitation: International Perspectives. Hillsdale, NJ: Lawrence Erlbaum Associates, 1994:281–291.
43. Kreutzer JS, Marwitz JH, Seel R, et al. Validation of a neurobehavioral functioning inventory for adults with traumatic brain injury. Arch Phys Med Rehabil 1996;77:116–124.
44. Lezak MD. Neuropsychological Assessment, 3rd ed. New York: Oxford University Press, 1995.
45. Teasdale TW, Christensen AL, Willmes K, et al. Subjective experience in brain-injured patients and their close relatives: a European Brain Injury Questionnaire study. Brain Inj 1997; 11:543–563.
46. Jennett B, Bond M. Assessment of outcome after severe brain damage. Lancet 1975;1:480–484.
47. Teasdale GM, Pettigrew LE, Wilson JT, et al. Analyzing outcome of treatment of severe head injury: a review and update on advancing the use of the Glasgow Outcome Scale. J Neurotrauma 1998;15:587–597.
48. Brooks DN, Hosie J, Bond MR, et al. Cognitive sequelae of severe head injury in relation to the Glasgow Outcome Scale. J Neurol Neurosurg Psychiatry 1986;49:549–553.
49. Maas AI, Braakman R, Schouten HJ, et al. Agreement between physicians on assessment of outcome following severe head injury. J Neurosurg 1983;58:321–325.
50. Wilson JT, Pettigrew LE, Teasdale GM. Structured interviews for the Glasgow Outcome Scale and the extended Glasgow Outcome Scale: guidelines for their use. J Neurotrauma 1998; 15:573–585.
51. Pettigrew LE, Wilson JT, Teasdale GM. Assessing disability after head injury: improved use of the Glasgow Outcome Scale. J Neurosurg 1998;89:939–943.
52. Hellawell DJ, Signorini DF. The Edinburgh Extended Glasgow Outcome Scale (EEGOS): rationale and pilot studies. Int J Rehabil Res 1997;20:345–354.
53. Crouchman M, Rossiter L, Colaco T, et al. A practical outcome scale for paediatric head injury. Arch Dis Child 2001;84:120–124.
54. Rappaport M, Hall KM, Hopkins K, et al. Disability rating scale for severe head trauma: coma to community. Arch Phys Med Rehabil 1982;63:118–123.
55. Gouvier WD, Blanton PD, LaPorte KK, et al. Reliability and validity of the Disability Rating Scale and the Levels of Cognitive Functioning Scale in monitoring recovery from severe head injury. Arch Phys Med Rehabil 1987;68:94–97.
56. Hall K, Cope DN, Rappaport M. Glasgow Outcome Scale and Disability Rating Scale: comparative usefulness in following recovery in traumatic head injury. Arch Phys Med Rehabil 1985;66:35–37.
57. Giacino JT, Kezmarsky MA, DeLuca J, et al. Monitoring rate of recovery to predict outcome in minimally responsive patients. Arch Phys Med Rehabil 1991;72:897–901.
58. Corrigan JD, Dickerson J, Fisher E, et al. The Neurobehavioural Rating Scale: replication in an acute, inpatient rehabilitation setting. Brain Inj 1990;4:215–222.
59. Vanier M, Mazaux JM, Lambert J, et al. Assessment of neuropsychologic impairments after head injury: interrater reliability and factorial and criterion validity of the Neurobehavioral Rating Scale-Revised. Arch Phys Med Rehabil 2000;81:796–806.
60. Levin HS, O'Donnell VM, Grossman RG. The Galveston Orientation and Amnesia Test: a practical scale to assess cognition after head injury. J Nerv Ment Dis 1979;167:675–684.
61. McDonald TW, Franzen MD: a validity study of the WAIT in closed head injury. Brain Inj 1999;13:331–346.
62. Ewing-Cobbs L, Levin HS, Fletcher JM, et al. The Children's Orientation and Amnesia Test: relationship to severity of acute head injury and to recovery of memory. Neurosurgery 1990;27: 683–691.
63. Livingston MG, Livingston HM. The Glasgow Assessment Schedule: clinical and research assessment of head injury outcome. Int Rehabil Med 1985;7:145–149.

3

What Is the Best Way to Assess and Classify Spinal Cord–Injured Patients?

Daniel K. Resnick and Nelson M. Oyesiku

This type of question does not lend itself to the standard class I, II, or III method of reviewing the literature. Although such methodology is appropriate for evaluating many kinds of studies, investigations of grading schemes do not readily lend themselves to that type of analysis. For the sake of consistency, the studies discussed in this chapter can be considered to report class III data, but the limitations of using such a classification scheme for this topic should be remembered.

Brief Answer

The American Spinal Injury Association (ASIA) spinal cord injury (SCI) assessment tool uses both disability-specific and functional independence measures. The ASIA assessment tool undergoes periodic review and is widely used in multicenter studies. It is considered the "gold standard" assessment tool for spinal cord–injured patients.

Background

SCI affects 12,000 to 14,000 people in the United States each year. Treatment of SCI currently consists of decompression of the spinal cord, stabilization of the spine, and administration of methylprednisolone. Despite these interventions, the functional consequences of a SCI remain severe, and new therapies are required for the treatment of SCI. Evaluation of these therapies requires the use of accurate and reliable functional outcome measures. Furthermore, the ability to provide accurate prognostic information in the early postinjury period is valuable for patient and family counseling. Finally, consistent and reproducible assessment scales are necessary to facilitate communication about patient status to other caregivers. This chapter describes the best clinical assessment tools available to the clinician responsible for the care of patients with SCIs.

Literature Review

A computerized search of the database of the National Library of Medicine from 1966 to December 2000 was performed. The search was limited to human studies in the English language. Searching the key words "spinal cord injuries" yielded 12,072 references. Limiting the search to papers dealing with "classification" yielded 152 references. The titles and abstracts of these 152 references were reviewed. Papers dealing with the assessment of both the acutely and the chronically injured patient were selected. The reference lists of these papers were also reviewed, and the additional references were included as needed. This resulted in the selection of the 32 references that form the basis of this review.

Numerous assessment scales have been used to describe patients with SCI. Scales may be divided into two general types. The first type is disability-specific and focuses on the neurologic deficits suffered as a result of SCI. These scales use the motor and sensory examination, as well as information regarding bowel and bladder function and reflex changes, to assign a numerical value or letter grade. The second type of scale focuses on overall functional outcome, such as the patient's ability to transfer, ambulate, or participate in personal hygiene. In general, the first type of scale is used for the acute assessment of patients with SCI, whereas both types are important for assessment and description of the chronically injured patient. The most widely used scales incorporate both disability-specific and functional outcome scores in their overall assessment.

Pearl

Use of any assessment tool in the acute period requires a nonpharmacologically paralyzed patient able to follow commands and communicate with at least a "yes" or "no."

Disability-specific scales for the assessment (both acute and long-term) of patients with SCI have existed for decades. Cheshire, Frankel, and Michaelis were early contributors to this effort,[1–3] and the Frankel scale (modified thereafter by several authors) was widely adopted for use in the 1970s. This scale consisted of a reported level and a rough assessment of the severity of injury based on motor and sensory function.[2] However, the Frankel grading system has been largely abandoned as an assessment tool or outcome measure because of its lack of sensitivity. For example, many authors felt that significant improvement in patient function could occur without the patient advancing a Frankel grade.[4] Modifications of the Frankel scale were made over time in an attempt to solve this shortcoming. A sensitive and specific instrument was required that could be reliably applied by investigators with a variety of backgrounds. Institutions and individuals proposed a variety of new assessment tools.[1,4–8] Additionally, a numerical scoring system that described the patient's neurologic examination was necessary to permit valid statistical analysis.

Pearl

Acute assessment may be impaired by associated injuries or by therapeutic restrictions.

In the late 1970s, Lucas and Ducker[7] developed a scoring system based on motor function at and below the level of injury and used this to characterize over 800 patients seen at the Maryland Institute for Emergency Medical Services. Using a relatively complex mathematical analysis, these authors were able to predict a motor outcome score based on the initial motor examination and an empirically derived understanding of the recovery rate of individual injury subtypes. The scoring system is limited in that many patients are excluded from the analysis (only 436 of over 800 patients were able to be analyzed), the standard deviation of the predicted recovery score is often large, and the calculations are cumbersome.[7] Bracken and others contemporaneously developed a scoring system that combined motor and sensory function and assigned specific values to the presence or absence of function in certain muscle groups and dermatomes.[9] This scale still suffered from the lumping of all patients into one of five possible motor scores and one of seven possible sensory scores.[9] In 1982 Tator et al[8] proposed a 10-point numerical scale for grading SCI function. This scale, commonly referred to as the Sunnybrook Cord Injury Scale, was essentially a Frankel scale with finer subdivisions.

Chehrazi et al[6] published what is now referred to as the Yale Scale in 1981. This is a comprehensive spinal cord function scale. This scale employs the British Medical Research Council's gradation of muscle strength (i.e., the widely used 0–5 scale) in a systematic fashion, using 10 selected muscle groups from each side of the body. Sensory function is also scored on a 0 to 58 point scale, but bowel and bladder function are not scored.[6] In 1992, Botsford and Esses[4] published a scale in which 15 muscle groups on each side of the body are examined and given a score of 0 to 5. The scores are divided by 2 to give a maximum possible motor score of 75. Sensory function is graded on a 0 to 10 scale, as is rectal tone. Normal bladder function is scored as 5 points. Thus, the maximum possible total score is 100. Botsford and Esses then applied this scale to a group of patients who had initially been evaluated by the Frankel scale. They found that their new scale was much more sensitive for the detection of improvement in function over time and as a result of intervention, which, in this case, was the surgical treatment of burst fractures.[4]

Pearl

Repeated observations may be required for an adequate assessment of functional loss due to SCI.

Functional outcome scales, also known as function-based scales, are nonspecific measures of how a person functions within society. The most commonly used scales for functional rating are the Modified Barthel Index and the Functional Independence Measure (FIM).[10–14] These scales attempt to quantify a patient's ability or inability to live independently. They are applicable to a wide range of nervous system disorders and are not specific for SCI. Another outcome

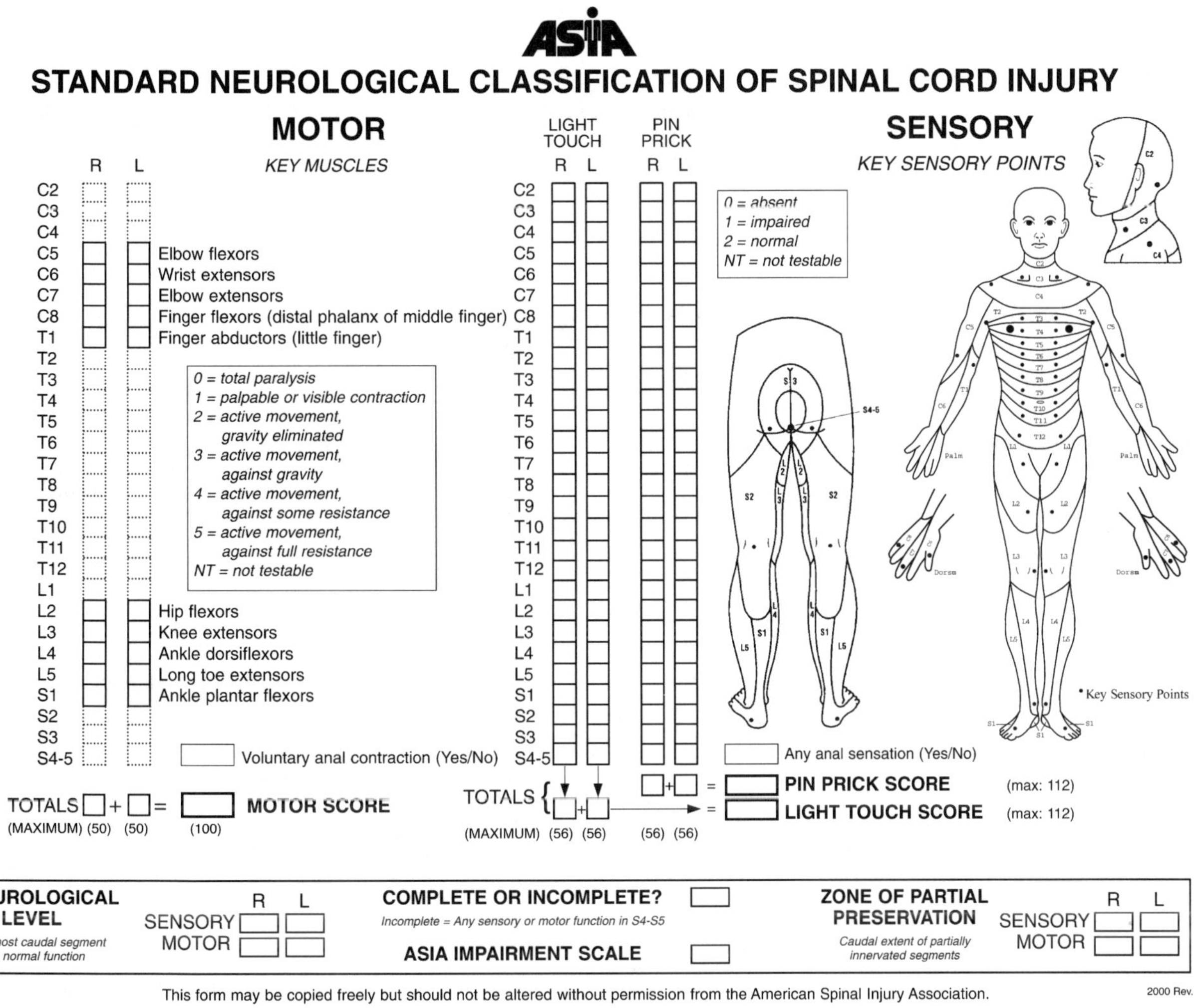

Figure 3-1 American Spinal Injury Association (ASIA) summary chart for determining motor and sensory scores.

measure, the Quadriplegic Index of Function,[15] is more specific for patients with spinal cord injuries. All of these scales have been successfully applied to the study of SCI.[15–19]

In 1982, ASIA published *Standards for the Neurological Classification of Spinal Injury Patients*.[20] These standards have undergone extensive revisions over the last several decades in response to input from multiple sources, including neurosurgeons, orthopedic surgeons, rehabilitation specialists, and basic scientists.[21–24] Repeated evaluation through reliability studies, training seminars, and statistical analysis has driven the evolution of this tool.[25–27] The current assessment tool incorporates a modified Frankel classification and a functional disability index.[24] The scale has been reviewed by numerous international organizations and, through a consortium effort, has been agreed upon as the "gold standard" classification tool. The scale defines 10 key muscle groups used for scoring, a six-point British Medical Research Council–based grading system for muscle strength, a modified Frankel scale (here called the "ASIA Impairment Scale"), and a version of the FIM. The ASIA scale was found to be more sensitive for improvement than the modified Frankel scale.[28] The ASIA scale has also been compared with other widely used comprehensive scales, such as the National Acute Spinal Cord Injury Study (NASCIS) scale used in the widely publicized methylprednisolone studies.[29] In one report, the ASIA motor scale and the NASCIS motor scale were not statistically different in terms of evaluating motor deficit and motor recovery; however, the ASIA scale is easier to apply because fewer muscle groups are tested.[30] The ASIA summary chart for determining motor and sensory scores is reproduced in Figure 3-1.

The ASIA board realizes that new information is being generated with regard to the ideal method used for classification of patients with spinal cord injuries. Revisions of the scale will be necessary as new outcome measures are evaluated, e.g., the Quadriplegia Index of Function and the Walking Index for Spinal Cord Injury.[31,32] For this purpose, the ASIA Board has established a standing committee charged with regular reevaluation of the literature.[24] Through this ongoing process, the ASIA scale will continue to evolve toward the ideal assessment/classification instrument for patients with spinal cord injuries.

Recommendations

Level II: By consensus, the International Standards for Neurological and Functional Classification of Spinal Cord Injury is the accepted "gold standard" assessment tool for the clinician involved in the care of SCI patients.

Level III: Numerous assessment tools are available for the evaluation of specific aspects of SCI. These tools may be useful in clinical studies of specific aspects of SCI.

References

1. Cheshire DJ. A classification of the functional end-results of injury to the cervical spinal cord. Paraplegia 1970;8:70–73.
2. Frankel HL, Hancock DO, Hyslop G, et al. The value of postural reduction in the initial management of closed injuries of the spine with paraplegia and tetraplegia. Paraplegia 1969;7:179–192.
3. Michaelis L. International inquiry on neurological terminology and prognosis in paraplegia and tetraplegia. Paraplegia 1969;7:1–5.
4. Botsford DJ, Esses SI. A new scale for the clinical assessment of spinal cord function. Orthopedics 1992;15:1309–1313.
5. Benzel E, Larson S. Functional recovery after decompressive operation for thoracic and lumbar spine fractures. Neurosurgery 1986;19:772–778.
6. Chehrazi B, Wagner FC Jr, Collins WF Jr, et al. A scale for the evaluation of spinal cord injury. J Neurosurg 1981;54:310–315.
7. Lucas JT, Ducker TB. Motor classification of spinal cord injuries with mobility, morbidity and recovery indices. Am Surg 1979;45:151–158.
8. Tator CH, Rowed DW, Schwartz ML. Sunnybrook Cord Injury Scales for assessing neurological injury and recovery. In: Tator CH, ed. Early Management of Acute Spinal Cord Injury. New York: Raven Press, 1982:7–24.
9. Bracken MB, Webb SB Jr, Wagner FC. Classification of the severity of acute spinal cord injury: implications for management. Paraplegia 1978;15:319–326.
10. Ditunno JF Jr. New spinal cord injury standards, 1992. Paraplegia 1992;30:90–91.
11. Hamilton BB, Granger CV, Sherwin FS. A uniform national data system for medical rehabilitation. In: Fuhrer MJ, ed. Rehabilitation Outcomes: Analysis and Measurement. Baltimore, MD: P.H. Brookes, 1987:137–147.
12. Hamilton BB, Laughlin JA, Fiedler RC, et al. Interrater agreement of the 7-level functional independence measure (FIM). Scand J Rehabil Med 1994;26:115–119.
13. Mahoney F, Barthel D. Functional evaluation: the Barthel index. Md State Med J 1965;14:61–65.
14. Yarkony GM, Roth E, Lovell L, et al. Rehabilitation outcomes in complete C5 quadriplegia. Am J Phys Med Rehabil 1988;67:73–76.
15. Gresham G, Labi M, Dittmar S, et al. The Quadriplegia Index of Function (QIF): sensitivity and reliability demonstrated in a study of thirty quadriplegic patients. Paraplegia 1986;24:38–44.
16. Ditunno JF Jr. Functional assessment measures in CNS trauma. J Neurotrauma 1992;9(S1):S301–S305.
17. Kucukdeveci AA, Yavuzer G, Tennant A, et al. Adaptation of the modified Barthel Index for use in physical medicine and rehabilitation in Turkey. Scand J Rehabil Med 2000;32:87–92.
18. Stineman MG, Marino RJ, Deutsch A, et al. A functional strategy for classifying patients after traumatic spinal cord injury. Spinal Cord 1999;37:717–725.
19. Wells JD, Nicosia S. Scoring acute spinal cord injury: a study of the utility and limitations of five different grading systems. J Spinal Cord Med 1995;18:33–41.
20. American Spinal Injury Association. Standards for the Neurological Classification of Spinal Injury Patients. Chicago: ASIA, 1982.
21. American Spinal Injury Association/International Medical Society of Paraplegia. International Standards for Neurological and Functional Classification of Spinal Cord Injury (revised 1992). Chicago: ASIA/IMSOP, 1992.
22. Ditunno JF Jr, Young W, Donovan WH, et al. The international standards booklet for neurological and functional classification of spinal cord injury. American Spinal Injury Association. Paraplegia 1994;32:70–80.
23. Ditunno JF Jr. American spinal injury standards for neurological and functional classification of spinal cord injury: past, present and future. 1992 Heiner Sell Lecture of the American Spinal Injury Association. J Am Paraplegia Soc 1994;17:7–11.
24. Maynard FM Jr, Bracken MB, Creasey G, et al. International Standards for Neurological and Functional Classification of Spinal Cord Injury. American Spinal Injury Association. Spinal Cord 1997;35:266–274.
25. Bode RK, Heinemann AW, Chen D. Measuring the impairment consequences of spinal cord injury. Am J Phys Med Rehabil 1999;78:582–594.
26. Cohen ME, Ditunno JF Jr, Donovan WH, et al. A test of the 1992 International Standards for Neurological and Functional Classification of Spinal Cord Injury. Spinal Cord 1998;36:554–560.
27. Priebe MM, Waring WP. The interobserver reliability of the revised American Spinal Injury Association standards for neurological classification of spinal injury patients. Am J Phys Med Rehabil 1991;70:268–270.
28. Capaul M, Zollinger H, Satz N, et al. Analyses of 94 consecutive spinal cord injury patients using ASIA definition and modified Frankel score classification. Paraplegia 1994;32:583–587.
29. Bracken MB, Shepard MJ, Holford TR, et al. Administration of methylprednisolone for 24 or 48 hours or tirilazad mesylate for 48 hours in the treatment of acute spinal cord injury. Results of the Third National Acute Spinal Cord Injury Randomized Controlled Trial. JAMA 1997;277:1597–1604.
30. El Masry WS, Tsubo M, Katoh S, et al. Validation of the American Spinal Injury Association (ASIA) motor score and the National Acute Spinal Cord Injury Study (NASCIS) motor score. Spine 1996;21:614–619.
31. Marino RJ, Rider-Foster D, Maissel G, et al. Superiority of motor level over single neurological level in categorizing tetraplegia. Paraplegia 1995;33:510–513.
32. Ditunno JF Jr, Ditunno PL, Graziani V, et al. Walking index for spinal cord injury (WISCI): an international multicenter validity and reliability study. Spinal Cord 2000;38:234–243.

◆ 4 ◆

When Are Computed Tomography Scans and Skull X-Rays Indicated for Patients with Minor Head Injury?

Sherman C. Stein and Mark G. Burnett

Brief Answer

The need for a computed tomography (CT) scan varies with injury severity. CT scanning should always be considered for mild or moderate head injury, but it is indicated only rarely for minimal head injury. Skull x-rays are seldom indicated for the evaluation of traumatic brain injury.

Background

Skull radiography has always been a questionable tool for the diagnosis of intracranial hematomas. The relationship between skull fractures and intracranial lesions is indirect, and the yield of routine skull radiography for minor head injury is low. Authorities have sought for years to limit its use. In contrast, a CT scan is quite accurate for detecting traumatic intracranial lesions. Although urgent CT scanning has long been routine for severe head injuries, concerns about price and availability have limited its use in minor head trauma.

There appears to be a wide range of risk of intracranial sequelae among patients with minor head injury. We have divided minor head injury into three subcategories, based on relative risk of intracranial injury. Table 4-1 shows the categories, their definitions, and relative incidences. We recently summarized the reasons for including patients with Glasgow Coma Scale (GCS) scores of 13 in the moderate head injury group.[1]

Literature Review

Class I evidence is quite sparse. There are very few prospective surveys and no controlled studies of any kind. At best, we can estimate the risks of intracranial lesions from pooled natural history data (mostly class III and some class II evidence) and compare the historical accuracy of different management schemes for the timely diagnosis of lesions. The observed outcomes of missed intracranial lesions in minor head injury populations allow a fair comparison of these management strategies. For the purposes of this chapter, we define an adverse outcome for a surgical lesion as a Glasgow Outcome Scale (GOS) score of severe disability or worse at 6 months. Adverse outcome for a nonsurgical lesion is less severe and is defined as subsequent return to the emergency department (ED) because of continued symptoms.

It is intuitively obvious that the risk of harboring a dangerous intracranial lesion is relatively low in minimal head injury and high in moderate injury. It is in the mild cases that the incidence of lesions and hence the indications for CT scanning are closest to threshold. Detailed analysis of this particular group would be most helpful in resolving differing opinions about the indications for scanning.

Table 4-2 reviews the evidence on the incidence of intracranial lesions in minor head injury and what proportion of these lesions require surgery. "Surgical" lesions are defined as evacuated hematomas or neurologic deterioration that caused an intracranial pressure (ICP) monitor to be inserted; elevation of fractures and

Table 4-1 Classification of Minor Closed Head Injury

Category	Definition	Relative Incidence (%)
Minimal	Glasgow Coma Scale (GCS) score = 15, plus no loss of consciousness (LOC) or amnesia; no neurologic deficit	82.2
Mild	GCS score = 14; or GCS score = 15 with brief (<5 minute) LOC, amnesia, or impaired alertness or memory	15.1
Moderate	GCS score = 9 to 13; or prolonged (>5 minute) LOC or focal neurological deficit	2.7

Source: Stein & Spettell.[36]

Table 4-2 Mild Closed Head Injury: Incidence of Complications

Published Series	No. of Pts.	% with CT	No. of Intracranial Lesions	No. of Surgical Lesions
Dacey et al. 1986[8]	592	11	?	12
Kraus & Nourjah 1988[12]	2265	?	453	Not reported
Livingston et al. 1991[42]	138	54	13/75	1
Mohanty et al. 1991[16]	322	100	12	0
Shackford et al. 1992[23]	2545	77	395	87 (2)
Mikhail et al. 1992[43]	85	41	8/35	3 (2)
Harad & Kerstein 1992[44]	291	100	52	≥8 (2)
Taheri et al. 1993[15]	310	59	76/184	5
Jeret 1993[17]	712	100	67	3 (2)
Cook et al. 1994[45]	107	100	9	2
Stein & Spettell 1995[36]	3558	100	405	29
Borczuk 1995[18]	1408	100	108	8 (2)
Dunham et al. 1996[19]	2123	91	134/1932 (5)	10
Culotta et al. 1996[9]	2934	100	213	23 (2), (3)
Servadei et al. 1995[46]	1221	19	82/230	21
Ingebrigsten & Romner 1996[32]	88	100	6	0
Miller et al. 1996[47]	1382	100	84	1 (2)
Arienta et al. 1997[24]	969	79	85/762	22 (2), (7)
Stiell et al. 1997[48]	1699	31	105/521	Not reported
Holmes et al. 1997[49]	264	100	35	2
Miller et al. 1997[21]	2143	100	138	5 (2)
Hsiang et al. 1997[20]	1315	61	49/797	33
Nagy et al. 1999[26]	1170	100	39	4
Tellier et al. 1999[50]	69	64	19/44	Not reported
Livingston et al. 2000[29]	2152	100	236	Not reported
Haydell et al. 2000[33]	1429	100	93	6
Vilke et al. 2000[30]	58	100	3	1
Inamasu et al. 2000[27]	1073	?	?	14
Viola et al. 2000[31]	672	100	44	6
Total	33094		2879/26698 = 10.8%	305/27654 = 1.1%

Table 4-3 Missed Diagnosis: Relative Accuracy of Management Strategies

	Management Strategy			
	Skull X-Ray Screen	**CT Screen**	**Prolonged ED**	**Universal Admission**
Missed nonsurgical lesions	61	Almost zero	25	Almost zero
Missed surgical lesions	40	0.028	63	100

Numbers represent rate of missed diagnosis (%)
See text for references on which these numbers are based.

scalp debridement are excluded. Variation exists among the patient populations studied in the quoted series (some include only GCS scores of 15, etc.), but the total of over 30,000 patients is large enough to minimize bias introduced by any single study. Although there has been considerable disagreement on how to interpret these figures, the incidence is remarkably consistent from study to study. We have chosen to compare the four alternative strategies for managing mild head injury suggested in the literature. These include *universal admission* (admit all to medical/surgical floor for 24 hours; CT only if condition worsens or symptoms persist),[2] *prolonged ED* (6-hour observation in ED; admission and CT only if condition worsens or symptoms persist),[3] *skull x-ray screen* (if fracture found, CT and admission; otherwise, discharge from ED with instruction sheet),[4] *CT screen* (CT all; discharge from ED with instruction sheet if normal).[5]

Pearl

Proposed strategies for managing mild head injury have included hospital admission for all patients, prolonged observation in the ED, skull radiography of all patients as a screening technique, and CT scanning of all patients.

Table 4-3 summarizes the evidence regarding the diagnostic accuracy of each management strategy. An entry of "almost zero" reflects a lack of documented diagnostic failures for a particular category; in terms of adverse outcomes or additions to baseline costs, it reflects a lack of unfavorable consequences. For the purposes of calculation, these categories count as rates of 0%. In a meta-analysis of the value of skull radiography in minor closed head injury (CHI), Hofman and associates[6] estimated that routine skull films would have missed 61% of intracranial hemorrhages. In another report, Miller et al[7] found that plain radiographs showed no fracture in 40% of patients whose missed hematomas later required evacuation (class III data). Although there have been a few case reports of surgical intracranial hematomas appearing after normal initial CT scans in mild CHI, only seven cases are recorded among the almost 25,000 scanned patients reported in the published series (class III data).[8,9] This yields an incidence of missed surgical lesions by CT screen of 0.028%. In a large series of pediatric patients with head injury, 63% of surgical lesions were not diagnosed within 5 hours of injury (class III data).[10] Prolonged observation in the ED would likely fail to diagnose them. We have observed that ~25% of patients harboring nonsurgical lesions become more symptomatic after 6 hours and would be "missed" by prolonged ED observation (Stein SC, unpublished data).

Prompt identification and evacuation of hematomas may prevent adverse outcomes (class III data),[11] some of which may be attributed to missed lesions. Regarding the consequences of missed lesions, Miller and associates[7] reviewed a series of patients with normal GCS scores who subsequently underwent operations for acute intracranial hematomas. The proportion of patients with poor outcomes was identical whether patients were observed until transfer to a neurosurgical unit or whether they were discharged and subsequently had to be readmitted (class III evidence). Hence the diagnosis can be considered to have been "missed" in all *universal admission* patients. Of the more than 2000 mild head injuries reported by Kraus and Nourjah,[12] 57% spent at least 2 days in the hospital; it could be argued that a similar proportion of patients with nonsurgical lesions would likely return to the ED for continued symptoms.

Pearl

Among neurologically normal patients who later underwent operations for acute intracranial hematomas, the rate of poor outcomes was the same in patients who were observed until transfer to a neurosurgical unit and in those who were discharged and subsequently had to be readmitted.

Adverse outcomes for a given management strategy can be calculated using the following formula:

% adverse outcomes = % *lesion incidence* × % *lesions missed by that strategy* × % *missed lesions resulting in adverse outcomes*

Table 4-4 Adverse Outcomes Due to Missed Diagnoses: Comparison of Management Strategies

	Management Strategy			
Adverse Outcomes (%)	**Skull X-Ray Screen**	**CT Screen**	**Prolonged ED**	**Universal Admission**
Nonsurgical lesions	3.4	Almost zero	1.4	Almost zero
Surgical lesions	0.10	0.00007	0.016	0.23

Table 4-5 Minor Head Injury Category and Relative Risk

Category	No. of Patients	% Intracranial Lesions	% with Surgery*
Minimal	70,920	?	0.01
Mild	37,712	10.8	1.1
Moderate	3121	34.1	11.7

*Craniotomies and ICP monitors only.

Using the above formula, Table 4-4 illustrates that routine CT scan screening yields the best outcomes in mild head injury for both surgical and nonsurgical lesions. For example, the incidence of nonsurgical lesions in mild head injury is 9.7% (total intracranial minus surgical lesions). According to Table 4-3, *skull x-ray screen* will miss 61% of these patients because they will not have skull fractures. Fifty-seven percent will return to the ED because of continued symptoms.[12] Thus, the percent adverse outcomes in patients with nonsurgical lesions and *skull x-ray screen* is 3.4% (9.7% × 61% × 57%). Outcomes utilizing *CT screen* are superior to the other management strategies by whole orders of magnitude; it is unlikely that minor adjustments in rates will alter this advantage.

Pearl

Outcomes from the strategy of obtaining CT scans on all patients are vastly superior to those obtained by the other management strategies.

Some authorities have considered the cost of routine scans excessive for mild head injury.[8,13–21] However, increasing availability of scanning has made it readily affordable in the U.S. and Europe.[22] Several centers have reported routine CT screening in recent years.[23–31] Taking cost factors into account, including the extra cost of false positives as well as missed diagnoses, *CT screen* appears to be the most cost-effective approach to mild head injury,[32] as well as the safest.

In a study of mild head injury reported by Livingston et al,[29] discharge of patients with normal CT scans from the ED was safe (class II). Haydel and associates[33] proposed clinical criteria for obtaining a head CT scan in mild head injury patients with GCS scores of 15 (class I data). They found that all patients with positive CT scans had at least one of the following seven findings: headache, vomiting, age >60 years, drug or alcohol intoxication, seizure, deficit in short-term memory, or physical evidence of trauma above the clavicles. Although these results await confirmation, limiting scans to patients with at least one of these findings would reduce scan rates by 20%.

Pearl

In terms of expense, including the extra costs of false positives as well as missed diagnoses, the CT screening strategy appears to be the most cost-effective approach to mild head injury, as well as the safest.

Employing the same techniques as in mild head injury, we analyzed management schemes for the minimal and moderate categories. Table 4-5 shows the incidences of intracranial and surgical lesions in all three categories. Of the more than 70,000 cases of minimal head injury reported in large series, the incidence of surgical lesions was less than 0.01%.[10,34–37] The number of nonsurgical intracranial lesions is unknown because no centers routinely perform CT scans on this group. The cost of routine CT or even plain radiography for minimal head injury is prohibitive for such a low yield. In contrast, the risks with moderate head injury far exceed those in the mild group. Of the more than 3000 cases reported,[24,36–40] over one third of patients harbored intracranial lesions, a third of which required surgery (Table 4-5). The high incidence of hematomas makes urgent CT scanning mandatory.[25] Delaying CT scanning until there has been clinical deterioration increases the risk of complications and therefore is ultimately more costly (Burnett MG et al, manuscript in preparation).

Pearl

For patients with moderate head injury, the high incidence of hematomas makes urgent CT scanning mandatory.

Recommendations

It is important to correct the misconception that all authorities mean the same thing when referring to "mild" head injury. By dividing "minor" head injury into three categories, we confine the term "mild" to a small and specific group. Over 80% of minor head injuries fall into the minimal category. The likelihood of surgical lesions in this group is vanishingly small unless complicating factors are present, such as associated injuries or medical conditions, extremes of age, suspected abuse, or other risk factors.[41] In contrast, risks are relatively high for the almost 3% of minor CHI patients in the "moderate" category. In summary, our recommendations for CT scans are as follows (Fig. 4-1):

> Minimal: safe to discharge from ED with instructions (level II)
>
> Mild: if CT normal, safe to discharge from ED with instructions (level II)
>
> Moderate: admit and obtain urgent CT (level I)

These recommendations, although evidence-based, must not be viewed as rigid standards of care. Special personnel or facilities may qualify a particular hospital's ED or inpatient ward to follow mild head injury patients so closely that estimates from the literature are inapplicable. Of course, it is not enough simply to order a CT. The images must be reviewed by a qualified physician, and abnormalities must be acted on without delay. Follow-up scans must be considered whenever a patient's clinical condition changes. Skull radiographs may be of some value in locating fragments after penetrating head wounds, but they are rarely indicated for closed head injury.

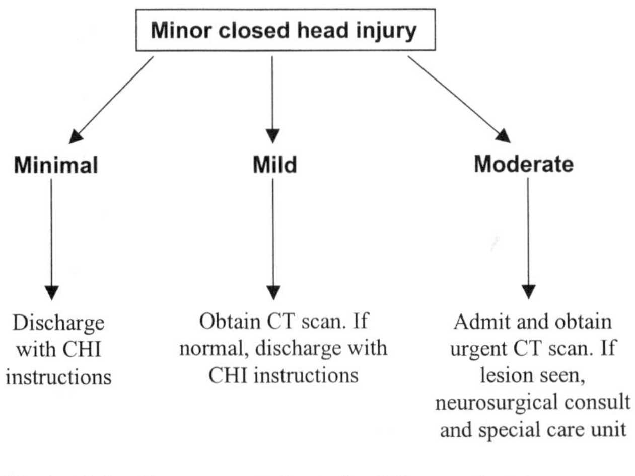

Figure 4-1 Recommendations for CT scans in minor closed head injury (see text for definitions).

References

1. Stein SC. Minor head injury: 13 is an unlucky number. J Trauma 2001;50:759–760.
2. Miller JD. Assessing patients with head injury. Br J Surg 1990;77:241–242.
3. Pitts LH. The role of neuroimaging in minor head injury. Ann Emerg Med 1991;20:1387–1388.
4. Ransohoff J, Fleischer A. Head injuries. JAMA 1975;234:861–864.
5. Stein SC, Ross SE. The value of computed tomographic scans in patients with low-risk head injuries. Neurosurgery 1990;26:638–640.
6. Hofman PA, Nelemans P, Kemerink GJ, et al. Value of radiological diagnosis of skull fracture in the management of mild head injury: meta-analysis. J Neurol Neurosurg Psychiatry 2000;68:416–422.
7. Miller JD, Murray LS, Teasdale GM. Development of a traumatic intracranial hematoma after a "minor" head injury. Neurosurgery 1990;27:669–673.
8. Dacey RG Jr, Alves WM, Rimel RW, et al. Neurosurgical complications after apparently minor head injury: assessment of risk in a series of 610 patients. J Neurosurg 1986;65:203–210.
9. Culotta VP, Sementilli ME, Gerold K, et al. Clinicopathological heterogeneity in the classification of mild head injury. Neurosurgery 1996;38:245–250.
10. Sainsbury CP, Sibert JR. How long do we need to observe head injuries in hospital? Arch Dis Child 1984;59:856–859.
11. Servadei F, Faccani G, Roccella P, et al. Asymptomatic extradural hematomas: results of a multicenter study of 158 cases in minor head injury. Acta Neurochir (Wien) 1989;96:39–45.
12. Kraus JF, Nourjah P. The epidemiology of mild, uncomplicated brain injury. J Trauma 1988;28:1637–1643.
13. Rimel RW, Jane JA. Minor head injury: management and outcome. In: Wilkins RH, Rengachary SS, eds. Neurosurgery. New York: McGraw-Hill, 1985:1608–1611.
14. Reinus WR, Wippold FJ II, Erickson KK. Practical selection criteria for noncontrast cranial computed tomography in patients with head trauma. Ann Emerg Med 1993;22:1148–1155.
15. Taheri PA, Karamanoukian H, Gibbons K, et al. Can patients with minor head injuries be safely discharged home? Arch Surg 1993;128:289–292.
16. Mohanty SK, Thompson W, Rakower S. Are CT scans for head injury patients always necessary? J Trauma 1991;31:801–805.
17. Jeret JS. Management of mild head injury. J Trauma 1993;35:490–491.
18. Borczuk P. Predictors of intracranial injury in patients with mild head trauma. Ann Emerg Med 1995;25:731–736.
19. Dunham CM, Coates S, Cooper C. Compelling evidence for discretionary brain computed tomographic imaging in those patients with mild cognitive impairment after blunt trauma. J Trauma 1996;41:679–686.
20. Hsiang JN, Yeung T, Yu AL, et al. High-risk mild head injury. J Neurosurg 1997;87:234–238.
21. Miller EC, Holmes JF, Derlet RW. Utilizing clinical factors to reduce head CT scan ordering for minor head trauma patients. J Emerg Med 1997;15:453–457.
22. Saini S, Sharma R, Levine LA, et al. Technical cost of CT examinations. Radiology 2001;218:172–175.
23. Shackford SR, Wald SL, Ross SE, et al. The clinical utility of computed tomographic scanning and neurologic examination in the management of patients with minor head injuries. J Trauma 1992;33:385–394.
24. Arienta C, Caroli M, Balbi S. Management of head-injured patients in the emergency department: a practical protocol. Surg Neurol 1997;48:213–219.
25. American College of Surgeons Committee on Trauma. Advanced Trauma Life Support Program For Physicians, Ed 6. Chicago: American College of Surgeons, 1997:193–194.
26. Nagy KK, Joseph KT, Krosner SM, et al. The utility of head computed tomography after minimal head injury. J Trauma 1999;46:268–270.
27. Inamasu J, Hori S, Aoki K, et al. CT scans essential after posttraumatic loss of consciousness. Am J Emerg Med 2000;18:810–811.

28. Ingebrigtsen T, Romner B, Kock-Jensen C. Scandinavian guidelines for initial management of minimal, mild, and moderate head injuries. The Scandinavian Neurotrauma Committee. J Trauma 2000;48:760–766.
29. Livingston DH, Lavery RF, Passannante MR, et al. Emergency department discharge of patients with a negative cranial computed tomography scan after minimal head injury. Ann Surg 2000;232:126–132.
30. Vilke GM, Chan TC, Guss DA. Use of a complete neurological examination to screen for significant intracranial abnormalities in minor head injury. Am J Emerg Med 2000;18:159–163.
31. Viola L, Zotta D, Martino V, et al. Minor head injuries: one year experience according to the new Italian guideline. Acta Neurochir (Wein) 2000;142:1281–1285.
32. Ingebrigtsen T, Romner B. Routine early CT-scan is cost saving after minor head injury. Acta Neurol Scand 1996;93: 207–210.
33. Haydel MJ, Preston CA, Mills TJ, et al. Indications for computed tomography in patients with minor head injury. N Engl J Med 2000;343:100–105.
34. Teasdale GM, Murray G, Anderson E, et al. Risks of acute traumatic intracranial haematoma in children and adults: implications for managing head injuries. BMJ 1990;300:363–367.
35. Chan KH, Yue CP, Mann KS. The risk of intracranial complications in pediatric head injury: results of multivariate analysis. Childs Nerv Syst 1990;6:27–29.
36. Stein SC, Spettell C. The Head Injury Severity Scale (HISS): a practical classification of closed-head injury. Brain Inj 1995;9: 437–444.
37. Stein SC, Doolin EJ. Management of minor head injury in children and adolescents. Pediatr Surg Int 1995;10:265–271.
38. Rimel RW, Giordani B, Barth JT, et al. Moderate head injury: completing the clinical spectrum of brain trauma. Neurosurgery 1982;11:344–351.
39. Tabaddor K, Mattis S, Zazula T. Cognitive sequelae and recovery course after moderate and severe head injury. Neurosurgery 1984;14:701–708.
40. Miller JD. Minor, moderate and severe head injury. Neurosurg Rev 1986;9:135–139.
41. Stein SC. Management of minor closed head injury. Neurosurg Q 1996;6:108–115.
42. Livingston DH, Loder PA, Koziol J, Hunt CD. The use of CT scanning to triage patients requiring admission following minimal head injury. J Trauma 1991;31:483–487.
43. Mikhail MG, Levitt MA, Christopher TA, et al. Intracranial injury following minor head trauma. Am J Emerg Med 1992;10: 24–26.
44. Harad FT, Kerstein MD. Inadequacy of bedside clinical indicators in identifying significant intracranial injury in trauma patients. J Trauma 1992;32:359–361.
45. Cook LS, Levitt MA, Simon B, et al. Identification of ethanol-intoxicated patients with minor head trauma requiring computed tomography scans. Acad Emerg Med 1994;1:227–234.
46. Servadei F, Ciucci G, Loroni L, et al. Diagnosis and management of minor head injury: a regional multicenter approach in Italy. J Trauma 1995;39:696–701.
47. Miller EC, Derlet RW, Kinser D. Minor head trauma: is computed tomography always necessary? Ann Emerg Med 1996; 27:290–294.
48. Stiell IG, Wells GA, Vandemheen K, et al. Variation in ED use of computed tomography for patients with minor head injury. Ann Emerg Med 1997;30:14–22.
49. Holmes JF, Baier ME, Derlet RW. Failure of the Miller criteria to predict significant intracranial injury in patients with a Glasgow Coma Scale score of 14 after minor head trauma. Acad Emerg Med 1997;4:788–792.
50. Tellier A, Della Malva LC, Cwinn A, et al. Mild head injury: a misnomer. Brain Inj 1999;13:463–475.

◆ 5 ◆

What Is the Best Way to Rule Out Spine or Spinal Cord Injury in a Trauma Patient, Especially When Head Injury Is Present?

Donald W. Marion

Brief Answer

After hemodynamic and pulmonary stabilization and treatment of all immediately life-threatening injuries in trauma patients, identification of cervical spine injuries can ideally be accomplished within 48 hours of admission. Patients who are alert and awake and who have no distracting pain, no midline neck pain, no neurologic deficits referable to the cervical spine, and no intoxication are extremely unlikely to have a significant cervical spine injury. They do not need either cervical spine x-rays or cervical spine precautions (level I recommendation). Patients with neck pain, neurologic deficits, or altered mental status should have anteroposterior, lateral, and open-mouth odontoid x-rays that clearly delineate the cervical spine from the occiput to T1. Axial computed tomography (CT) images should be obtained from the occiput to C2. In addition, if the lower cervical spine is not clearly visualized on lateral x-rays, axial CT scanning should be performed through this area, as well as through any areas that appear suspicious or questionable on the plain films. If all studies are normal, patients with neck pain should have flexion/extension x-rays (level II recommendation). Patients with neurologic deficits should have a magnetic resonance imaging (MRI) scan of the cervical spine (level II recommendation). For those with impaired consciousness, plain x-rays with CT supplementation as described above will identify significant cervical spine instability in 99% of cases.

Background

In 2000, the Cervical Spine Clearance ad hoc committee of the Eastern Association for the Surgery of Trauma (EAST) updated the evidence-based guidelines that it had produced in 1998.[1] The committee had identified two groups of trauma patients for whom clearing the cervical spine was difficult: individuals who were alert and awake, with normal mental status not altered by drugs or alcohol, and with no painful injuries that might distract their attention from possible cervical spine injuries; and those who had an altered mental status, most commonly due to a closed head injury. The former group was capable of describing the presence or absence of neck pain, whereas the latter group was not. The literature indicates that the ability to verify the presence or absence of neck pain in a reliable manner is very useful in identifying significant cervical spine injuries. A large amount of prospectively collected data (over 6000 trauma patients) suggests that no patient who was alert and awake at the time of evaluation and who was free of distracting pain had a clinically significant cervical spine injury in the absence of neck pain. The committee, therefore, concluded that cervical spine radiographs were not necessary for clearance of the cervical spine in these patients. However, debate persists about the most appropriate studies for clearance of the cervical spine for those patients who are unable to reliably describe the presence or absence of neck pain.

Pearl

The ability to verify the presence or absence of neck pain in a reliable manner is very useful in identifying significant cervical spine injuries.

This review focuses on articles that have been published subsequent to the literature review conducted during the formulation of the original EAST guidelines. One hundred five publications that have appeared since 1995 were retrieved through a search of the National Library of Medicine using the search terms "cervical spine" and "trauma." Studies that were relevant to the issue of radiographically identifying cervical spine injuries were reviewed and are summarized below.

Literature Review

Clearance of the Cervical Spine in Alert, Awake Trauma Patients

Several large studies published since 1995 support the original recommendations of the EAST guidelines regarding clearance of the cervical spine in alert, awake patients. Velmahos et al[2] reported a prospective study of 549 consecutive alert, oriented, and clinically nonintoxicated blunt trauma victims with no symptoms of neck injury (class II data). In all patients, three-view plain radiographs were supplemented by axial CT through suspicious or inadequately visualized areas of the lower cervical spine. No patient was found to have a significant cervical spine injury. In a retrospective study of 267 nonintoxicated, fully oriented trauma patients, Ersoy et al[3] found that no patient without neck pain or tenderness had a cervical spine injury (class III data). In a prospective study of 118 patients, Mahadevan et al[4] documented relatively good interrater reliability (87.7%) of emergency medicine physicians for identifying altered mental status, intoxication, posterior midline tenderness, and distracting pain as clinical risk factors for cervical spine injury (class II data). Hoffman et al[5] conducted a prospective, observational, multicenter study of 34,069 patients to determine the ability of a decision instrument employing the five criteria of no midline cervical tenderness; no focal neurologic deficit; normal alertness; no intoxication; and no painful, distracting injury to identify those blunt trauma patients who do not require cervical spine radiography. The decision instrument incorrectly identified only two patients as unlikely to have a clinically significant cervical spine injury (99.6% sensitivity, 99.9% negative predictive value); only one of these two patients underwent surgery (class I data). Despite disparities between emergency medical technicians and emergency medicine physicians in identification of those trauma patients who do not need prehospital cervical spine immobilization,[6] there seems to be increasing support for using criteria of this type to determine which patients may be treated safely without prehospital spinal immobilization.[7,8]

Clearance of the Cervical Spine in Obtunded or Comatose Patients

The recent literature provides further support for the recommendation that the upper cervical spine (C1-C2) be routinely imaged with axial CT scanning during the initial CT evaluation of the cranium (class III data).[9] In a study of 202 patients with traumatic brain injury (TBI), Link et al[10] found that 5.4% had C1 or C2 fractures that were not visualized on three-view radiographs and 4.0% had occipital condyle fractures that were not visualized by plain radiography (class II data). Blacksin and Lee[11] evaluated 100 consecutive trauma patients and found an 8% incidence of fractures of either the occipital condyle (3%) or C1-C2 (5%) not detected on cross-table lateral cervical spine radiographs (class II data). Further evidence also supports the conclusion that three views of the cervical spine (lateral, anteroposterior, and open-mouth odontoid) are more likely to detect cervical spine fractures than is a single lateral view (class II data).[12]

Pearl

Routine imaging of the upper cervical spine (C1-C2) should be performed during the initial CT evaluation of the cranium.

No prospective study has clearly defined the incidence of missed cervical spine injuries in obtunded patients. Although most trauma centers routinely obtain three-view cervical spine radiographs for all trauma patients admitted to the hospital, none has reported the results of follow-up imaging studies obtained at some interval after the initial three-view studies in all of these patients. As a result, the true incidence of occult instability cannot be reliably determined.

Several authors have attempted to determine the incidence of occult ligamentous instability in TBI patients with impaired consciousness. Ajani et al[13] prospectively studied 100 trauma patients with standard three-view plain radiographs as well as a swimmer's view if needed to visualize C7-T1 (class II data). Patients also underwent CT scanning and/or MRI for further evaluation of actual or suspected abnormalities on plain radiographs. If these studies were interpreted as normal, the patients had flexion and extension radiographs. Of the 91 patients who survived long enough for data collection, six were found to have "unstable" cervical spine injuries. In five patients, the instability was identified by the screening radiographs, but in one patient it was detected only with passive flexion/extension radiographs (although the authors also state that thin cut CT scan of the entire cervical spine would likely have been an adequate substitute for flexion/extension radiographs in this patient, who had an abnormal neurologic examination). Sees et al[14] reported a retrospective study of 20 obtunded trauma patients evaluated with flexion/extension fluoroscopy (class III data). All 20 patients had technically acceptable three-view cervical spine radiographs that were interpreted as normal prior to the flexion/extension studies. The complete cervical spine could not be visualized with flexion/extension studies in six patients. The flexion/extension studies identified subluxation at C4–5 in one of the 20 patients.

Beirne et al[15] attempted to determine prospectively the incidence of cervical spine injury in 582 patients with facial fractures who presented to their trauma center over a 1-year period (class II data). Six patients were found to have cervical spine injuries, but the injuries were identifiable on three-view radiographs in only two of the six. In two patients, the injuries could be detected only with flexion/extension radiographs. Davis et al[16] prospectively evaluated the utility of dynamic flexion and extension cervical spine studies performed via fluoroscopy in 301 patients with a Glasgow Coma Scale score <13 for greater than 48 hours (class II data). All patients were initially thought to have normal and adequate five-view cervical spine films, supplemented with axial CT images through any suspicious areas identified on plain films and, in the more recently enrolled patients, through the occiput-C2 region. Only two patients (0.7%) demonstrated significant instability on fluoroscopic evaluation. Another patient had a false-negative evaluation. In that case, the fluoroscopic examination visualized only C1-C6. Despite the inadequacy of the fluoroscopic study, cervical spine precautions were discontinued in that patient. She was allowed to sit up in a chair, whereupon she became quadriplegic from C6–7 and C7-T1 subluxations. Review of her initial cervical spine x-rays revealed that they had been incorrectly misinterpreted as normal even though subluxations were present at C6–7 and at C7-T1.

In three of the four studies cited above, it is possible to determine the total number of trauma patients who had flexion/extension radiographs.[13,14,16] Meta-analysis of these three studies reveals an incidence of 5/412 (1.2%) of occult cervical spine injury not identified with three-view radiographs plus CT supplementation. It is important to note that spinal cord injury was not caused by passive flexion/extension in any of these patients.

A practical difficulty that is commonly encountered during attempted fluoroscopic flexion and extension cervical spine studies in the supine position is inability to visualize the lower cervical spine. Bolinger et al[17] described their attempts to perform fluoroscopic flexion/extension cervical spine studies in a series of 56 consecutive, comatose, pharmacologically paralyzed head-injured patients (class II data). They were able to visualize the entire cervical spine in only two of these 56 patients. In such cases in which the lower cervical spine cannot be visualized by bedside fluoroscopy, the best alternative may be MRI. Unfortunately, although MRI is very sensitive for detecting soft tissue injuries, particularly within the first 48 hours of injury (class II and class III data),[18–21] there exists no good evidence to show that minor injuries detected with MRI represent true instability. In fact, it has been stated that MRI may overestimate true instability in as many as 25 to 40% of patients (class III data).[22]

Pearl

One study found that fluoroscopic flexion/extension studies could visualize the entire cervical spine in only two of 56 patients (3.6%).

Pearl

MRI may overestimate the presence of cervical spine instability in as many as 25 to 40% of patients.

Recommendations

Trauma patients can be categorized by their clinical presentations into four categories of risk for cervical spine injury. The following guidelines are presented by category of patient, and recommendations specific to that category are provided.

1. Alert, awake, not intoxicated, neurologically normal, and no midline neck pain or tenderness even with full range of motion of neck and palpation of cervical spine

Level I recommendation: Cervical spine x-rays are not necessary.

Attending-level physicians (from emergency medicine, trauma surgery, orthopedic spine surgery, or neurosurgery) may make this determination, document it in the medical record, and remove the cervical collar. Prehospital spine immobilization is indicated in the trauma patient who has sustained an injury with a mechanism having the potential to cause a spine injury and who has at least one of the following:

a. Altered mental status
b. Evidence of intoxication
c. A distracting painful injury (e.g., long bone extremity fracture)
d. Neurologic deficits
e. Spinal pain or tenderness to palpation

2. Alert, awake, complains of neck pain

Level II recommendations: Obtain three-view cervical spine x-rays supplemented with axial CT images at 3-mm intervals through suspicious areas on three-view cervical spine x-rays. If lower cervical spine is not adequately visualized on lateral cervical spine x-ray, obtain swimmer's view. If swimmer's view is inadequate, obtain axial CT images with sagittal reconstruction through lower cervical spine at 3-mm intervals.

If above studies are normal, remove the cervical collar and obtain flexion/extension lateral cervical spine x-rays with the patient sitting and voluntarily flexing and extending his or her neck. Voluntary and painless excursion must exceed 30 degrees. Flexion/extension x-rays may be obtained by the radiology technician under the supervision of the radiologist. No other physician or nurse needs to be present while they are obtained.

If voluntary, painless excursion during flexion/extension does not exceed 30 degrees, the cervical spine collar should be replaced and flexion/extension lateral cervical spine x-rays repeated in 2 weeks.

3. Neurologic deficits referable to a spine injury

Level II recommendations: Obtain plain films and CT images as described in item 2 above and also obtain MRI of the cervical spine.

4. Altered mental status and return of normal mental status not anticipated for 2 days or longer, e.g., severe traumatic, hypoxic, or ischemic brain injury

Level II recommendations: Obtain plain films and CT images as described in item 2 above. In addition, obtain axial CT images at 3-mm intervals with sagittal reconstruction from the base of the occiput through C2.

Level III recommendations (may detect occult instability in ~1% of patients): If above studies (under item 4) are normal, perform flexion/extension lateral cervical spine fluoroscopy with static images obtained at extremes of flexion and extension. Excursion of the neck is done by housestaff or attendings of trauma surgery, neurosurgery, or orthopedic spine surgery. If the entire cervical spine cannot be visualized with flexion/extension lateral cervical spine fluoroscopy, MRI of the cervical spine is recommended.

Addenda

A. Radiologic clearance of the cervical spine should occur only after hemodynamic, respiratory, and surgical stabilization of a patient. During such stabilization, the cervical spine should be kept immobilized in an approved cervical spine collar.

B. Three-view cervical spine x-rays are defined as follows:

Lateral cervical spine radiograph: must be of good quality and must adequately delineate the entire cervical spine, from the base of the occiput to the upper part of the first thoracic vertebra.

Anteroposterior cervical spine radiograph: must reveal the spinous processes of C2 to C7.

Open-mouth odontoid radiograph: must visualize the entire dens and the lateral masses of C1.

C. For patients with neurologic deficits referable to a cervical spine injury, it is extremely important to obtain an MRI scan as soon as possible after the patient arrives at the emergency department, particularly when plain radiographs are normal (level III). High-dose methylprednisolone therapy started within, but not after, 8 hours of injury has been associated with neurologic improvement. Early decompression of mass lesions such as traumatic herniated disks or epidural hematomas may also improve neurologic outcome.

D. The ultimate evaluation of all radiographic studies is the responsibility of attending radiologists. However, attending physicians from trauma surgery, emergency medicine, neurosurgery, and orthopedic spine surgery are considered qualified to interpret cervical spine radiographs properly. Based on that interpretation and on their clinical evaluation of the patient, they may "clear" the cervical spine and remove the cervical spine collar after proper documentation in the patient's medical record.

Acknowledgment

This chapter was adapted, with permission, from the Trauma Practice Guideline "Practice Management Guidelines for Identifying Cervical Spine Injuries Following Trauma," © 2000 by the Eastern Association for the Surgery of Trauma; available at *www.east.org*.

References

1. Marion DW, Domeier RM, Dunham CM, et al. Determination of cervical spine stability in trauma patients. Eastern Association for the Surgery of Trauma website. Available at *http://www.east.org/tpg/chap3u.pdf.*
2. Velmahos GC, Theodorou D, Tatevossian R, et al. Radiographic cervical spine evaluation in the alert asymptomatic blunt trauma victim: much ado about nothing. J Trauma 1996;40:768–774.
3. Ersoy G, Karcioglu O, Enginbas Y, et al. Are cervical spine x-rays mandatory in all blunt trauma patients? Eur J Emerg Med 1995;2:191–195.
4. Mahadevan S, Mower WR, Hoffman JR, et al. Interrater reliability of cervical spine injury criteria in patients with blunt trauma. Ann Emerg Med 1998;31:197–201.
5. Hoffman JR, Mower WR, Wolfson AB. Validity of a set of clinical criteria to rule out injury to the cervical spine in patients with blunt trauma. N Engl J Med 2000;343:94–99.
6. Meldon SW, Brant TA, Cydulka RK, et al. Out-of-hospital cervical spine clearance: agreement between emergency medical technicians and emergency physicians. J Trauma 1998;45:1058–1061.
7. Domeier RM. Indications for prehospital spinal immobilization. National Association of EMS Physicians Standards and Clinical Practice Committee. Prehosp Emerg Care 1999;3:251–253.
8. Domeier RM, Evans RW, Swor RA, et al. Prospective validation of out-of-hospital spinal clearance criteria: a preliminary report. Acad Emerg Med 1997;4:643–646.
9. Nunez DB Jr, Zuluaga A, Fuentes-Bernardo DA, et al. Cervical spine trauma: how much more do we learn by routinely using helical CT? Radiographics 1996;16:1307–1318.
10. Link TM, Schuierer G, Hufendiek A, et al. Substantial head trauma: value of routine CT examination of the cervicocranium. Radiology 1995;196:741–745.
11. Blacksin MF, Lee HJ. Frequency and significance of fractures of the upper cervical spine detected by CT in patients with severe neck trauma. AJR 1995;165:1201–1204.
12. West OC, Anbari MM, Pilgram TK, et al. Acute cervical spine trauma: diagnostic performance of single-view versus three-view radiographic screening. Radiology 1997;204:819–823.
13. Ajani AE, Cooper DJ, Scheinkestel CD, et al. Optimal assessment of cervical spine trauma in critically ill patients: a prospective evaluation. Anaesth Intensive Care 1998;26:487–491.
14. Sees DW, Rodriguez Cruz LR, Flaherty SF, et al. The use of bedside fluoroscopy to evaluate the cervical spine in obtunded trauma patients. J Trauma 1998;45:768–771.
15. Beirne JC, Butler PE, Brady FA. Cervical spine injuries in patients with facial fractures: a 1-year prospective study. Int J Oral Maxillofac Surg 1995;24:26–29.
16. Davis JW, Kaups KL, Cunningham MA, et al. Routine evaluation of the cervical spine in head-injured patients with dynamic fluoroscopy: a reappraisal. J Trauma 2001;50:1044–1047.
17. Bolinger B, Shartz M, Marion DW. Bedside fluoroscopic flexion and extension cervical spine x-rays for clearance of the cervical spine in comatose trauma patients. J Trauma 2004;56:132–136.
18. Benzel EC, Hart BL, Ball PA, et al. Magnetic resonance imaging for the evaluation of patients with occult cervical spine injury. J Neurosurg 1996;85:824–829.
19. D'Alise MD, Benzel EC, Hart BL. Magnetic resonance imaging of the cervical spine in the comatose or obtunded trauma patient. J Neurosurg 1999;91:54–59.
20. Emery SE, Pathria MN, Wilber RG, et al. Magnetic resonance imaging of posttraumatic spinal ligament injury. J Spinal Disord 1989;2:229–233.
21. Katzberg RW, Benedetti PF, Drake CM, et al. Acute cervical spine injuries: prospective MR imaging assessment at a level one trauma center. Radiology 1999;213:203–212.
22. Hadley MN, Walters BC, Grabb PA, et al. Guidelines for the management of acute cervical spine and spinal cord injuries. Clin Neurosurg 2002;49:407–498.

◆ 6 ◆

How Can I Decide That a Head-Injured Patient Can't Be Salvaged?

Donald W. Marion

Brief Answer

Decisions regarding "salvageability" of the severely brain-injured patient and decisions to terminate life-support measures are complicated by physicians' inability to be certain about prognosis, by the concerns of patients' families, particularly regarding the level of long-term disability they are willing to accept, and by concerns regarding organ donation. Prospective cohort studies do indicate, as a level II recommendation, that patients with traumatic brain injury (TBI) who are older than 60 years, who are flaccid or posturing, and who have at least one non-reactive pupil after cardiopulmonary resuscitation, at 24 hours after injury will not achieve a good outcome [Glasgow Outcome Scale (GOS) score of 4 or 5]. Patients of any age who have sustained a gunshot wound that penetrates the brainstem or basal ganglia, who have no large intracranial mass lesion, and who have a similar neurologic examination (posturing, fixed pupil) also will not achieve a GOS of 4 or 5.

Background

The ability to predict within hours after injury that a patient with severe TBI will die or remain in a persistent vegetative state despite our best treatment efforts is desirable for several reasons. Modern intensive care can sustain vital functions in most patients indefinitely, and persistent vegetative survival may last for months or years, causing prolonged grieving of family members. Medical care of TBI patients has been estimated to cost as much as $84 million per year, with the majority of the money spent on those with the most severe injuries, who are unlikely to attain a meaningful recovery. Early and accurate prediction of outcomes could allow for redistribution of health care dollars to those who are most likely to benefit.

During the last 20 to 30 years, more than 60 published studies have examined the sensitivity and specificity of various early prognostic indicators. Specific components of the physical and radiologic examination, demographic factors, electrophysiologic findings, and chemical and metabolic profiles of the brain as inferred from jugular venous blood or cerebrospinal fluid (CSF) analysis have been evaluated as potential prognostic indicators. Most studies conclude that a combination of these measures provides the most accurate prediction of outcome and that reevaluation 24 hours after injury significantly improves predictive sensitivity.

Clinical Determination of Brain Death

The diagnosis of brain death implies that no brain function is detectable and, most importantly, that this condition is irreversible. The most widely accepted criteria for this diagnosis include (1) establishing the cause; (2) ruling out or correcting medical conditions that can depress the neurologic examination (e.g., severe electrolyte, acid-base, or endocrine abnormalities; hypothermia; hypotension; drug intoxication; poisoning; ingestion of systemic neuromuscular paralytic agents); (3) computed tomography (CT) findings that confirm severe brain injury or swelling, and (4) a careful neurologic examination that confirms the absence of cortical and brainstem function.[1] The Glasgow Coma Scale (GCS) score should be 3, and the pupils nonreactive to light. No oculocephalic, corneal, or cough reflex is present, and cold caloric stimulation does not cause tonic deviation of the eyes. An apnea test may be done to confirm absence of respiratory effort even when the $PaCO_2$ reaches 60 mmHg. Confirmatory tests advocated by some, and recommended for children, include the atropine test (no change in heart rate after intravenous infusion of 1 mg of atropine), electroencephalography (EEG) (no activity at levels higher than 2 μV for 30 minutes of recording, with sensitivity set at 2 μV/mm), cerebral angiography (no intracranial blood flow), transcranial Doppler (absence of diastolic flow or reverberating flow), and nuclear imaging (absence of intracerebral uptake of tracer). Some also advocate repeating a test after 6 to 24 hours.

Literature Review: Early Prognostic Indicators

Physical Examination and Age

Pearl

Patient age, the motor component of the GCS score, and pupillary size and reactivity are consistently found to correlate independently with the severity of brain injury and therefore with outcome.

Patient age and two elements of the physical examination (the motor component of the GCS score and pupillary size and reactivity) are consistently found to independently correlate with the severity of brain injury and therefore with outcome. Choi et al[2] reviewed the 12-month outcomes of 555 patients with severe TBI who were prospectively included in their TBI database (class II data). Among 23 prognostic indicators, they found that age, GCS motor score, and pupillary reactivity were the most important prognostic indicators and could be used in combination to predict death or vegetative survival with an accuracy rate of 90%. However, 12 of 121 patients predicted to have a poor outcome were neurologically normal or had only moderate disabilities at 12 months. Mamelak et al[3] developed a predictive model by using stepwise logistic regression analysis to define the clinical variables most important for predicting 6-month outcome in 672 TBI patients entered prospectively into a database. The authors then applied the model to 108 patients randomly selected from the database to determine its predictive accuracy (class II data). They, too, found that age, best motor score, and pupillary reactivity were the most significant predictors of outcome. These elements were included in their model, which had a sensitivity of 100%; in the 108 patients in whom it was tested, the model correctly identified all survivors and made no false-negative predictions of nonsurvival in patients who actually survived. However, when applied during the first 6 hours after injury, its specificity was only 43%; 57% of patients who were predicted to have a good outcome actually died or were vegetative by 6 months after injury. When applied at 24 hours after injury, the model demonstrated an increase in specificity to 73%. In a later report, Lang et al[4] reanalyzed 1066 patients from the same database and included hypotension as an independent predictor in their model (class II data). They also concluded that the 24-hour evaluation was more accurate, but the sensitivity of their model (as defined above) was only 89.6%, and the specificity was 76%.

Pearl

Prognostication is more accurate at 24 hours after injury than at only a few hours after injury.

Such models are important for emphasizing that accurately predicting the likelihood of favorable outcomes in all patients with severe TBI is impossible, either at admission or at 24 hours after injury. Furthermore, these models are complex and not easily applied by most physicians caring for TBI patients. In a more practical report, Quigley et al[5] examined the influence of age, GCS, and pupillary reactivity on outcomes (at least 6 months after injury) of 380 patients with an admission GCS score of 3 to 5 (class II data). All of their 80 patients aged 60 and older were either dead or vegetative at follow-up. When one or both pupils were nonreactive, all 96 patients older than 50 years and all but one of 121 patients older than 40 years were either dead or vegetative. This study also found that among those less than 20 years of age, 27% (24/88) achieved a functional recovery. In the subset with one or both pupils nonreactive, 15% (11/72) had a functional recovery.

For patients with gunshot wounds to the head, outcomes appear to be more closely related to the initial GCS and pupillary reactivity and less related to age. Polin et al[6] reviewed eight outcome studies of cranial gunshot wounds and found that only 8.1% of 431 patients with an initial GCS score of 3 to 5 survived (class III data). Survival for all patients with an admission GCS score of 3 to 8 was only 12.7%.

Computed Tomography Findings

Marshall et al[7] identified several CT characteristics that are most closely correlated with outcomes following severe nonpenetrating TBI when they reviewed the CT scans from 746 patients enrolled in the Traumatic Coma Data Bank (TCDB).[7] They determined that compression of the basal cisterns, the presence and size of hematomas or contusions, and shift of the midline structures were most important for predicting outcome, and they developed a classification system that used the presence or absence of these CT findings to grade the severity of injury (class II data). When applied to the patients in the TCDB, 94% of those with the worst findings on CT (diffuse injury IV: midline shift >5 mm, no high- or mixed-density lesion >25 cc) were found to have poor outcomes (GOS score 1–3), and their mortality rate was 56%. If the cisterns were compressed or absent and there were no large mass lesions (diffuse injury III), the mortality rate was 34%. If there was a large mass lesion not surgically evacuated, the mortality rate was 53%, and only 11% of these patients achieved a good outcome (GOS score 4 or 5). These investigators found that combining the CT findings with age and GCS motor score increased the sensitivity of their outcome prediction model by 6% compared with a model that included only age and motor score, though it did not increase the specificity of the model. In a subsequent study of 72 patients with severe TBI, Kido et al[8] emphasized the importance of the size of the lesion for predicting outcomes (class II data). They found a twofold greater risk of poor outcomes in patients who harbored clots or contusions greater than 41 mL in volume compared with those who did not, but they found no correlation between lesion location or skull fracture and outcome.

Sophisticated prehospital trauma triage and transport systems have dramatically decreased the time from injury to CT evaluation of trauma patients, and such ultra-early CT images may not accurately reflect the ultimate severity of the brain injuries. Servadei et al[9] found that 16% of 384 patients with diffuse injuries on their initial CT scans had worse injuries on follow-up CT scans. In 74% of these patients the second scan revealed a mass lesion not apparent on the first scan. The likelihood of a poor outcome was 62% for those in whom a mass lesion evolved, compared with 38% for those without a subsequent mass lesion (class II data).

Pearl

Ultra-early CT scanning may not accurately reflect the ultimate severity of brain injury because mass lesions may not appear until several hours after the traumatic event.

For cranial gunshot wounds, no study has reported a functional outcome in patients of any age in whom a bullet has penetrated the brainstem or basal ganglia. In a meta-analysis of the effects of bullet traversal of the midsagittal plane, Polin et al[6] reviewed the results of six series (totaling 343 patients) and noted that the mortality rate was 87% if the bullet track crossed the midsagittal plane, i.e., was bihemispheric (class III data).

Pearl

No study has reported a functional outcome in a patient in whom a bullet has traversed the brainstem or basal ganglia.

Electrophysiologic Findings

The most widely used electrophysiologic techniques for early prediction of outcome following severe TBI are EEG and somatosensory evoked potentials (SEPs). EEG has not been shown to reliably predict outcome except in the case of absent EEG activity at high voltage gain in a nonsedated, normotensive patient, in which case it virtually always indicates brain death. However, by combining EEG with analysis of the central conduction time of SEPs in a study of 50 TBI patients, Gutling et al[10] were able to predict good (GOS 4 or 5) versus poor outcomes in all but one patient (98% accuracy) (class II data). In a study of early SEPs in 31 consecutive patients with severe TBI but no large mass lesions, Claassen and Hansen[11] found that bilateral absence of cortical responses was 100% predictive of death or vegetative survival at 3 months after injury (class II data). Judson et al[12] studied 100 patients with SEPs and found that the presence of cortical potentials (even if abnormal) predicted favorable outcomes with a sensitivity of 95% and a specificity of 73%. If cortical responses were absent at any time on one or both sides, the sensitivity for predicting death, vegetative survival, or severe disability was 73%, and the specificity was 95% (class II data).

Other Prognostic Indicators

Several physiologic and metabolic abnormalities commonly observed after severe TBI have been used in attempts to identify reliable early prognostic indicators. Intracranial pressure (ICP) has been extensively studied, and there clearly is a correlation between sustained ICPs above 20 mmHg and poor outcomes. Intracranial hypertension refractory to treatment bears an even stronger association with death or vegetative survival (class III data).[13] However, Resnick et al[14] found no influence of early intracranial hypertension on outcome at one year after injury in young patients with an initial GCS >5 (class II data).[14] Molecular markers of brain injury in the serum or CSF, such as neuron-specific enolase and S-100 protein, also have been evaluated as early prognostic indicators but have not been found to be reliable independent predictors of outcome (class II data).[15,16] Serum levels of S-100 protein may be more closely related to the severity of musculoskeletal injury than to brain injury (class II data).[17]

Recommendations

Level II

1. Closed head injury: Patients who have severe TBI with age >60 years, postresuscitation GCS motor score of 1 to 3, and at least one nonreactive pupil at 24 hours postinjury will not achieve a good outcome (GOS 4 or 5) and will likely either die or survive in a vegetative state.
2. Gunshot wounds: Patients with a postresuscitation GCS motor score of 1 to 3, at least one nonreactive pupil, no large intracranial mass lesion, and a bullet trajectory that traverses the brainstem or basal ganglia will not achieve a good outcome (GOS 4 or 5).
3. Among patients with the most severe penetrating and nonpenetrating TBI, it is not possible to reliably predict who will die and who will remain in a vegetative state based on early prognostic indicators analyzed singly or in combination unless the patients meet the criteria for brain death.

References

1. Wijdicks EF. The diagnosis of brain death. N Engl J Med 2001;344:1215–1221.
2. Choi SC, Muizelaar JP, Barnes TY, et al. Prediction tree for severely head-injured patients. J Neurosurg 1991;75:251–255.
3. Mamelak AN, Pitts LH, Damron S. Predicting survival from head trauma 24 hours after injury: a practical method with therapeutic implications. J Trauma 1996;41:91–99.
4. Lang EW, Pitts LH, Damron SL, et al. Outcome after severe head injury: an analysis of prediction based upon comparison of neural network versus logistic regression analysis. Neurol Res 1997;19:274–280.
5. Quigley MR, Vidovich D, Cantella D, et al. Defining the limits of survivorship after very severe head injury. J Trauma 1997; 42:7–10.
6. Polin RS, Shaffrey ME, Phillips CD, et al. Multivariate analysis and prediction of outcome following penetrating head injury. Neurosurg Clin North Am 1995;6:689–699.
7. Marshall LF, Marshall SB, Klauber MR, et al. A new classification of head injury based on computerized tomography. J Neurosurg 1991;75:S14–S20.
8. Kido DK, Cox C, Hamill RW, et al. Traumatic brain injuries: predictive usefulness of CT. Radiology 1992;182:777–781.
9. Servadei F, Murray GD, Penny K, et al. The value of the "worst" computed tomographic scan in clinical studies of moderate and severe head injury. European Brain Injury Consortium. Neurosurgery 2000;46:70–75.
10. Gutling E, Gonser A, Imhof HG, et al. EEG reactivity in the prognosis of severe head injury. Neurology 1995;45:915–918.
11. Claassen J, Hansen HC. Early recovery after closed traumatic head injury: somatosensory evoked potentials and clinical findings. Crit Care Med 2001;29:494–502.
12. Judson JA, Cant BR, Shaw NA. Early prediction of outcome from cerebral trauma by somatosensory evoked potentials. Crit Care Med 1990;18:363–368.
13. Prat R, Calatayud-Maldonado V. Prognostic factors in postraumatic severe diffuse brain injury. Acta Neurochir (Wien) 1998; 140:1257–1260.
14. Resnick DK, Marion DW, Carlier P. Outcome analysis of patients with severe head injuries and prolonged intracranial hypertension. J Trauma 1997;42:1108–1111.
15. Ross SA, Cunningham RT, Johnston CF, et al. Neuron-specific enolase as an aid to outcome prediction in head injury. Br J Neurosurg 1996;10:471–476.
16. Romner B, Ingebrigtsen T, Kongstad P, et al. Traumatic brain damage: serum S-100 protein measurements related to neuroradiological findings. J Neurotrauma 2000;17:641–647.
17. Anderson RE, Hansson LO, Nilsson O, et al. High serum S100B levels for trauma patients without head injuries. Neurosurgery 2001;48:1255–1258.

♦ Part II ♦

Issues Common to Head Injury and Spinal Cord Injury

◆ 7 ◆

Can Special Beds Reduce the Incidence of Complications in Head-Injured and Spinal Cord–Injured Patients?

Jeff W. Chen

Brief Answer

The prolonged immobility caused by traumatic brain injury (TBI) and spinal cord injury (SCI) renders patients with these conditions especially vulnerable to skin breakdown and to impairments in pulmonary function. Specially designed beds are particularly helpful in dealing with these problems. Class I, II, and III data demonstrate that beds that provide automatic side-to-side rotation improve pulmonary function and decrease the incidence of pulmonary complications. Class I data also indicate that low-air-loss beds decrease the incidence of, and expedite the healing of, pressure ulcers. However, not all studies have demonstrated such benefits, probably because of differences in design and implementation of the investigational protocols of the various studies. The effects of kinetic therapy on intracranial pressure (ICP) have not been studied as rigorously, but modest elevations of ICP that have sometimes been reported to occur with rotational therapy do not seem to be clinically significant, especially if rotation is not performed toward the side of a cerebral mass lesion.

Background

Rationale for Patient Mobilization

Nosocomial pneumonia is a major problem in the critically ill patient. Its estimated prevalence is 5 to 10 per 1000 hospital admissions. The risk of pneumonia increases fourfold in patients receiving mechanical ventilation.[1] Furthermore, the recumbent position is associated with decreases in tidal volume and in mucociliary transport, which in turn lead to atelectasis.

In the 1960s, it became apparent that the established practices of bed rest and immobilization in the treatment of seriously ill patients increased their susceptibility to pulmonary complications and to loss of skin integrity. Thus, early use of kinetic therapy came to be recommended. *Kinetic therapy* is a general term used to describe the movement of immobilized patients. This movement is provided generally with the patient in the supine position and is directed at improving the perfusion of the lungs, decreasing atelectasis, and mobilizing secretions. Extrapulmonary benefits include reduction in venous stasis and prevention of skin and subcutaneous tissue breakdown.

For many years, periodic changing of body position in critically ill patients has been accomplished by nurses physically positioning and turning patients every 2 hours. These efforts result in improved pulmonary blood flow, ventilation, and mobilization of bronchopulmonary secretions.[2] This most basic form of kinetic therapy continues to be part of standard practice in many intensive care units.[3] Notable adverse effects of this turning of patients, however, include cardiac arrhythmias, inadvertent removal of intravascular access and monitoring lines, significant manpower requirements, and job-related injuries.[2] Furthermore, patients with head or spinal cord injury are especially difficult to mobilize readily. These negative aspects of an otherwise important treatment

Table 7-1 Selected Studies of Rotational Therapy

Study	Issue Addressed	Type of Study	Number of Patients	Class of Evidence
Bein et al, 1998[9]	Pulmonary function	Prospective	10	I
deBoisblanc et al, 1993[20]	Incidence of pneumonia	Prospective, randomized	124	I
Choi and Nelson, 1992[11]	Pulmonary complications, pressure ulcers, mortality, length of stay, decubitus ulcers	Meta-analysis	419	Meta-analysis
Ferrell et al, 1993[16]	Pressure ulcer healing	Prospective, randomized	84	I
Gentilello et al, 1988[7]	Pneumonia and atelectasis	Prospective, randomized	65	I
Gonzalez-Arias et al, 1983[14]	ICP	Retrospective	10	II
Inman et al, 1993[17]	Prevention of pressure ulcers	Prospective, randomized	100	I
Reines and Harris, 1987[15]	Pulmonary complications in SCI patients	Retrospective	123 (20 on rotating beds)	III

modality served as the impetus for the development of automated kinetic beds.

Definitions and Types of Specialty Beds

The first form of automated rotational therapy was introduced in 1967 by Keane.[4] This bed was the forerunner of the current Roto Rest bed (Kinetic Concepts, Inc., San Antonio, TX). It consisted of a firm surface with surrounding pads that allowed side-to-side tilting of patients with maintenance of their supine position. Keane proposed that improved mobilization of secretions by such therapy could decrease pulmonary complications.

The Roto Rest beds rotate from side to side through an arc of up to 62 degrees from the horizontal in each direction (total arc 124 degrees). Because these beds employ a rigid platform, they maintain immobilization of patients with unstable spines, and cervical traction may be applied. A disadvantage of these beds is that they are large, cumbersome, and very difficult to move. These considerations become important if a patient requires frequent transport for operative procedures or radiologic studies. Furthermore, use of such beds may be unnecessary in patients with stable spines. Kinetic therapy may also be administered via a Biodyne-type bed (Kinetic Concepts, Inc., San Antonio, TX). These beds are filled with multiple pockets of air that sequentially inflate and deflate to permit patient rotation through a large arc.[5]

Literature Review

Scope of Studies

Numerous studies have examined the effects of patient positioning and kinetic therapy on cardiopulmonary function. The results provide evidence for improved oxygenation and decreased atelectasis. Other investigations have assessed the effects of kinetic therapy on functional improvement, decubitus ulcer formation, and wound healing. Several of these reports provide class I or II evidence. Table 7-1 summarizes some representative studies of the effects of kinetic beds on pulmonary function, wound healing, and ICP in patients with head or spinal cord injury.

Kinetic Therapy and Pulmonary Function

Several prospective studies have compared mechanical rotational therapy to standard turning of patients every 2 hours by nursing staff. Kelley et al[6] performed a prospective randomized study of 53 patients who had suffered an acute stroke that left them drowsy, stuporous, or lightly comatose (class I data). Pneumonia occurred in 13 of 25 patients (52%) in the standard hospital bed and in five of 18 (28%) in the rotational bed ($p = .20$) (author's calculation). Despite this trend toward a lower rate of pneumonia in patients in the rotating beds, the mortality rate was slightly increased in the study group: six of 18 (33%) versus five of 25 (20%) in patients in the standard hospital beds ($p = .48$) (author's calculation). Of further concern is that all patients who died of transtentorial herniation had been treated with rotating beds, including two patients enrolled in the study and three who were disqualified because of their short lengths of survival.

In another study, Gentilello et al[7] prospectively randomized 65 critically ill patients to treatment in a conventional hospital bed ($n = 38$) or to mechanical kinetic therapy ($n = 27$) (class I data). These patients suffered from head injury, spinal injury, or orthopedic injury requiring traction. Baseline data indicated that the two groups were comparable in terms of gender distribution and percentages with pulmonary contusion, spinal cord injury, and need for traction. Patients in the study group were rotated through an arc of 124 degrees every 7 minutes. The proportion of patients with major pulmonary complications (either atelectasis or pneumonia) was higher in the control group (66%) than in the study group (33%) ($p < .01$).

Summer et al[2] performed a randomized prospective study of continuous mechanical turning on 83 patients with the following illnesses: sepsis (30), chronic obstructive pulmonary disease/asthma (16), drug overdose (11), metabolic coma (12), stroke/neuromuscular (14) (class I data). Patients were randomized either to standard turning every 2 hours by nurses or to rotational therapy. The kinetic therapy group tended to have a shorter length of stay in the intensive care unit (ICU) (6.7 days for the kinetic therapy group versus 11.6 days for the control group; difference not significant). In a small study that used a historical control group, Pape et al[8] concluded that bed rotation to 62 degrees significantly improved lung function compared with conventional supine positioning (class II data).

Bein et al[9] conducted a prospective investigational study to examine the effect of continuous rotational therapy with a Roto Rest bed on ventilation-perfusion inequality in 10 patients with acute lung injury (class I data). The etiologies of lung injury included lung contusion, polytrauma, pneumonia, and aspiration. These authors used the multiple inert gas elimination technique to assess ventilation-perfusion relationships. Each patient served as his or her own control, and supine measurements were compared with measurements performed while rotating. Continuous rotation led to an acute reduction in ventilation-perfusion mismatch when lung injury was mild to moderate, but not when it was more advanced. No significant differences were found in cardiac index, mean arterial pressure, or heart rate during continuous rotation versus the supine position. The authors hypothesized that the change in intrapulmonary shunting occurred as a result of redistribution of pulmonary blood flow from nonventilated to well-ventilated lung units. They also speculated that continuous movement on a rotating bed seemed to be of greater benefit than intermittent semidecubitus positioning.

Dolovich and colleagues[10] used a radiolabeled aerosol to investigate the effect of continuous lateral rotational therapy on lung mucus transport in 13 mechanically ventilated patients (class I data). The intent of this study was to determine if continuous rotation altered mucus transport in critically ill, intubated patients. Prior reviews had suggested that rotational therapy was associated with a decrease in pulmonary complications, possibly from improved clearance of secretions.[1,11] Dolovich et al found that, in comparison to the supine position, continuous lateral rotational therapy to 30 degrees in each direction was associated with a slight but not significant increase in mucus clearance. It is possible that use of a greater depth of angle of rotation, i.e., rotation beyond 30 degrees, might have demonstrated significant improvements in clearance of mucus and diminution of atelectasis.

Pearl

Some investigators have found that rotational therapy improves pulmonary function and reduces pulmonary complications, but others have failed to find any benefit. Differences in study design and in bed rotation protocols may account for many of these differences.

MacIntyre et al[3] conducted a multicenter, prospective, randomized study to test the hypothesis that automated rotational therapy reduces the incidence of lower respiratory tract inflammatory syndrome (LRIS) (class I data). One hundred four patients were entered into the study over a 2-year period at four university hospitals. Patients in the study group were rotated through an arc of 32 degrees from the horizontal in each direction on beds that used computer-controlled inflation of different sections of the mattress rather than tilting of the bed frame. The incidence of LRIS was 17% in the rotational therapy group versus 26% in the control group, a difference that was not statistically significant ($p = .15$). Similarly, Traver et al,[12] in a prospective randomized study of 103 patients, found that the incidence of pneumonia and the length of hospital stay were not significantly affected by the use of an oscillating bed in comparison to manual turning every 2 hours (class I data). In this study, the patients were rotated 25.5 degrees in each direction on the Biodyne bed. This result again raises questions about the degree of turning required to achieve a significant effect. The authors noted that a larger arc of rotation might be needed to achieve the beneficial effects reported in some other studies of rotational therapy.

Pearl

An arc of rotation of less than 40 degrees to each side may be inadequate to achieve the potential benefits of rotational therapy.

In summary, although several high-quality studies have found that rotational therapy improves pulmonary function and decreases pulmonary complications in high-risk patients, other class I investigations have not demonstrated significant benefit from continuous rotational therapy. Differences among published studies in such parameters as the magnitude of rotation, the timing of initiation of rotational therapy, and the duration of such therapy may account for much of the variability of these results.

Specific Studies on Patients with Increased Intracranial Pressure

Tillett and colleagues[13] prospectively examined the effects on ICP of turning in a Roto Rest bed (class I data). Fifty-eight patients with severe brain injury [Glasgow Coma Scale (GCS) <10] were placed in a Roto Rest bed with side-to-side rotation maintained at 40 degrees from the center. Because ICP during rotation was compared with ICP in the nonrotated position, each patient served as his or her own control. In addition, ICP during rotation was analyzed to determine the effect of angulation on ICP. The ICPs were followed for a mean of 5.7 days of rotational therapy. Turning from right/center/left positions was associated with minimal differences in ICP (1–2 mmHg). However, when patients with a unilateral intracranial lesion were rotated to the side of the lesion, ICP increased up to 6.5 mmHg ($p = .12$). No changes in ICP management were prompted by the rotational therapy. The authors recommended that when unilateral mass lesions are present, consideration be given to rotating patients only in the flat and contralateral directions to avoid potential elevations of ICP.

Gonzalez-Arias et al[14] also examined the effects of kinetic therapy on ICP (class II data). Ten patients who required ICP monitoring were maintained in constant rotation in a Roto Rest bed. These patients included four with head injury (GCS score <7), three with brain tumors, two with cerebral aneurysms, and one with a posterior fossa abscess; these latter three had evidence of hydrocephalus. ICP was measured by ventriculostomy (five patients), subdural catheter (one patient), or subarachnoid bolt (four patients; two later changed to ventriculostomy). Fiberoptic ICP monitoring technology had not yet been introduced. The bed was rotated through an arc of 124 degrees every 3.5 minutes. The maximum difference between mean ICP during rotation to the right, mean ICP when supine, and mean ICP during rotation to the left was 4.4 mmHg. No worsening of ICP was appreciated as a result of the bed rotation. Limitations of this study include the small sample size and the heterogeneity of the patient population.

Pearl

Small elevations of ICP that have been associated with rotational therapy do not appear to be clinically significant, but potential safety concerns suggest that consideration should be given to avoiding rotation toward the side of a cerebral mass lesion.

The above studies do not mention any major adverse effects of rotational therapy on control of ICP. However, one potential drawback of most of the beds used for rotational therapy is the limited degree to which the head may be elevated above the rest of the body. Because of the bed's inherent design and because of the frequent need to maintain neutrality of the spine, the maximal elevation of the head of the bed is generally limited to roughly 15 to 20 degrees.

As discussed earlier, Gentilello et al[7] examined the effects of the use of rotational therapy in 65 patients with head injury, spinal injury, or orthopedic injury requiring traction (class I data). They reported a statistically significant decrease in the incidence of combined pulmonary complications (i.e., pneumonia and atelectasis) in the treatment group. One patient was excluded because of problems with ICP control. In another study that was discussed earlier, Kelley et al[6] found that the incidence of pneumonia in patients with stroke tended to be lower in those receiving rotational therapy, even though the mortality rate of that group was slightly higher than that of the control group ($p = .48$) (class I data). Of interest, deaths from transtentorial herniation occurred only in patients receiving rotational therapy.

Further studies that focus on the effects of kinetic beds on ICP and on cerebral perfusion pressure are needed. The author has observed that ICP in his patients is clearly affected by patient positioning. Close monitoring and, when appropriate, aggressive intervention may be able to obviate catastrophic increases in ICP that may conceivably be set in motion by kinetic therapy.

Specific Studies on Patients with Spinal Cord Injury

Reines and Harris[15] performed a retrospective chart review of 123 patients with acute spinal cord injury treated over a 10-year period (class III data). Overall, 53 pulmonary complications were noted in 44 patients (36%) during the first month of hospitalization. Use of the Roto Rest bed was not instituted until the 6th year of the study period. Twenty patients were treated with rotational therapy for a mean of 12 ± 5 days. Pulmonary complications were found in only two (10%) of these patients while they received rotational therapy, but 55% of them developed pulmonary complications when removed from the bed.

Specific Studies on the Effect of Specialty Beds on Wound Healing

In their meta-analysis of six independent studies (419 patients), Choi and Nelson[11] did not find that kinetic therapy had any statistically significant effect on pressure ulcers. In a randomized controlled trial, Ferrell et al[16] found that low-air-loss beds were associated with a significant improvement in the healing of pressure ulcers when compared with foam mattresses (class I data). These beds (KinAir bed, Kinetic Concepts Inc., San Antonio, TX) consist of multiple inflatable fabric pillows. The pillows are buoyed by heated air that gradually flows through the mattress and sheets to the patient's skin. The resultant reduction in moisture and temperature may reduce skin maceration and improve patient comfort. These beds have been shown to reduce skin surface pressures to levels near or even below capillary filling pressures.[16]

In a randomized controlled study of 100 patients, Inman et al[17] found that patients who were maintained on air suspension beds had a statistically significant decrease in incidence of single ($p = .0001$), multiple ($p = .007$), or severe ($p = .0005$) pressure ulcers (class I data). The control group was treated with side-to-side turning in a standard ICU bed every 2 hours. The patients in this study had initial Acute Physiology and Chronic Health Evaluation II[18] scores >15, an expected length of ICU stay of at least 3 days, and an age of at least 17 years.

Pearl

Low-air-loss suspension beds may prevent pressure ulcers and may facilitate the healing of existing ulcers.

Cost Analysis

Many hospital administrators have limited the use of specialty beds because of their high rental costs. Summer et al[2] evaluated the financial impact of the reduction in ICU days and improvements in pulmonary care associated with the use of rotating beds. They estimated that overall ICU costs could be reduced by up to 35% in specific groups of patients. Another cost-benefit analysis of the economic impact of the Roto Rest bed suggested that appropriate use of these beds could result in an average savings of thousands of dollars per patient, largely through a reduced incidence of pulmonary complications.[5]

Effect of Prone Positioning

One might expect that the next step in attempting to improve outcomes through use of novel approaches to patient positioning would call for the use of the prone position. Prone positioning has been shown to significantly improve gas exchange in patients with adult respiratory distress syndrome (ARDS) and has been used for up to 20 hours per day for several days (class I data).[19] We routinely use the prone position at our institution for patients with ARDS. We agree with Fridrich et al[19] that unstable cervical spine injuries and intracranial hypertension are contraindications to the use of the prone position. We have found that the prone position is associated with a slight increase (~5 mmHg) in ICP, most likely from increased intrathoracic pressure in the prone position.

Recommendations

1. Continuous kinetic therapy provided by special beds may improve pulmonary function and reduce pulmonary complications (level I).
2. Continuous kinetic therapy provided by special beds may be used in patients with head injury and spinal cord injury without adverse neurologic effects (level II).
3. Low-air-loss beds may decrease the incidence of decubitus ulcers and facilitate the healing of existing ulcers (level I).

References

1. Sahn SA. Continuous lateral rotational therapy and nosocomial pneumonia. Chest 1991;99:1263–1267.
2. Summer WR, Curry P, Haponik EF, et al. Continuous mechanical turning of intensive care unit patients shortens length of stay in some diagnostic-related groups. J Crit Care 1989;4:45–53.
3. MacIntyre NR, Helms M, Wunderink R, et al. Automated rotational therapy for the prevention of respiratory complications during mechanical ventilation. Respir Care 1999;44:1447–1451.
4. Keane FX. Roto-rest. BMJ 1967;3:731–733.
5. Basham KA, Vollman KM, Miller AC. To everything turn, turn, turn . . . an overview of continuous lateral rotational therapy. Respir Care Clin North Am 1997;3:109–134.
6. Kelley RE, Vibulsreth S, Bell L, et al. Evaluation of kinetic therapy in the prevention of complications of prolonged bed rest secondary to stroke. Stroke 1987;18:638–642.
7. Gentilello L, Thompson DA, Tonnesen AS, et al. Effect of a rotating bed on the incidence of pulmonary complications in critically ill patients. Crit Care Med 1988;16:783–786.
8. Pape HC, Regel G, Borgmann W, et al. The effects of kinetic positioning on lung function and pulmonary haemodynamics in posttraumatic ARDS: a clinical study. Injury 1994;25:51–57.
9. Bein T, Reber A, Metz C, et al. Acute effects of continuous rotational therapy on ventilation-perfusion inequality in lung injury. Intensive Care Med 1998;24:132–137.
10. Dolovich M, Rushbrook J, Churchill E, et al. Effect of continuous lateral rotational therapy on lung mucus transport in mechanically ventilated patients. J Crit Care 1998;13:119–125.
11. Choi SC, Nelson LD. Kinetic therapy in critically ill patients: combined results based on meta-analysis. J Crit Care 1992;7:57–62.

12. Traver GA, Tyler ML, Hudson LD, et al. Continuous oscillation: outcome in critically ill patients. J Crit Care 1995;10: 97–103.
13. Tillett JM, Marmarou A, Agnew JP, et al. Effect of continuous rotational therapy on intracranial pressure in the severely brain-injured patient. Crit Care Med 1993;21:1005–1011.
14. Gonzalez-Arias SM, Goldberg ML, Baumgartner R, et al. Analysis of the effect of kinetic therapy on intracranial pressure in comatose neurosurgical patients. Neurosurgery 1983; 13:654–656.
15. Reines HD, Harris RC. Pulmonary complications of acute spinal cord injuries. Neurosurgery 1987;21:193–196.
16. Ferrell BA, Osterweil D, Christenson P. A randomized trial of low-air-loss beds for treatment of pressure ulcers. JAMA 1993; 269:494–497.
17. Inman KJ, Sibbald WJ, Rutledge FS, et al. Clinical utility and cost-effectiveness of an air suspension bed in the prevention of pressure ulcers. JAMA 1993;269:1139–1143.
18. Knaus WA, Draper EA, Wagner DP, et al. APACHE II: a severity of disease classification system. Crit Care Med 1985;13: 818–829.
19. Fridrich P, Krafft P, Hochleuthner H, et al. The effects of long-term prone positioning in patients with trauma-induced adult respiratory distress syndrome. Anesth Analg 1996;83:1206–1211.
20. deBoisblanc BP, Castro M, Everret B, et al. Effect of air-supported, continuous, postural oscillation on the risk of early ICU pneumonia in non-traumatic critical illness. Chest 1993; 103:1543–1547.

◆ 8 ◆

What Is the Safest Way to Prevent Deep Venous Thrombosis and Pulmonary Embolism After Head or Spinal Cord Injury? How Soon After Surgery or Injury Can I Anticoagulate My Patients Who Develop Deep Venous Thrombosis?

R. Loch Macdonald

What is the Safest Way to Prevent Deep Venous Thrombosis and Pulmonary Embolism After Head or Spinal Cord Injury?

Brief Answer

For patients with spinal cord injury, low-molecular-weight heparin (LMWH) is the recommended method of deep venous thrombosis (DVT) prophylaxis. This treatment should be delayed for 24 to 72 hours in patients with incomplete injuries. Treatment should continue for 3 months, perhaps with more aggressive anticoagulation after 2 weeks. Thigh-high intermittent pneumatic compression (IPC) may be instituted immediately and may be used in conjunction with pharmacologic measures. For head-injured patients, IPC is the initial method of choice for DVT prophylaxis. If desired, LMWH can probably be used in place of IPC after the first 2 or 3 days. Treatment should probably be continued until discharge to home or to rehabilitation. Prophylactic use of inferior vena cava filters is not recommended. These recommendations may need to be modified for patients with lower extremity injuries, coagulopathy, anticipated future surgery or invasive procedures, etc.

Background

The goals of venous thromboembolism (VTE) prophylaxis are to prevent complications of pulmonary embolism (PE) (especially death) and to prevent the complications of DVT, the most important being the postphlebitic syndrome. Two different approaches have been advocated. One is to screen patients for subclinical DVT and institute therapy whenever DVT is detected. The second is primary prophylaxis to prevent development of VTE. Primary prophylaxis is the most viable option at this time because it is more effective and less expensive and because screening tests such as duplex ultrasound have only moderate sensitivity and positive predictive value for detecting DVT in asymptomatic, high-risk patients.[1] It must be emphasized that clinical features of DVT are useless as screening tools. Only three of 201 trauma patients (1.5%) with venogram-proven DVT had clinical signs or symptoms before venography (class II data).[2] These figures likely hold true for other patient populations.

Risk Factors

Risk factors for VTE can be classified as a triad, described by Virchow as abnormalities in blood coagulation, in blood flow, and in the vein wall. Common risk factors are increasing age, obesity, varicose veins, immobility, paresis or plegia of the limbs, systemic infection, pregnancy and the puerperium, estrogen therapy, previous VTE, malignancy, deficiency of antithrombin 3, protein C or protein S, activated protein C resistance (factor 5 Leiden), prothrombin variant 20210A, lupus anticoagulant, antiphospholipid antibody syndrome, heparin-induced thrombocytopenia, trauma (especially spinal cord injury and fractures of the pelvis and lower limb), heart failure, systemic infection, indwelling central venous catheters, and surgery.

In patients undergoing surgery, the risk is higher with certain types of surgery. Intracranial surgery has a greater risk than spinal surgery, and major orthopedic surgery of the lower limbs and of the pelvis has a high risk that increases with the number of fractures repaired. Risk increases with longer times of anesthesia, with general anesthesia as compared with spinal or local anesthesia, and with postoperative patient immobilization.[3]

The risk of VTE can be estimated from these factors. This is important since prophylaxis itself may carry risk, which has to be balanced against the risk that a patient will develop VTE. Low-risk patients include those with isolated spinal fractures but not cord injury. They have a risk of calf DVT of <10%. Moderate-risk patients have a calf DVT risk of 10 to 40% and include patients with isolated lower limb fractures who are under 40 years old. High-risk patients have a calf DVT risk of 40 to 80% and include most patients with spinal cord injury, multiple trauma, elective intracranial neurosurgery, major orthopedic surgery of the lower limbs, or prior VTE.

Methods of DVT Prophylaxis

Prophylaxis for prevention of VTE may be mechanical and/or pharmacologic. Mechanical methods include graduated compression stockings, IPC of the lower limbs (usually the calves), rotating tables, and electrical stimulation of the calf muscles. Pharmacologic methods include low-dose unfractionated heparin, LMWH, adjusted-dose heparin, or warfarin.

In general, the greater the degree of pharmacologic anticoagulation that is achieved, the lower the risk of VTE and the higher the risk of bleeding. Meta-analysis of numerous large randomized clinical trials suggests that there is no increase (or only a small increase) in wound bleeding in patients treated with low-dose unfractionated heparin or LMWH.[1] This is of more concern in neurosurgical patients than other surgical patients and is carefully considered in the recommendations that are made in this chapter (Table 8-1). Mechanical methods of prophylaxis avoid this risk but may be impractical in many trauma patients because of lower limb injuries. It has been suggested that a systemic fibrinolytic state can be induced by intermittent

Table 8-1 Recommendations for Prophylaxis of VTE Patients with Head or Spinal Cord Injury

	Spinal Cord Injury		Head Injury	
Prophylaxis	**Evidence Class**	**Recommendation Level**	**Evidence Class**	**Recommendation Level**
Graduated compression stockings	III	II	III	I (when pharmacologic prophylaxis is delayed)
Intermittent pneumatic compression	II	II	I	I (when pharmacologic prophylaxis is delayed)
Low-dose subcutaneous heparin	II	II	II	III
Low-molecular-weight heparin	I	I	I	I (when considered safe)
Combined mechanical + pharmacologic	II	II	III	III
Other Issues				
When to initiate after injury	Immediately for mechanical methods; may start pharmacologic prophylaxis immediately, or may delay 24 to 72 hours in patients who are incomplete or have multiple other injuries or ongoing bleeding		Immediately for mechanical methods; may start pharmacologic prophylaxis immediately or may delay in patients with intracranial hemorrhage or ongoing bleeding	
	II	II	II	II
Duration of prophylaxis	3 months	Until discharge or ambulating		
	III	III	III	III
Other considerations	Risk of bleeding with low-molecular-weight heparin needs to be studied further.			

Table 8-2 Randomized Trials of Prophylaxis in Patients with Spinal Cord Injury

Reference	Number	Groups	DVT Detection	Outcome
Green, 1982[10]	28	IPC vs IPC + aspirin 300 mg twice a day + dipyridamole 75 mg 3 times a day	^{125}I-labeled fibrinogen and impedance plethysmography	6/15 (40%) IPC and 3/12 (25%) IPC + antiplatelet drugs had DVT ($p < .1$); DVT incidence lower than historical controls
Green, 1988[11]	75	Heparin, 5000 U twice daily vs adjusted-dose heparin to prolong partial thromboplastin time (PTT) to 1.5 times normal	Impedance plethysmography or duplex ultrasound	9/29 (31%) fixed-dose and 2/29 (7%) adjusted-dose heparin had DVT ($p < .05$); bleeding complications in 24% on adjusted-dose heparin and none in fixed-dose group
Merli, 1988[6]	48	Placebo vs heparin 5000 U 3 times a day vs heparin + electrical stimulation of calves	^{125}I-labeled fibrinogen	8/17 (47%) placebo, 8/16 (50%) heparin and 1/15 (7%) heparin + electrical stimulation developed DVT ($p < .05$ for heparin + electrical stimulation compared with other groups)
Green, 1990[12]	41	Heparin 5000 U 3 times a day vs tinzaparin 3500 anti-Xa units once daily	Impedance plethysmography, duplex ultrasound	5/21 (24%) with standard heparin developed VTE, including two fatal PE, versus 0/20 with tinzaparin ($p < .01$); two severe bleeding complications in heparin group and none with tinzaparin
Geerts, 1996[18] & 2001[1]	23	Heparin 5000 U or enoxaparin 30 mg daily	Venography	10/15 (67%) heparin and 4/8 (50%) enoxaparin patients had DVT (subgroup analysis of larger study cited in Table 8-3)

DVT, deep venous thrombosis; IPC, intermittent pneumatic compression.

compression even of the upper limbs or feet, but efficacy has not been proven in randomized trials. Other limitations of mechanical methods are that they may not be as efficacious in high-risk patients or in routine practice, where compliance may be lower than in a clinical trial.

It is recommended that pharmacologic prophylaxis be withheld the morning of surgery and resumed 24 hours later in the absence of ongoing bleeding. Patients who are exposed to heparin in any dose, even as a flush in intravascular catheters, should have their platelet count measured every 2 days or so for the first 14 days of exposure to detect heparin-induced thrombocytopenia. This complication is less common in patients receiving LMWH.

Pearl

Patients with any exposure to heparin (even as a flush in intravascular catheters) should have their platelet count measured frequently to detect heparin-induced thrombocytopenia. This occurs less commonly in patients receiving LMWH.

Data reviewed below are from randomized trials in trauma and spinal cord injury patients. If no such trials have been conducted, prospectively and retrospectively collected data are reviewed. The neurosurgical literature contains five trials of mechanical and seven of pharmacological prophylaxis, but trauma patients were entered into only one, which showed lack of efficacy of an antiplatelet agent.

Literature Review: Spinal Cord Injury

Spinal cord injury carries one of the highest risks of VTE. A multicenter study of 1419 patients with acute spinal cord injury noted that 15% developed symptomatic DVT and 5% developed clinically evident PE (class III data).[4] The incidence of DVT in observational studies and in the untreated control groups of randomized trials of patients studied acutely after spinal cord injury was 71% [45/63 patients in five trials (class I–III data), range 47% to 100%] as detected by ^{125}I-labeled fibrinogen[5–9] and 81% (21/26 patients in one trial) as detected by venography (class I data).[2]

Pearl

Antiplatelet drugs are generally not efficacious for VTE prophylaxis, and their use for this purpose is not recommended.

Randomized trials have been conducted in patients with spinal cord injury (Table 8-2). Interpretation is hampered by small numbers of patients, lack of inclusion of placebo groups, lack of venography as an end point, and use of many different regimens. A randomized comparison of IPC alone versus IPC plus aspirin and dipyridamole noted no significant difference between the groups (class I data).[10] Antiplatelet drugs are generally not efficacious for VTE prophylaxis in any setting, and their use is not recommended.

Retrospective and prospective observational studies of patients treated with low-dose heparin yield conflicting results. They seem to suggest that heparin only slightly reduced the risk of DVT, with no increase in bleeding.[1] Comparison of low-dose heparin to placebo and to heparin plus electrical stimulation of the calf muscles found that heparin alone was ineffective but that combined treatment was beneficial.[6] Since low-dose heparin alone seemed inadequate, adjusted-dose heparin administered to elevate the partial thromboplastin time to 1.5 times normal was compared with low-dose heparin and was found to be more effective, but with a significant increase in bleeding complications (class I data).[11] A randomized trial comparing the LMWH tinzaparin to heparin noted that tinzaparin significantly reduced DVT without increasing bleeding (class I data).[12] Uncontrolled data from 60 selected patients treated with tinzaparin for 8 weeks found an incidence of DVT of 18% and bleeding in 3% (class III data).[13] Patients with head injury, hemothorax, and long bone fractures were excluded. In another report, enoxaparin prophylaxis in 105 patients was associated with a 10% risk of bleeding and with no DVTs in the 60 patients screened with ultrasound (class II data).[14]

Pearl

Prophylactic use of inferior vena cava filters in patients with spinal cord injury is not recommended as a first-line means of preventing PE.

Inferior vena cava filters may be used for prophylaxis and treatment of VTE. No randomized trials of their use in prophylaxis were found. One study used a two-by-two design to randomize patients with proximal DVT (with or without PE) to filter placement or no filter placement and to LMWH or unfractionated heparin. Filter placement was associated with an early reduction in PE, but also a long-term increase in recurrent DVT; there was no effect on mortality (class II data).[15] Thus, prophylactic use of filters is not recommended. Current indications for vena cava filters for treatment of VTE include a contraindication to anticoagulant therapy, recurrent PE while on anticoagulants, major bleeding necessitating cessation of anticoagulation, and recent surgical pulmonary embolectomy.[16] Complications include thrombosis of the inferior vena cava with or without lower extremity swelling, migration, retroperitoneal hematoma, and incorrect placement.

Conclusions and Recommendations: Spinal Cord Injury

Patients with acute spinal cord injury should receive DVT prophylaxis with LMWH (level I)[1] (although a reduction in PE has not been documented with this treatment). Low-dose heparin, elastic stockings, and IPC are relatively ineffective, but mechanical methods are indicated for patients in whom the risk of bleeding is believed to contraindicate anticoagulants (see also next section) (level II). Prophylactic vena cava filters are not recommended (level II). Pharmacologic prophylaxis should be delayed for 24 to 72 hours in patients whose injuries are incomplete to reduce the risk of early bleeding that might cause neurologic compromise and that might also complicate emergency surgery in the event of neurologic deterioration (level III). It seems unlikely to this reviewer that there is any specific benefit from LMWH compared with unfractionated heparin other than a reduced incidence of thrombocytopenia. Furthermore, the improved protection of LMWH seems to be due to increased or more reliable anticoagulant effect, which also would theoretically be associated with a higher risk of bleeding. The peak risk of VTE is within the first 2 weeks of injury, although a substantial risk persists during rehabilitation, and it is recommended that pharmacological prophylaxis be continued for 3 months (level III).[1,17] After 14 days, higher levels of anticoagulation, such as with LMWH or full-dose warfarin to an international normalized ratio of two to three, have been recommended (level III). A high likelihood of further surgery in the acute postinjury period impacts on these decisions.

Pearl

Pharmacologic prophylaxis should be delayed for 24 to 72 hours in patients with incomplete spinal cord injury.

Literature Review: Head Injury

Fatal PE occurs in 0.4 to 2% of trauma patients and is the third most common cause of death in patients surviving beyond 1 day.[1] Geerts and colleagues[2] performed serial impedance plethysmography and lower-extremity contrast venography on 716 patients who did not undergo VTE prophylaxis after admission to a regional trauma unit (class II data). Of 349 patients who had adequate venography, 201 (58%) had DVTs. Multivariate analysis found that DVT was more likely with increasing age, blood transfusion, need for surgery, femur or tibia fracture, and spinal cord injury. The patients entered were severely injured victims with a mean Injury Severity Score of 27. Sixty-four percent were injured in motor vehicle accidents and 15% in pedestrian accidents. The site of major injury was the head in 26%; the face, chest, or abdomen in 37%; and the spine in 19%.

Table 8-3 Randomized Trials of Prophylaxis in Trauma Patients

Reference	Number	Groups	DVT Detection	Outcome
Geerts, 1996[18]	344	Heparin 5000 U or enoxaparin 30 mg every 12 hours	Venography	60/136 (44%) heparin and 40/129 (31%) enoxaparin had DVT ($p = .014$); one major hemorrhage in the heparin group (1%) and five in the enoxaparin group (4%) (not significant); excluded patients with frank intracranial bleeding but not with contusions, petechial hemorrhage, or diffuse axonal injury; treatment began within 36 hours of injury
Haentjens, 1996[20]	283	Nadroparin 3075 anti-Xa IU vs adjusted dose regimen	B-mode ultrasound	1/142 (1%) fixed dose and 4/141 (3%) variable dose patients had DVT (not significant); 1/142 (1%) fixed dose and 2/141 (1%) variable dose patients developed PE (not significant); five patients in each group developed major hemorrhage; patients had only pelvic, spinal, or lower limb fractures.
Knudson, 1996[21]	372	Enoxaparin 30 mg every 12 hours vs IPC or arteriovenous impulse device	Duplex ultrasound	Only 202 randomized; 1/120 (1%) enoxaparin and 2/82 (2%) patients developed DVT (not significant); randomized patients did not have severe head injury or spinal cord injury; 6/120 (5%) treated with enoxaparin and none with IPC developed bleeding
Elliott, 1999[19]	149	Thigh-length IPC vs plantar IPC	Ultrasound	13/62 (21%) plantar IPC and 4/62 (6%) thigh-high IPC had DVT ($p = .009$); 83% of patients had severe head injury

DVT, deep venous thrombosis; IPC, intermittent pneumatic compression.

Several randomized trials of pharmacological and/or mechanical prophylaxis have been conducted in trauma patients (Table 8-3).[18–21] Only one used venography, which is the gold standard for diagnosis of DVT (class I data).[18] The studies are difficult to interpret because of differences in patient populations, use of many different prophylactic regimes, and lack of placebo groups. Randomized studies of mechanical prophylaxis found that thigh-high IPC significantly lowered the incidence of DVT compared with plantar venous compression devices in a trauma population that included many patients with severe head injury (class I data).[19] In trauma patients without severe head injury, IPC was as effective as LMWH (class II data).[21] A consensus conference noted that nonrandomized studies had produced conflicting results as to the efficacy of IPC so that such treatment could not be recommended for trauma patients.[1] This report favored pharmacologic prophylaxis based on a single study conducted by an author of the consensus conference report, but it acknowledged that IPC might be indicated for patients who could not be given anticoagulants early, such as those with head injury. The largest and only study using venography included patients with head injury without major intracranial bleeding.[18] Significantly more patients treated with heparin (44%) developed DVT compared with those treated with enoxaparin (31%). Five times as many patients given enoxaparin experienced major bleeding (five versus only one treated with heparin), but this was not statistically significant. It was concluded that both interventions were safe and that enoxaparin was more efficacious.

Pearl

In a trauma population that included many patients with severe head injury, thigh-high IPC significantly lowers the incidence of DVT compared to plantar venous compression devices.

Pearl

Prophylactic doses of anticoagulants probably carry only a small risk of bleeding by 2 or 3 days after injury.

Conclusions and Recommendations: Head Injury

This reviewer recommends mechanical prophylaxis with IPC in head-injured patients in whom use of such devices is possible (level I). Heparin has not been compared with placebo or with mechanical prophylaxis in patients with severe head injury. Enoxaparin is efficacious in selected patients with head injury, but it seems possible that studies conducted thus far have not been large enough to determine reliably whether enoxaparin significantly increases the risk of bleeding.

Heparin (level III) or LMWH (level I) may be used within 36 hours of multiple trauma in patients who do not have intracranial bleeding, incomplete spinal cord injury, ongoing uncontrolled bleeding, and/or uncorrected coagulopathy. In these groups, heparin or LMWH may be used when the risk of bleeding has passed. The exact time at which this occurs is unknown, but the data reviewed below suggest that prophylactic doses of anticoagulants probably carry only a small risk of bleeding by 2 or 3 days after injury (level III). Prophylactic insertion of vena cava filters is discussed above and cannot be recommended at this time (level II). How long prophylaxis should be continued has not been studied in detail. It is recommended that it be continued until the patient is discharged from hospital to home or rehabilitation (level III).

How Soon After Surgery of Injury Can I Anticoagulate My Patients Who Develop Deep Venous Thrombosis?

Brief Answer

Therapeutic anticoagulation should probably be withheld for the first 5 to 7 days after trauma. An IVC should be inserted if VTE develops during this interval.

Background and Literature Review

The usual recommendation is to wait for 7 days after intracranial surgery. However, there are no randomized trials or prospective reports in head or spinal cord injury. In one review of retrospectively collected data from a series of neurosurgical patients with gliomas, subarachnoid hemorrhage, intracerebral hemorrhage, or nonoperative head injury, two of seven patients anticoagulated for PE within 5 days of surgery suffered intracranial hemorrhage at the operative site, whereas none of the nine patients in whom anticoagulation was reported to have begun after 5 days experienced operative site hemorrhage (class III data).[22] In 26 anticoagulated patients with mechanical heart valves who survived after sustaining an intracranial hemorrhage, anticoagulation was restarted a median of 8 days after the ictus (range: 2 days to 3 months), and no patient rebled (class III data).[23] Another study of 27 anticoagulated patients with intracranial hemorrhage found no intracranial rebleeding among operated patients who were restarted on anticoagulation therapy within 3 days of bleeding (class III data).[24]

The lack of data on neurosurgical patients led to a review of anticoagulation after other types of surgery.[25] Patients who required anticoagulation because of prosthetic cardiac valves who underwent nonneurological surgery were reported in two series. No bleeding occurred when anticoagulation was resumed 3 to 5 days postoperatively, but it has been estimated that major postoperative bleeding, almost always at the operative site, would occur at a rate of 3% in patients anticoagulated for the first 48 hours after surgery.[26] These authors concluded that patients with recent VTE are at high risk of mortality from recurrent thromboembolic events. If they require neurosurgical procedures, they should have filters placed in the inferior vena cava, with low-dose heparin or anticoagulation started 3 to 5 days after surgery (class III). There are no other available data. All other reports of anticoagulation of head- and spinal cord—injured patients either do not indicate how long after injury anticoagulation was started or start anticoagulation after 7 days.

Pearl

If patients with recent VTE require neurosurgical procedures, they should have filters placed in the inferior vena cava, with low-dose heparin or anticoagulation started 3 to 5 days after surgery.

Knowledge of risks and benefits would be helpful in formulating a rational answer to the question.[26] Unfortunately, most of these are not accurately known. The risk of death from recurrent PE in a patient presenting with PE approaches 25% acutely. The risk of recurrent VTE after DVT is 40% in the absence of anticoagulation in the first month, but these data are from patients who were first treated with therapeutic heparin for 2 weeks, followed by low-dose heparin. Therefore, the risk of recurrence may be higher when no treatment is given. Less than 6% of recurrent episodes are fatal. The risk of major bleeding in patients anticoagulated for DVT was 1.6 to 4.2% in the first 12 days (depending on whether LMWH or unfractionated heparin was used) (class I data)[15] and 11% in the first 5 days in another series of patients at high risk of bleeding because of recent surgery, although the exact time from surgery was not stated.[26] The risk of bleeding is much higher immediately after surgery. Fifty-three percent of 15 patients with tissue trauma or vascular damage bled (usually at the site of trauma) when anticoagulated within 7 days of the trauma, compared with 18% of 65 patients without trauma (class II data).[27] Anticoagulant-related intracranial hemorrhage was fatal in a third of patients in one series.[23]

Conclusions and Recommendations

It is recommended, therefore, that because the risk of fatal PE is low on a daily basis even acutely after VTE, and because the risk of fatal bleeding due to anticoagulation is high immediately after surgery or trauma, treatment be delayed for 5 to 7 days after trauma. If VTE develops during this period, a filter should be placed, and pharmacologic prophylaxis should be continued or increased (level II). If further surgery is needed or anticipated, a filter may be preferred. If heparin or anticoagulants cannot be used because of risk of bleeding, and VTE has occurred within the preceding 2 weeks, then a filter should be considered.

References

1. Geerts WH, Heit JA, Clagett GP, et al. Prevention of venous thromboembolism. Chest 2001;119:132S–175S.
2. Geerts WH, Code KI, Jay RM, et al. A prospective study of venous thromboembolism after major trauma. N Engl J Med 1994;331:1601–1606.
3. Hamilton MG, Hull RD, Pineo GF. Venous thromboembolism in neurosurgery and neurology patients: a review. Neurosurgery 1994;34:280–296.
4. Waring WP, Karunas RS. Acute spinal cord injuries and the incidence of clinically occurring thromboembolic disease. Paraplegia 1991;29:8–16.
5. Brach BB, Moser KM, Cedar L, et al. Venous thrombosis in acute spinal cord paralysis. J Trauma 1977;17:289–292.
6. Merli GJ, Herbison GJ, Ditunno JF, et al. Deep vein thrombosis: prophylaxis in acute spinal cord injured patients. Arch Phys Med Rehabil 1988;69:661–664.
7. Myllynen P, Kammonen M, Rokkanen P, et al. Deep venous thrombosis and pulmonary embolism in patients with acute spinal cord injury: a comparison with nonparalyzed patients immobilized due to spinal fractures. J Trauma 1985;25:541–543.
8. Petaja J, Myllynen P, Rokkanen P, et al. Fibrinolysis and spinal injury: relationship to post-traumatic deep vein thrombosis. Acta Chir Scand 1989;155:241–246.
9. Rossi EC, Green D, Rosen JS, et al. Sequential changes in factor VIII and platelets preceding deep vein thrombosis in patients with spinal cord injury. Br J Haematol 1980;45:143–151.
10. Green D, Rossi EC, Yao JS, et al. Deep vein thrombosis in spinal cord injury: effect of prophylaxis with calf compression, aspirin, and dipyridamole. Paraplegia 1982;20:227–234.
11. Green D, Lee MY, Ito VY, et al. Fixed- vs adjusted-dose heparin in the prophylaxis of thromboembolism in spinal cord injury. JAMA 1988;260:1255–1258.
12. Green D, Lee MY, Lim AC, et al. Prevention of thromboembolism after spinal cord injury using low-molecular-weight heparin. Ann Intern Med 1990;113:571–574.
13. Green D, Chen D, Chmiel JS, et al. Prevention of thromboembolism in spinal cord injury: role of low molecular weight heparin. Arch Phys Med Rehabil 1994;75:290–292.
14. Harris S, Chen D, Green D. Enoxaparin for thromboembolism prophylaxis in spinal injury: preliminary report on experience with 105 patients. Am J Phys Med Rehabil 1996;75:326–327.
15. Decousus H, Leizorovicz A, Parent F, et al. A clinical trial of vena cava filters in the prevention of pulmonary embolism in patients with proximal deep-vein thrombosis: Prevention du Risque d'Embolie Pulmonaire par Interruption Cave Study Group. N Engl J Med 1998;338:409–415.
16. Merli GJ. Management of deep vein thrombosis in spinal cord injury. Chest 1992;102:652S–657S.
17. Green D. Prophylaxis of thromboembolism in spinal cord-injured patients. Chest 1992;102:649S–651S.
18. Geerts WH, Jay RM, Code KI, et al. A comparison of low-dose heparin with low-molecular-weight heparin as prophylaxis against venous thromboembolism after major trauma. N Engl J Med 1996;335:701–707.
19. Elliott CG, Dudney TM, Egger M, et al. Calf-thigh sequential pneumatic compression compared with plantar venous pneumatic compression to prevent deep-vein thrombosis after nonlower extremity trauma. J Trauma 1999;47:25–32.
20. Haentjens P. Thromboembolic prophylaxis in orthopaedic trauma patients: a comparison between a fixed dose and an individually adjusted dose of a low molecular weight heparin (nadroparin calcium). Injury 1996;27:385–390.
21. Knudson MM, Morabito D, Paiement GD, et al. Use of low molecular weight heparin in preventing thromboembolism in trauma patients. J Trauma 1996;41:446–459.
22. Ricco G, Marini C, Rindi M, et al. Pulmonary embolism in neurosurgical patients: diagnosis and treatment. J Neurosurg 1984;60:972–975.
23. Wijdicks EF, Schievink WI, Brown RD, et al. The dilemma of discontinuation of anticoagulation therapy for patients with intracranial hemorrhage and mechanical heart valves. Neurosurgery 1998;42:769–773.
24. Kawamata T, Takeshita M, Kubo O, et al. Management of intracranial hemorrhage associated with anticoagulant therapy. Surg Neurol 1995;44:438–442.
25. Lazio BE, Simard JM. Anticoagulation in neurosurgical patients. Neurosurgery 1999;45:838–847.
26. Kearon C, Hirsh J. Management of anticoagulation before and after elective surgery. N Engl J Med 1997;336:1506–1511.
27. Wilson JR, Lampman J. Heparin therapy: a randomized prospective study. Am Heart J 1979;97:155–158.

◆ Part III ◆

Brain Injury

Monitoring

◆ 9 ◆

When and How Should I Monitor Intracranial Pressure?

Jonas J. Gopez, Richard J. Meagher, and Raj K. Narayan

Brief Answer

The literature cannot support a level I recommendation regarding the use of intracranial pressure (ICP) monitoring in patients with traumatic brain injury (TBI). However, sufficient evidence exists to support a level II recommendation for ICP monitoring in patients with severe head injury [Glasgow Coma Scale (GCS) score 3–8] with an abnormal admission computed tomography (CT) scan that reveals hematomas, contusions, edema, or compressed basal cisterns. Evidence also supports a level II recommendation to monitor ICP in patients with severe head injury with a normal admission CT scan if two or more of the following are present: age >40 years, unilateral or bilateral motor posturing, and systolic blood pressure (SBP) <90 mmHg. A level II recommendation supports the use of ICP monitoring in certain selected conscious patients with traumatic mass lesions who are felt to be at risk for deterioration, although ICP monitoring is not routinely indicated in patients with mild to moderate head injury. Finally, although assessment of ICP monitoring technology does not lend itself to classification by levels of recommendation, the available data support the use of a ventricular catheter connected to an external strain gauge as the preferred ICP monitoring device.

Background

ICP monitoring was first introduced by Lundberg et al[1] in the early 1960s. Because such monitoring requires the expenditure of some resources, increases the work involved, and carries some risk of complications, documentation of its efficacy would be desirable. To date, there has been no prospective randomized trial proving that ICP monitoring improves outcome in patients with severe head injury. A study of this nature has not been conducted primarily because of ethical issues surrounding the need for a control group that would be treated empirically, without ICP monitoring. In addition, such a study would require approximately 349 patients in each treatment arm to demonstrate a 10% decrease in mortality [with an alpha (probability of a type I error, or erroneously rejecting a null hypothesis that is really true) of 5% and a beta (probability of a type II error, or erroneously failing to reject a null hypothesis that is false) of 20%] and cost over $5 million. In fact, a proposal for such a study in head-injured patients was submitted to the National Institutes of Health several years ago but did not receive funding.

Enthusiasm for ICP monitoring has grown because of a large body of clinical experience and anecdotal and historical evidence that it facilitates rational management, provides prognostic information, and improves outcomes. In 1991, Marmarou et al[2] (class II data) reported the results of an analysis of 428 severely head-injured patients from the Traumatic Coma Data Bank (TCDB). They noted that one of the strongest predictors of outcome in patients with severe head injury was the percentage of time ICP exceeded 20 mmHg. Specifically, as the amount of time ICP remained above 20 mmHg increased, poor outcomes became more likely, whereas favorable outcomes became less likely. Further evidence in favor of ICP monitoring has also come from studies focusing on cerebral perfusion pressure (CPP) (class II data), which is defined as mean arterial pressure minus ICP.[3] Of course, treating elevated ICP and maintaining adequate CPP are impossible without continuous monitoring of blood pressure and ICP.

Pearl

One of the strongest predictors of outcome in patients with severe head injury was the percentage of time ICP exceeded 20 mmHg.

Most experts in the field of neurotrauma agree that ICP monitoring should be an integral part of the management of patients with severe TBI. However, when Ghajar et al[4] (class III data) conducted a survey of 219 randomly selected trauma centers in 1991, they found that ICP monitoring was routinely used in the management of patients with severe TBI in only 28% of these centers, and 7% never used ICP monitoring, even though all surveyed hospitals indicated that they provided care for severely head-injured patients. Thus, in the early 1990s, the majority of trauma centers were not routinely treating their severe TBI patients in ways that could potentially improve outcome. These statistics improved after the publication of the *Guidelines for the Management of Severe Head Injury*[5] (*Guidelines*) in 1995. In 1997, Marion and Spiegel[6] (class III data) reported a survey of 3156 neurosurgeons who were surveyed by the American Board of Neurological Surgery. Of the 1262 respondents, 83% felt that ICP monitoring should be performed in patients with severe head injury.

Literature Review: Indications for Intracranial Pressure Monitoring

Normal ICP is 0 to 10 mmHg (0–135 mmH_2O), and most centers use 20 mmHg as the upper limit beyond which treatment is initiated. TBI patients with a GCS of 8 or less appear to be at risk for developing intracranial hypertension (ICH). Because accurate prediction of ICP based solely on the neurologic examination is not possible, measurement of ICP in patients with severe TBI gives the clinician objective data that may profoundly influence management. In 1979, Marshall et al[7] (class III data) reported the results of 100 consecutive patients with severe head injury treated with a standard aggressive protocol that included ICP monitoring. They found that ICP exceeded 15 mmHg in 55% of patients, causing them to recommend ICP monitoring in patients with severe head injury. In 1982, in a prospective series of 207 consecutive patients with severe closed head injury, Narayan et al[8] (class III data) reported that the incidence of ICH was 53 to 63% in comatose patients with an abnormal CT scan. Only 13% of patients with a normal admission CT scan developed ICH. However, if a patient had a normal admission CT scan but demonstrated at least two of three adverse features (age over 40 years, unilateral or bilateral motor posturing, or SBP $<$90 mmHg), the risk of developing ICH was similar to that of patients with abnormal CT scans (60%). Thus, head-injured patients who do not obey commands are at increased risk of developing ICH if their admission CT scans are abnormal or if they exhibit at least two of the adverse features listed above despite a normal admission CT scan.

On the other hand, patients with mild to moderate head injury (GCS 9–15), that is, those who are generally able to follow simple commands, are believed to have a relatively low risk for ICH and can be followed with serial neurologic exams. Less than 3% of patients with mild head injury (GCS 13–15) and approximately 10 to 20% of those with moderate head injury (GCS 9–12) will deteriorate into coma.[9] Therefore, ICP monitoring is not indicated in most patients with mild to moderate head injury, although physicians may opt to place an ICP monitor in certain conscious patients with traumatic mass lesions.[9]

Pearl

Less than 3% of patients with mild head injury (GCS 13–15) and approximately 10 to 20% of those with moderate head injury (GCS 9–12) will deteriorate into coma.

At some centers, therapies to reduce ICP have been initiated routinely even though ICP was not being measured. However, several of the therapies used to control ICP, including hyperventilation, mannitol, sedation, and paralysis, may have deleterious side effects.[9] For example, in 1991, Muizelaar et al[10] (class II data) reported the results of a prospective randomized study that found that severe prolonged hyperventilation resulted in poorer outcomes in patients with severe head injury. Regarding mannitol treatment, Kaufmann et al[11] in 1992 reported the results of a laboratory study that demonstrated that cumulative doses of mannitol can worsen cerebral edema by leaking into the interstitium. Lastly, although sedation, analgesia, and chemical paralysis reduce blood pressure elevations and ICP surges, their use makes it nearly impossible to follow and interpret the clinical exam. In such situations, ICP monitoring would be most valuable to allow early detection of brain swelling or intracranial hematoma formation.[9] Furthermore, because the routine use of paralytic agents may increase the risk of pulmonary complications (class II data),[12] it has been recommended that paralysis be used to control ICP only if sedation is inadequate. ICP monitoring can eliminate unnecessary interventions and their potentially adverse effects.

Pearl

Because therapies used to control ICP may have deleterious side effects, their empiric use in patients without ICP monitors is discouraged.

ICP data are useful not only for guiding therapy, but also for predicting outcome. In 1981, Narayan et al[13] (class II data) reported that patients with normal ICPs have a better prognosis than those who demonstrate elevated ICP requiring therapy either early in the monitoring period, late in the monitoring period, or throughout their course. Numerous other authors have reported similar associations. This information helps the clinician counsel patients' families and may even allow for a more appropriate allocation of resources.

Several class II studies provide evidence to support the notion that ICP monitoring might improve outcome. In 1977, Becker et al[14] (class II data) reported results in a series of 160 patients with severe head injury treated by an aggressive management protocol that included ICP monitoring. They reported a 30% mortality rate. In comparison, Jennett et al[15] (class II data) reported in the same year a 50% mortality rate in comatose head-injured patients who were treated without ICP monitoring. In 1982, Saul and Ducker[16] (class III data) reported the results of a study comparing a historical control group of 127 severe TBI patients who were treated for ICP >20–25 mmHg with mannitol and cerebrospinal fluid (CSF) drainage to a group of 106 patients treated in a similar manner at a lower ICP threshold of 15 mmHg. The mortality rate was 46% in the group with an ICP treatment threshold of 20 to 25 mmHg, compared to a rate of only 28% for the patients treated at the lower ICP threshold.

Further evidence came in 1991, when the TCDB investigators reported a mortality rate of 36% (compared to 50% reported by Jennett et al[15]) in head-injured patients with a GCS of 8 or less (class II data).[17] The four trauma centers that composed the TCDB all routinely used ICP monitoring in the care of patients with severe TBI. In 1993, Ghajar et al[18] (class III data) reported the results of a study of ICP monitoring in head-injured patients with a GCS of 7 or less. They compared 34 patients treated with ICP monitoring and drainage of CSF when ICP exceeded 15 mmHg to 15 patients who did not receive ICP monitors and were not treated for ICH. They reported a mortality rate in the monitored patients of 12%, as compared to 53% in the unmonitored patients. This study was limited by its small size and nonrandomized nature. In 1996, Ghajar[19] reported a meta-analysis of 14 series of head-injured patients. He found a mortality rate of 21% in series that used CSF drainage routinely, as compared to 35% in those that used it sometimes and 43% in those that never used CSF drainage. Most recently, a report from a community setting (class III data) concluded that the application of head injury management guidelines did reduce mortality.[20]

Pearl

Several class II studies provide evidence to support the notion that ICP monitoring might improve outcome.

Conclusions: Indications for Intracranial Pressure Monitoring

Because the efficacy of ICP monitoring in improving outcome in patients with severe head injury has never been proven in a prospective randomized clinical trial, there are insufficient data to support its use as a level I recommendation. However, there exists a large body of published clinical experience that indicates that severe TBI patients (GCS 3–8) are at increased risk of developing elevated ICP in comparison to patients with mild to moderate TBI. In addition, evidence shows that ICP monitoring may have the following benefits: early detection of expanding intracranial mass lesions; reduction of the indiscriminate use of ICP-lowering therapies, which may have adverse effects; improved prognostication; and possible improvement in outcomes. For these reasons, we concur with the recommendations of the *Guidelines*.[9]

Recommendations: Indications for Intracranial Pressure Monitoring

1. ICP monitoring is appropriate in patients with severe head injury (GCS 3–8) with an abnormal admission CT scan that reveals hematomas, contusions, edema, or compressed basal cisterns (level II).
2. ICP monitoring is appropriate in patients with severe head injury with a normal admission CT scan if two or more of the following are present: age >40 years, unilateral or bilateral motor posturing, or SBP <90 mmHg (level II).
3. ICP monitoring is not routinely indicated in patients with mild to moderate head injury, but a physician may opt to monitor ICP in certain conscious patients with traumatic mass lesions (level II).

Literature Review: Types of Monitoring Devices

Once the decision has been made to monitor ICP, a particular monitoring device must be selected from the many that are available. Ventricular, parenchymal, subarachnoid, and epidural monitors have all been used, with varying degrees of success. The ideal monitor should be durable, accurate, and inexpensive. Although no device is perfect, several are acceptable.

The pressure transduction mechanism of each monitor is an important consideration. Each type is associated with its own pros and cons. Devices that transduce pressure through an external strain gauge are coupled to the patient via fluid-filled tubing. Advantages of this type of device include the ability to recalibrate and, in general, a high degree of accuracy. However, such devices must be maintained at a fixed reference point (zero point) relative to the patient's head. Changes in the position of the transducer without corresponding changes in the position of the patient's head can lead to erroneous measurements of ICP. Inaccurate ICP readings may also be caused by obstruction within the fluid-filled tubing, which may be recognized by a dampened waveform.

Pearl

Fluid-coupled ICP monitoring systems allow drainage of CSF and frequent recalibration, but obstruction within the fluid-filled tubing may cause ICP readings to be inaccurate.

In contrast to external strain gauge devices, intracranial strain gauge or fiberoptic devices are not limited by fixed reference points. However, they tend to become less accurate over time due to "drift." Furthermore, they cannot be recalibrated once inserted. In a study of 15 adults and five children whose ICP was monitored simultaneously with a parenchymal fiberoptic device and a fluid-coupled ventricular catheter, Ostrup et al[21] found a measurement drift of up to 1 mmHg per day with the fiberoptic device. Piek and Bock[22] observed a drift of up to 4 mmHg in the first day of monitoring in 13 patients in whom measurements from a parenchymal strain gauge device were compared to simultaneous readings from a fluid-coupled ventricular catheter. In a prospective study of 101 subdural and ventricular fiberoptic devices by Bavetta et al,[23] an average drift of −3.3 mmHg per day for up to 5 days was observed. Even devices that transduce pressure through similar mechanisms can show wide variability in ICP readings if they are used in different ways. Barlow et al[24] found that only 44% of ICP readings from a subdural fluid-coupled device were within a 10 mmHg range of readings obtained by a ventricular catheter in 10 patients monitored simultaneously with both devices.

Because a particular type of monitor might not be the best choice for all patients, the clinical circumstances of each patient must be considered when deciding which type of monitor to use. For example, when ICP monitoring is performed in conscious patients, a device that does not penetrate the parenchyma, such as a subdural monitor, might suffice. In patients with collapsed ventricles, insertion of a ventricular catheter might be difficult, necessitating use of a parenchymal device. In coagulopathic patients in whom ICP monitoring is necessary, the least invasive device is preferred.

Compared to other types of monitors, a ventricular catheter has the added advantage of allowing CSF drainage. It can thus be used as a therapeutic tool in patients with elevated ICP. The potential therapeutic value of ventricular catheters makes them the preferred type of monitoring device in most patients. Intraventricular pressure as recorded by an intraventricular catheter has also been accepted as the gold standard against which other types of monitors are compared.

The potential risks of the various monitoring devices must be considered. These include infection, intracranial hemorrhage, poor positioning, and malfunction. To develop recommendations for ICP monitoring technology, the authors of the *Guidelines* performed a Medline search using the key words "monitor" and "intracranial pressure." Clinically relevant articles were used; case reports were excluded. Regarding infection rates of the various types of monitors, the *Guidelines* pointed out that most studies defined *infection* as positive CSF cultures or positive cultures of the device. The *Guidelines* favored the term *colonization* instead of *infection* because most reported infections did not reflect clinically significant events. Ventriculostomies were associated with an average colonization rate of 5%.[25] Subarachnoid and subdural monitors were also associated with an average colonization rate of 5%. Monitors placed into the parenchyma were associated with an average colonization rate of 14%. The overall incidence of hematomas with all devices was 1.4%, with a range from 0 for subarachnoid bolts, subdural catheters, and catheter-tip strain gauge devices to 2.8% for fiberoptic parenchymal devices.[25] Ventriculostomies were associated with an average incidence of hematomas of 1.1%. Malfunction rates of fiberoptic devices ranged from 9 to 40%.[25] Malfunction rates of fluid-coupled ventricular catheters, subarachnoid bolts, and subdural catheters were reported as 6.3%, 16%, and 10.5%, respectively.[24,26,27] Three percent of patients with ventricular catheters underwent revision of the catheters because of malposition.[25] Ventriculostomies thus compare favorably to other types of ICP monitors in rates of colonization, hemorrhage, and malfunction, although they might be slightly more difficult to insert.

Pearl

Reported malfunction rates range from 9 to 40% for fiberoptic devices, whereas fluid-coupled ventricular catheters have a reported malfunction rate of 6.3%.

The cost-effectiveness of monitoring devices is another important consideration. Fiberoptic and catheter-tip strain gauge devices require additional hardware that can cost in the thousands of dollars. The implanted devices themselves often cost more than $350 each. Fluid-coupled systems are substantially cheaper.

Pearl

Although fluid-coupled systems are much less expensive than most other types of ICP monitors, they may be more difficult to insert.

Recommendations: Types of Monitoring Devices

The authors of the *Guidelines* ranked ICP monitoring devices based on their accuracy, stability, and ability to drain CSF. Intraventricular catheters that are fluid-coupled to an external strain gauge are ranked first.[25] They are considered the most reliable type of ICP monitoring device, and they can be used therapeutically. Parenchymal, subdural, subarachnoid, and epidural devices are ranked second through fifth, respectively.[25] Ventriculostomies have a low complication rate and are more cost-effective than most other ICP monitoring devices. However, a ventricular catheter might not be the best monitoring device for all patients, and the particular ICP monitoring device chosen for each patient should be tailored to the particular circumstances of that patient.

References

1. Lundberg N, Troupp H, Lorin H. Continuous recording of the ventricular-fluid pressure in patients with severe acute traumatic brain injury: a preliminary report. J Neurosurg 1965;22: 581–590.
2. Marmarou A, Anderson RL, Ward JD, et al. Impact of ICP instability and hypotension on outcome in patients with severe head trauma. J Neurosurg 1991;75:S59–S66.
3. Rosner MJ, Rosner SD, Johnson AH. Cerebral perfusion pressure: management protocol and clinical results. J Neurosurg 1995;83:949–962.
4. Ghajar J, Hariri RJ, Narayan RK, et al. Survey of critical care management of comatose, head-injured patients in the United States. Crit Care Med 1995;23:560–567.
5. Brain Trauma Foundation, American Association of Neurological Surgeons, Joint Section on Neurotrauma and Critical Care. Guidelines for the management of severe head injury. J Neurotrauma 1996;13:641–734.
6. Marion DW, Spiegel TP. Changes in the management of severe traumatic brain injury: 1991–1997. Crit Care Med 2000;28: 16–18.
7. Marshall LF, Smith RW, Shapiro HM. The outcome with aggressive treatment in severe head injuries, I: the significance of intracranial pressure monitoring. J Neurosurg 1979;50:20–25.
8. Narayan RK, Kishore PR, Becker DP, et al. Intracranial pressure: to monitor or not to monitor? A review of our experience with severe head injury. J Neurosurg 1982;56:650–659.
9. Brain Trauma Foundation, American Association of Neurological Surgeons, Joint Section on Neurotrauma and Critical Care. Guidelines for the management of severe traumatic brain injury: indications for intracranial pressure monitoring. J Neurotrauma 2000;17:479–491.
10. Muizelaar JP, Marmarou A, Ward JD, et al. Adverse effects of prolonged hyperventilation in patients with severe head injury: a randomized clinical trial. J Neurosurg 1991;75:731–739.
11. Kaufmann AM, Cardoso ER. Aggravation of vasogenic cerebral edema by multiple-dose mannitol. J Neurosurg 1992;77: 584–589.
12. Hsiang JK, Chesnut RM, Crisp CB, et al. Early, routine paralysis for intracranial pressure control in severe head injury: is it necessary? Crit Care Med 1994;22:1471–1476.
13. Narayan RK, Greenberg RP, Miller JD, et al. Improved confidence of outcome prediction in severe head injury: a comparative analysis of the clinical examination, multimodality evoked potentials, CT scanning, and intracranial pressure. J Neurosurg 1981;54:751–762.
14. Becker DP, Miller JD, Ward JD, et al. The outcome from severe head injury with early diagnosis and intensive management. J Neurosurg 1977;47:491–502.
15. Jennett B, Teasdale G, Galbraith S, et al. Severe head injuries in three countries. J Neurol Neurosurg Psychiatry 1977;40:291–298.
16. Saul TG, Ducker TB. Effect of intracranial pressure monitoring and aggressive treatment on mortality in severe head injury. J Neurosurg 1982;56:498–503.
17. Marshall LF, Gautille T, Klauber MR, et al. The outcome of severe closed head injury. J Neurosurg 1991;75:S28–S36.
18. Ghajar JB, Hariri RJ, Patterson RH. Improved outcome from traumatic coma using only ventricular cerebrospinal fluid drainage for intracranial pressure control. Adv Neurosurg 1993;21:173–177.
19. Ghajar JB. Variability of neurotrauma care in hospitals. In: Narayan RK, Wilberger JE Jr, Povlishock JT, eds. Neurotrauma. New York: McGraw-Hill, 1996:1007–1017.
20. Palmer S, Bader MK, Qureshi A, et al. The impact on outcomes in a community hospital setting of using the AANS traumatic brain injury guidelines. J Trauma 2001;50:657–664.
21. Ostrup RC, Luerssen TG, Marshall LF, et al. Continuous monitoring of intracranial pressure with a miniaturized fiberoptic device. J Neurosurg 1987;67:206–209.
22. Piek J, Bock WJ. Continuous monitoring of cerebral tissue pressure in neurosurgical practice—experiences with 100 patients. Intensive Care Med 1990;16:184–188.
23. Bavetta S, Norris JS, Wyatt M, et al. Prospective study of zero drift in fiberoptic pressure monitors used in clinical practice. J Neurosurg 1997;86:927–930.
24. Barlow P, Mendelow AD, Lawrence AE, et al. Clinical evaluation of two methods of subdural pressure monitoring. J Neurosurg 1985;63:578–582.
25. Brain Trauma Foundation, American Association of Neurological Surgeons, Joint Section on Neurotrauma and Critical Care. Management and prognosis of severe traumatic brain injury. Recommendations for intracranial pressure monitoring technology. J Neurotrauma 2000;17: 497–506.
26. Bavetta S, Sutcliffe JC, Sparrow OC, et al. A prospective comparison of fibre-optic and fluid-filled single lumen bolt subdural pressure transducers in ventilated neurosurgical patients. Br J Neurosurg 1996;10:279–284.
27. North B, Reilly P. Comparison among three methods of intracranial pressure recording. Neurosurgery 1986;18:730–732.

◆ 10 ◆

Should I Monitor Jugular Venous Oxygen Saturation?

Nino Stocchetti

Brief Answer

Yes. Any time the adequacy of the global oxygen supply to the brain is of interest, and better systems are not available, measurement of jugular venous oxygen saturation ($SjvO_2$) is useful. This technique requires constant attention, and data interpretation may sometimes be complex, but $SjvO_2$ monitoring can provide important information that directly influences our management of head injury.

Background

Pathophysiology

A normal adult human brain has a mean cerebral blood flow (CBF) of around 50 to 60 mL/100 g/min. If its normal hemoglobin (Hgb) content is fully saturated with oxygen, arterial blood carries ~20 mL of oxygen per deciliter (dL). The oxygen content of venous blood draining the brain varies. Under normal conditions, internal jugular (IJ) hemoglobin oxygen saturation ranges between 55% and 69%. Therefore, the normal arteriojugular difference in O_2 content ($AJDO_2$) is 6.3 ± 2.4 mL/dL. According to the Fick principle, $AJDO_2$ is proportional to cerebral metabolic rate of oxygen consumption ($CMRO_2$) and inversely proportional to CBF.[1–4]

Under normal conditions, $AJDO_2$ remains stable. If flow decreases or $CMRO_2$ increases, $AJDO_2$ rises as well, indicating that the brain is extracting more oxygen from the blood flowing through the cerebral circulation. When flow increases relative to cerebral oxygen consumption, $AJDO_2$ drops. High $AJDO_2$ (and, somewhat less accurately, low $SjvO_2$) has thus been interpreted as synonymous with cerebral ischemia, whereas low $AJDO_2$ is taken as a clear indicator of hyperemia. However, this is an oversimplification, and some points need to be clarified.

Pearl

The normal arteriojugular difference in O_2 content ($AJDO_2$) is 6.3 ± 2.4 mL/dL.

$AJDO_2$, Not Simply $SjvO_2$, Is Related to Flow and Metabolism

Although it is easier to use $SjvO_2$ instead of $AJDO_2$ for estimating the relationship between $CMRO_2$ and CBF, jugular saturation also depends on the Hgb concentration. Therefore, IJ saturation cannot be used independently of the Hgb value for estimating the status of cerebral metabolism, and $AJDO_2$ must be calculated. For example, low levels of jugular saturation may simply indicate anemia (in which the brain may extract more oxygen from the diluted blood), not inadequate flow.

Pearl

$SjvO_2$ cannot be used independently of the hemoglobin concentration to estimate the status of cerebral metabolism.

$AJDO_2$ Estimates the Global Relationship Between Flow and Metabolism

There are heterogeneities in the distribution of flow and in oxygen consumption in the brain. $AJDO_2$ cannot detect problems in small areas of the brain, and it can miss important events, such as cerebral infarction, when they are of limited extent (class III data).[5]

Oxygen May Still Be Needed Even If It Is Not Extracted

There are limits to the brain's ability to extract oxygen. When these capabilities are exhausted, no more oxygen can be removed from the blood, so $AJDO_2$ does not rise further. That does not imply there is no need for more oxygen. In this situation, $AJDO_2$ does not increase, and ischemia develops.

Oxygen extraction may be impaired, as in cases of mitochondrial dysfunction. $AJDO_2$ may be very low in this situation, or when a large portion of the brain does not extract oxygen at all (as in cerebral infarction).

For all these reasons, the simple extrapolation "low $AJDO_2$ indicates hyperemia" is simply not true.

Pearl

If cerebral oxygen extraction is impaired after brain injury, $AJDO_2$ may be very low, and $SjvO_2$ may be high.

Literature Review

Since the landmark paper by Obrist et al[6] and further work by Robertson et al,[2] $AJDO_2$ has been used increasingly in monitoring severe head injury. It has been both praised as the optimal monitoring guide in head injury management[7] and rejected as still unproven and experimental.[8]

Technical Aspects of Monitoring Jugular Saturation

On Which Side Should the Jugular Catheter Be Inserted?

Jugular saturation may vary depending on whether the jugular catheter is positioned on the right or left side. Bilateral sampling has confirmed that the two sides generally provide comparable data. Nevertheless, differences that may sometimes be clinically relevant have been detected in a substantial percentage of patients (class II data).[9]

Such differences, which arise from drainage of cerebral areas with different values for blood flow and $CMRO_2$, likely occur more frequently when focal masses are present. For this reason, some clinicians choose to insert $SjvO_2$ catheters on the side of predominant intracerebral pathology.

For cases of diffuse damage, however, use of the larger jugular vein or "dominant IJ" has been proposed. Cannulation of the dominant IJ should guarantee that sampling takes place on the side of greater cerebral venous drainage. Different methods of identifying the dominant IJ have been reported, including unilateral compression of the neck during intracranial pressure (ICP) recording, with the side of the larger ICP increase considered to be the side of predominant venous drainage,[3] or identification by computed tomography (CT) scan of the side with the larger jugular foramen.[9,10] In a randomized trial, ultrasound measurement was found useful for increasing the likelihood of successful jugular vein cannulation (class I data).[11] Although this study tested the IJ for central venous catheter placement, the findings can probably be applied to the retrograde jugular cannulation necessary for determining $AJDO_2$.

Where Should the Tip of the Jugular Catheter Be Placed?

The tip of the catheter must be in the upper portion of the superior jugular bulb. When the tip lies too inferiorly, samples are contaminated with blood draining the neck and the face, rather than the brain. On the other hand, even if the tip is advanced too far, reliable $AJDO_2$ data can still be obtained. A lateral skull radiograph is helpful for determining the location of the catheter tip.

Venous oxygen saturation in the sinuses is generally slightly lower than that in the jugular bulb.[9] If a catheter is erroneously positioned in the inferior petrosal sinus, it may produce misleading data. The inferior petrosal sinus has a higher Hgb saturation than the jugular bulb, probably because it drains the anterior pituitary lobe and carries some extracranial blood, for example, from the superior ophthalmic vein.[12]

Thus, in practical terms, two aspects must be considered. When conspicuous unilateral damage exists, it may be reasonable to attempt to cannulate the ipsilateral jugular vein; this is not the case with diffuse damage (level III recommendation). The second crucial point is that after placement of the catheter, the position of its tip should be checked by x-ray.[13]

Slow Sampling Is Necessary for Accurate Measurement of Saturation

When intermittent samples are used, the rate of blood withdrawal may affect IJ saturation. With fast withdrawal, higher saturations are detected, probably as a result of extracranial contamination (class II data). Thus, blood samples should be withdrawn slowly (level II recommendation).[14]

Intermittent Sampling or Continuous Measurement?

Jugular saturation can be monitored by two techniques. Intermittent sampling can be done through standard intravenous catheters. Continuous measurement requires fiberoptic catheters.

When optical catheters are used for continuous reading, they provide reliable data only if carefully maintained. Close attention must be paid to their position, light intensity, and other details. Although optical catheters have been reported to give a very low percentage of reliable data in some centers, others have described higher levels of confidence.[4,15]

Complications

Complications of jugular venous monitoring are rare (class III data). Carotid puncture has an incidence of 1 to 4.5%.[4,16] Infection is very rare, and no cases of severe infection due to jugular cannulation for jugular venous monitoring have been reported. Damage to the vein is more difficult to assess and to quantify, perhaps explaining the paucity of reports of this complication. In 20 patients systematically investigated with ultrasonography, eight (40%) had nonobstructive subclinical internal jugular vein thrombi after jugular bulb catheter monitoring (95% confidence interval, 19–61%). In this single series, therefore, the incidence of subclinical internal jugular vein thrombosis after jugular bulb catheter monitoring was considerable.[16]

Clinical Use of Jugular Saturation

Jugular Saturation in the Early Postinjury Phase

Episodes of high $AJDO_2$ are usually detected during the early phases after head injury. Although $CMRO_2$ is likely to be low during this period, CBF is depressed by an even greater extent. Hyperventilation is also frequently used, sometimes inadvertently.[17] During rescue and transport to the trauma center, in fact, ventilation is not likely to be carefully titrated. Due to the combination of intra- and extracranial injuries, anemia is also frequent and lowers jugular saturation even if CBF is preserved.

Expansion of intracranial masses that cause intracranial hypertension and reduced cerebral perfusion can be detected by $SjvO_2$ monitoring. In 25 severely head-injured patients who underwent removal of intracranial traumatic hematomas, jugular saturation was low preoperatively but improved after surgical evacuation (class II data).[18]

Hyperventilation

Hyperventilation is a powerful tool for controlling increased intracranial pressure. It lowers the intracranial blood volume by reducing cerebral blood flow. Since avoiding cerebral ischemia is essential in head-injured patients, there seems to be conflict between the potential improvement in cerebral perfusion pressure obtained by hypocapnia and the undesirable side effect of flow reduction. Because $AJDO_2$ is very sensitive to changes in cerebrovascular resistance induced by hypocapnia, jugular vein monitoring may reveal inappropriate reductions of CBF caused by hyperventilation. Therefore, $SjvO_2$ monitoring should be used for titrating the level of hyperventilation (level III recommendation).[19]

Arteriovenous Fistulas

Because arteriovenous fistulas are characterized by a rapid transit of arterial blood to the venous circulation, $AJDO_2$ measurements are not useful in such cases. However, extremely high values of jugular venous oxygen saturation, approaching arterial levels, have prompted cerebral angiography to confirm clinical suspicions that traumatic carotid-cavernous fistulas were present.[20,21]

Jugular Saturation, $AJDO_2$, and Their Association with Outcome

Jugular venous desaturation (to less than 50%) has been correlated with poor outcome (class II data).[22] If desaturation occurs while $AJDO_2$ is high, flow may be inadequate. It seems reasonable, therefore, to attempt to relate inadequacy of flow and brain damage. In fact, repeated episodes of jugular desaturation have been found to correlate with unfavorable outcome.[22] However, when cerebral metabolism is very depressed, as in cases with profound damage to neuronal cells, oxygen consumption is very low.[23] In this situation $AJDO_2$ is very low too, suggesting impaired cerebral activity rather than excessive flow. Patients with unfavorable outcome have a lower $AJDO_2$ than patients with good results (class II data).[24,25]

Pearl

Jugular venous desaturation (to less than 50%) has been correlated with poor outcome.

Brain Death

$AJDO_2$ values undergo a characteristic pattern during the progression toward brain death. As ischemia develops, $AJDO_2$ typically increases, followed by a steep reduction down to almost zero oxygen extraction from the brain. The explanation for this pattern is that, shortly before brain death, blood flow through the brain is very low. The remaining living tissue extracts oxygen maximally from the residual flow, producing a very low $SjvO_2$. When flow ceases in the brain, the blood flowing through the jugular vein no longer comes from the brain. Instead, it merely represents venous drainage from the face and neck. In this situation, $AJDO_2$ is extremely low.

Recommendations (Level III)

The maintenance of a blood flow closely related to the metabolic needs of cerebral tissue is a key goal of intensive care after acute brain injury. The monitoring of parameters related to this coupling seems sound, especially if such monitoring can be performed continuously.

Jugular saturation may indicate the adequacy of CBF, especially when CBF may be modified by therapeutic manipulation, such as hyperventilation. This valuable information can be obtained at low cost and without significant complications.

To ensure accurate sampling of the venous cerebral drainage, a decision must be made about the best side to cannulate. X-ray verification is used to check the position of the catheter tip.

$AJDO_2$ data require careful interpretation so that knowledge of the status of oxygen extraction becomes a useful part of the routine management of patients. This may seem cumbersome, and it is, but so are most meaningful parameters monitored in intensive care.

References

1. Gibbs EL, Lennox WG, Nims LF, et al. Arterial and cerebral venous blood: arterial-venous differences in man. J Biol Chem 1942;144:325–332.
2. Robertson CS, Narayan RK, Gokaslan ZL, et al. Cerebral arteriovenous oxygen difference as an estimate of cerebral blood flow in comatose patients. J Neurosurg 1989;70:222–230.
3. Dearden NM. Jugular bulb venous oxygen saturation in the management of severe head injury. Curr Opin Anaesthesiol 1991;4:279–286.
4. Macmillan CS, Andrews PJ. Cerebrovenous oxygen saturation monitoring: practical considerations and clinical relevance. Intensive Care Med 2000;26:1028–1036.
5. Andrews PJ, Murugavel S, Deehan S. Conventional multimodality monitoring and failure to detect ischemic cerebral blood flow. J Neurosurg Anesthesiol 1996;8:220–226.
6. Obrist WD, Langfitt TW, Jaggi JL, et al. Cerebral blood flow and metabolism in comatose patients with acute head injury: relationship to intracranial hypertension. J Neurosurg 1984; 61:241–253.
7. Cruz J. The first decade of continuous monitoring of jugular bulb oxyhemoglobin saturation: management strategies and clinical outcome. Crit Care Med 1998;26:344–351.
8. Latronico N, Beindorf AE, Rasulo FA, et al. Limits of intermittent jugular bulb oxygen saturation monitoring in the management of severe head trauma patients. Neurosurgery 2000; 46:1131–1139.
9. Stocchetti N, Paparella A, Bridelli F, et al. Cerebral venous oxygen saturation studied with bilateral samples in the internal jugular veins. Neurosurgery 1994;34:38–44.
10. Metz C, Holzschuh M, Bein T, et al. Monitoring of cerebral oxygen metabolism in the jugular bulb: reliability of unilateral measurements in severe head injury. J Cereb Blood Flow Metab 1998;18:332–343.
11. Mallory DL, McGee WT, Shawker TH, et al. Ultrasound guidance improves the success rate of internal jugular vein cannulation: a prospective, randomized trial. Chest 1990;98:157–160.
12. Targa L, Chieregato A, Calzolari F, et al. Inferior petrosal sinus and internal jugular vein: possible sources of contamination of sampling for jugular bulb oxygen saturation monitoring. Proceedings of the 8th European Congress of Intensive Care Medicine, Monduzzi Bologna 1995;891–894.
13. Bankier AA, Fleischmann D, Windisch A, et al. Position of jugular oxygen saturation catheter in patients with head trauma: assessment by use of plain films. AJR 1995;164:437–441.
14. Matta BF, Lam AM. The rate of blood withdrawal affects the accuracy of jugular venous bulb: oxygen saturation measurements. Anesthesiology 1997;86:806–808.
15. Rossi S, Cormio M, Marmarou A. Internal jugular vein oxygen saturation: clinical usefulness and limitations in the management of head-injured patients. Crit Rev Neurosurg 1996;6: 202–208.
16. Coplin WM, O'Keefe GE, Grady MS, et al. Thrombotic, infectious, and procedural complications of the jugular bulb catheter in the intensive care unit. Neurosurgery 1997;41:101–109.
17. Schneider GH, von Helden A, Lanksch WR, et al. Continuous monitoring of jugular bulb oxygen saturation in comatose patients: therapeutic implications. Acta Neurochir (Wien) 1995;134:71–75.
18. Gopinath SP, Cormio M, Ziegler J, et al. Intraoperative jugular desaturation during surgery for traumatic intracranial hematomas. Anesth Analg 1996;83:1014–1021.
19. Brain Trauma Foundation, American Association of Neurological Surgeons, Joint Section on Neurotrauma and Critical Care. Guidelines for the management of severe traumatic brain injury: hyperventilation. J Neurotrauma 2000;17:513–520.
20. Chieregato A, Veronesi V, Calzolari F, et al. Prematurely detected traumatic carotid-cavernous sinus fistula, by means of unintentional contralateral inferior petrosal sinus catheterization: bilateral jugular bulb oxygen saturation finding. J Neurosurg Anesthesiol 1998;10:16–21.
21. Komiyama M, Kan M, Shigemoto T. Marked regional heterogeneity in venous oxygen saturation in severe head injury studied by superselective intracranial venous sampling: case report. Neurosurgery 1999;45:1469–1473.
22. Gopinath SP, Robertson CS, Contant CF, et al. Jugular venous desaturation and outcome after head injury. J Neurol Neurosurg Psychiatry 1994;57:717–723.
23. Cormio M, Valadka AB, Robertson CS. Elevated jugular venous oxygen saturation after severe head injury. J Neurosurg 1999;90:9–15.
24. Macmillan CS, Andrews PJ, Easton VJ. Increased jugular bulb saturation is associated with poor outcome in traumatic brain injury. J Neurol Neurosurg Psychiatry 2001;70:101–104.
25. Cruz J. Relationship between early patterns of cerebral extraction of oxygen and outcome from severe acute traumatic brain swelling: cerebral ischemia or cerebral viability? Crit Care Med 1996;24:953–956.

◆ 11 ◆

Should I Monitor Brain Tissue PO_2?

Karl L. Kiening, Asita S. Sarrafzadeh, John F. Stover, and Andreas W. Unterberg

Brief Answer

Continuous monitoring of brain tissue oxygen tension ($PbtO_2$) can reveal unique information about the status of cerebral metabolism. $PbtO_2$ monitoring can reveal not only impending metabolic collapse, but also the efficacy of therapeutic interventions on improving cerebral metabolism. However, because no studies have demonstrated improvements in outcome as a result of $PbtO_2$ monitoring, use of this technology can be advocated only as a level III recommendation. Prospective, randomized, controlled studies are needed to clarify the role of $PbtO_2$ monitoring in head-injured patients. Care must also be taken not to assume that $PbtO_2$ data, which are obtained from a very small volume of tissue, always reflect the state of global cerebral metabolism; when considerable regional heterogeneity of cerebral metabolism is present, such extrapolations may lead to markedly incorrect conclusions.

Background

Importance of Posttraumatic Cerebral $PbtO_2$

Patients with severe traumatic brain injury (TBI) are at risk of developing inadequate cerebral perfusion pressure (CPP) and consequent secondary cerebral ischemic damage, most commonly because of intracranial hypertension or arterial hypotension. Low CPP, in turn, may compromise cerebral blood flow (CBF) and tissue oxygenation, potentially contributing to evolving structural and functional tissue damage and thus negatively affecting the final neurologic outcome. Consequently, maintenance of an adequate CPP, either by reducing elevated intracranial pressure (ICP) or increasing mean arterial blood pressure (MAP), is a widely accepted recommendation of the evidence-based *Guidelines for the Management of Severe Traumatic Brain Injury* produced by the Brain Trauma Foundation, the American Association of Neurological Surgeons (AANS), and the AANS/Congress of Neurological Surgeons (CNS) Section on Neurotrauma and Critical Care (class III data).[1]

In healthy individuals, tissue oxygenation and cerebral perfusion show a critical and mutual interdependence (class II data).[2] The existence of a strict perfusion-dependent increase in tissue oxygenation in activated human cortex underlines the importance of oxidative metabolism for meeting activation-induced increases in energy demands. Consequently, any decrease in cerebral perfusion may impair oxygen supply and oxidative metabolism. As shown in clinical (class II data)[3,4] as well as experimental[5] pathophysiologic studies, changes in $PbtO_2$ can be used to reliably monitor evolving disturbances of tissue metabolism. Because the mammalian brain is not equipped with sufficient oxygen and energy depots and because the activity of many key enzymes is regulated by $PbtO_2$ (class III data),[6] tissue oxygenation must be maintained within physiologic limits to prevent additional cell damage.

Recent experience has taught us that local cerebral hypoxia may develop under conditions of normal ICP, CPP, and MAP, stressing the importance of targeted monitoring within the tissue of interest. Such episodes of local cerebral hypoxia may be caused by hyperventilation-induced hypocapnia (class II data),[3,7] by insufficient arterial oxygenation (class II data),[3] or by a mismatch between oxygen delivery, that is, CBF, and cerebral metabolic rate of oxygen ($CMRO_2$) (class III data).[8]

Pearl

Local cerebral hypoxia may develop under conditions of normal ICP, CPP, and MAP.

Techniques for Monitoring Cerebral Oxygenation

Given the overriding importance of oxygen in maintaining energetic and ionic homeostasis and in preserving the integrity of cellular and subcellular function and structure, early detection of any decrease in cerebral oxygenation is likely to be necessary to guide adequate therapy. Real-time monitoring of cerebral oxygenation can be performed by tracking changes in jugular venous oxygen saturation ($SjvO_2$) via jugular bulb oximetry (class II data),[9] which measures global cerebral oxygenation. Cerebral partial pressure of oxygen can also be measured with intraparenchymal oxygen sensors (class II data),[10] which indicate local cerebral oxygenation.

Despite the strength of its scientific background (class II data),[9,11] $SjvO_2$ monitoring is not widely used because it can be cumbersome and because it is prone to artifact and to other potential problems with poor data quality (class II and III data).[12,13] On the other hand, monitoring of $PbtO_2$ has steadily increased in popularity because of its reliability and safety (class II data).[14] Currently, two main $PbtO_2$ monitoring systems are commercially available: the Licox (Integra Neuroscience, Plainsboro, NJ) and the Neurotrend (Diametrics Medical, St. Paul, MN). The Neurotrend system is a multiparameter sensor that measures brain PCO_2, pH, and temperature in addition to $PbtO_2$. The Licox system measures only $PbtO_2$ (insertion of a separate temperature probe is usually performed as well).

Initially, both systems were based on the polarographic technique (modified "Cark-type" electrodes).[15] In 1998, Neurotrend performed significant technical modifications and switched from a polarographic to a colorimetric method, utilizing optical fluorescence in combination with fiberoptics to measure changes in $PbtO_2$. In the latest Licox system design, the catheters are precalibrated and therefore suitable for immediate insertion, whereas in the Neurotrend system bedside calibration to a defined concentration of oxygen is necessary. Moreover, these systems cannot be compared because of differences in insertion depth, in accuracy of measurements at the zero point (Licox: 0.3 ± 0.3 mmHg; Neurotrend: 7.0 ± 1.4 mmHg) (class II data)[16] and, in particular, differences in reported cerebral ischemic thresholds [Licox: 10 mmHg (class II data)[17]; Neurotrend: 19 mmHg (class II data)].[18] In addition, the change in the type of PO_2 monitoring technology used in the Neurotrend catheter makes it difficult to perform a direct comparison of $PbtO_2$ data obtained with the old versus new Neurotrend sensors.

Where to Measure $PbtO_2$

Experimental studies have demonstrated that tissue oxygenation has a very heterogeneous distribution. The $PbtO_2$ value that is measured depends in part on the surrounding cell density and on the proximity of the inserted electrodes to blood vessels. The highest $PbtO_2$ levels are found close to penetrating vessels and in neuron-rich areas, for example, cortex and hippocampus, as opposed to white matter tracts that consist predominantly of axons (class III data).[6]

To date, no consensus has been reached as to the ideal placement of $PbtO_2$ monitors relative to different traumatic brain lesions; for example, focal/unilateral versus multiple/bilateral versus diffuse brain injury versus generalized edema. The $PbtO_2$ values that are measured in brain-injured patients are strongly influenced by the positioning of the catheter relative to cerebral contusions, with $PbtO_2$ values close to a lesion being significantly lower than those in areas in which a computed tomography scan reveals no injury (class II data).[19]

In clinical practice, parenchymal oxygen sensors are often placed in white matter that is contralateral to a focal lesion ("uninjured"). The assumption underlying this strategy is that a reduction in $PbtO_2$ in the uninjured hemisphere is indicative of widespread, global energetic perturbation caused by such events as a decrease in arterial oxygenation, an increase in ICP, impairment of cerebral perfusion, use of uncontrolled hyperventilation, or similar event. When bilateral lesions are present, those who use this approach prefer to monitor $PbtO_2$ in the hemisphere with the least injury. Some investigators, however, recommend the opposite approach. They suggest that it may be wiser to monitor $PbtO_2$ in the pericontusional zone, concentrating on the tissue that is at high risk of death (comparable to the penumbra in stroke).

Pearl

No consensus has been reached as to the ideal positioning of $PbtO_2$ monitors relative to the location of different types of brain lesions; that is, whether monitors should be adjacent to a lesion or remote from (or even contralateral to) it.

Literature Review: Can $PbtO_2$ Monitoring Be Recommended Based on the Existing Literature?

Methodology of Literature Review

None of the published investigations describing cerebral oxygen measurements have been performed in large, prospective, randomized trials (class I evidence). Thus, the goal of this chapter is to determine, based on class II and class III evidence, if $PbtO_2$ monitoring can be recommended for routine use in severe TBI.

A PubMed search was performed covering the period from 1996 (first clinical report on this topic[10]) to July 2002. Using the key word "brain tissue PO_2," 141 references were generated, whereas the headings "cerebral oxygenation" and "head injury" resulted in 105 papers. After eliminating duplicates, experimental articles, nontrauma papers, non-$PbtO_2$ papers, reviews, and papers with purely technical issues, the 45 remaining papers dealt with clinical head injury and invasive monitoring of brain tissue PO_2 by one of the two fundamentally different monitoring systems described above.

In the following discussion, we focus on the Licox catheter, which is more commonly used and which provides a larger scientific background (30 articles) than the published papers that employed the Neurotrend catheter ($n = 15$). Only four papers compared both catheters.

As mentioned above, none of the Licox or Neurotrend papers contains data from a prospective, blinded, controlled, randomized study. Consequently, no class I evidence is available on which to base a "gold standard" recommendation. The clinical papers related to the Licox catheter (30 papers) deal with studies that employed prospective data collection and retrospective analyses, making them class II evidence at best. A further elimination of papers with only a small sample size ($n \leq 10$), or in which $PbtO_2$ was not major parameter of interest, reduces the number to 24 eligible studies. These papers mainly focus on hypoxic thresholds ($n = 3$), clinical outcome ($n = 8$), hyperventilation therapy ($n = 9$), CPP therapy ($n = 7$), metabolic monitoring via microdialysis ($n = 3$), and hypothermia ($n = 1$) (some papers address more than one of these topics).

Critical $PbtO_2$ Thresholds and Neurologic Outcome

$PbtO_2$ monitoring has been validated in severe TBI patients by comparison to other established methods like $SjvO_2$ monitoring, in which a decrease in oxygen saturation to below 50% is indicative of cerebral ischemia. In one study, this critical threshold for jugular venous oxygen saturation was found to correspond to a $PbtO_2$ of 8.5 mmHg (class II data).[13] Other clinical (class II data)[3] and experimental[20] studies also suggest that the $PbtO_2$ threshold below which ischemic damage develops is 8 to 10 mmHg.

Pearl

The critical $PbtO_2$ threshold below which ischemic damage develops seems to be 8 to 10 mmHg (measured with a Licox catheter).

Other methods to establish clinically relevant $PbtO_2$ thresholds have concentrated on neurologic outcome of severe TBI patients in relation to different $PbtO_2$ levels (class II data).[4,10,14,16,21–24] Clinical data reveal that important indicators of poor prognosis include decreases in $PbtO_2$ values <10 mmHg within the first week after TBI (and especially within the first 24 hours) and a total time of more than 300 minutes of $PbtO_2$ <10 mmHg during the monitoring period (class II data).[4,21–23] In a series of 22 severely head-injured patients, van Santbrink and colleagues[10] reported that four out of five patients with $PbtO_2$ values ≤5 mmHg during the first 24 hours died (class II data), a finding that was underlined by the same group later in a larger subsequent series ($n = 101$) in which mortality approached 50% if $PbtO_2$ remained ≤5 mmHg for 30 minutes or longer (class II data).[14] A few years earlier Valadka and colleagues[16] had reported increased mortality after severe TBI with any decrease in $PbtO_2$ ≤6 mmHg (class II data).

Overall, the critical $PbtO_2$ threshold of 10 mmHg is adequately substantiated by the literature and confirmed by neurochemical findings (see below) (class II data).[17,25]

$PbtO_2$ and Hyperventilation

Recent studies have shown that in most patients hyperventilation decreases $PbtO_2$ because of decreased CBF (3% change in CBF per 1 mmHg change in arterial PCO_2) (class II data),[4,7,24,26–30] which offsets its potential benefit of reducing ICP and improving CPP. Patients are at especially high risk of suffering cerebral hypoxia during pronounced hyperventilation ($PaCO_2$ ≤30 mmHg) (class III data for this particular question)[26] or during hyperventilation that is employed within the first 24 hours after TBI (class III data for this particular question)[26,27] because of potential aggravation of a reduction in CBF that occurs commonly after TBI (class II data).[31] Even during moderate hyperventilation (average $PaCO_2$ of 29.4 mmHg), critically low $PbtO_2$ levels (<10 mmHg) were reported in ~17% of head-injured patients in one study (class II data).[7] Because individual responses in terms of the extent and trend of $PbtO_2$ changes during hyperventilation are rather variable, $PbtO_2$ monitoring can guide such therapeutic interventions.

Recently performed positron emission tomography studies in severe TBI patients have found a substantial reduction in global and regional mean CBF during forced hyperventilation, sometimes to below 10 mL/100 g/min. However, global and regional mean $CMRO_2$ remained unchanged in these sedated patients (class II data).[32,33] These results were interpreted as indicating that cerebral oxygenation remained sufficient during hyperventilation, despite the drop in CBF to ischemic values. Although the mean $CMRO_2$ in these studies did not change significantly, the potential for individual variability in the response of $CMRO_2$ to hyperventilation emphasizes the necessity of closely monitoring each individual patient.

$PbtO_2$ and CPP

Although the 2000 edition of the *Guidelines for the Management of Severe Traumatic Brain Injury*[1] recommend maintenance of CPP >70 mmHg as an option, this threshold has been questioned, and recent evidence suggests that a threshold of 60 mmHg may be more appropriate. This change is based on results from several studies that suggest that a CPP >60 mmHg is generally sufficient for adequate cerebral oxygenation (class II and class III data).[4,13,30,34,35] A low CPP (<60 mmHg) was found to be significantly related to low $PbtO_2$ (<10 mmHg) (class II data),[4,30,36] and $PbtO_2$ was not influenced by changes in CPP as long as CPP remained above the threshold of 60 mmHg (class II data).[4,13,30]

Even though the studies cited above highlight the importance of a stable CPP for maintaining sufficient cerebral oxygenation after severe TBI in general, this relationship may not necessarily hold true for low $PbtO_2$ caused by traumatic vasospasm (class II data),[34] a diagnosis that is difficult to establish clinically. It remains unclear whether decreases in $PbtO_2$ that occur during traumatic vasospasm can be treated successfully by raising CPP, as is commonly done for aneurysmal vasospasm.

$PbtO_2$ and Neurochemical Monitoring

Recent reports (class II data)[17,25,37] have shown that combining $PbtO_2$ monitoring and microdialysis measurements may allow detailed characterization of the nature of energetic perturbation (anaerobic versus oxidative glucose metabolism) following TBI by simultaneous determination of changes in tissue oxygenation and metabolic parameters. For this purpose, $PbtO_2$ and microdialysis catheters are usually placed adjacent to each other.

Simultaneous monitoring of $SjvO_2$, $PbtO_2$, and cerebral extracellular lactate and glucose in patients with severe TBI has revealed a tight relationship between changes in tissue oxygenation and metabolic deterioration (class II data).[25] Episodes of both global as well as local hypoxia as reflected by decreases in $SvjO_2$ <50% and/or in $PbtO_2 \leq 5$ mmHg coincided with a significant increase in extracellular lactate. In a follow-up study, the same group reported a significant increase in lactate and nonsignificant decrease in glucose during transient cerebral ischemia ($SjvO_2 < 50\%$; median $PbtO_2$ decreased to 10 mmHg) (class II data).[37] These in vivo results nicely demonstrate that changes in $PbtO_2$ are extremely helpful in detecting anaerobic glycolysis. Changes in lactate and glucose alone can also be taken as indicators of the state of oxidative glucose metabolism.

Following severe TBI, decreases in $PbtO_2$ below the ischemic threshold (<10 mmHg) have been reported to coincide in most cases with pathologically elevated lactate/pyruvate ratios and with normal or elevated levels of extracellular glutamate.[17]

Thus, microdialysis measurements may provide valuable information about the impact of local cerebral hypoxia on energy metabolism, thereby substantiating the validity of $PbtO_2$ measurements.

When to Start $PbtO_2$ Monitoring

Because CBF is already significantly reduced during the first few hours after severe TBI (class II data),[31] and because the brain is highly vulnerable to secondary insults during this period, initiation of extensive multimodal monitoring consisting of $PbtO_2$, ICP, CPP, and MAP measurements is indicated. Such efforts are justified because cerebral viability is at stake. Early decreases in $PbtO_2$ point to a worse prognosis (class II data)[10,14,22,23] and serve as an early warning system for the initiation and guidance of therapeutic interventions. Although monitoring $PbtO_2$ as early as possible is most desirable, early $PbtO_2$ monitoring is limited by the rather long stabilization time of 2 to 6 hours after probe insertion (class II data).[3,14] During this period, therapeutic decisions cannot be based on the $PbtO_2$ readings. This period of lack of reliable data collection and inability to interpret observed $PbtO_2$ alterations is a major disadvantage.

Pearl

Monitoring of $PbtO_2$ should be initiated as soon as possible after injury because early decreases in $PbtO_2$ (which can be detected and treated only with early monitoring) are associated with a worse prognosis.

Recommendations

Taken together, although available $PbtO_2$ data reflect predominantly class II evidence, the general recommendation to use $PbtO_2$ monitoring in severe TBI patients, particularly to guide hyperventilation and CPP therapy, must be considered to be a level III recommendation because of the lack of solid evidence showing that such $PbtO_2$-guided therapy results in better neurologic outcomes. Similarly, although continuous $PbtO_2$ monitoring may reveal acute changes suggestive of impending ischemic and energetic deterioration and may therefore guide therapeutic interventions aimed at preventing evolving tissue injury and potential neurologic impairment, it remains to be clarifed whether use of this information in these situations leads to improved outcomes.

One conflicting technical issue is related to the "correct" positioning of the oxygen sensor. Since this sensor can only determine changes within a small radius of tissue surrounding the probe, the "true" validity of this technique is limited to the small area of monitored tissue. In other words, extrapolating local $PbtO_2$ data to the oxygenation status of one hemisphere or of the whole brain carries the risk that regional or global ischemia may evolve undetected despite normal $PbtO_2$ values in the monitored region.

A major drawback of past studies is the rather "uncontrolled" nature in which equally important concomitant and possibly conflicting variables have been managed; for example, sedation, analgesia, pharmacologic paralysis, fluid therapy, ICP, CPP, etc. These intercenter differences in basic management practices need to be considered as important independent variables and have to be tightly controlled in an urgently needed, prospective, randomized study to determine the role of $PbtO_2$-guided therapy.

Acknowledgment

The authors thank Dr. Roger Härtl, Department of Neurological Surgery, Weill Medical College of Cornell University, New York, for valuable discussions.

References

1. Brain Trauma Foundation, American Association of Neurological Surgeons, Joint Section on Neurotrauma and Critical Care. Guidelines for the management of severe traumatic brain injury. J Neurotrauma 2000;17:507–511.
2. Hoge RD, Atkinson J, Gill B, et al. Linear coupling between cerebral blood flow and oxygen consumption in activated human cortex. Proc Natl Acad Sci USA 1999;96:9403–9408.
3. Gopinath SP, Valadka AB, Uzura M, et al. Comparison of jugular venous oxygen saturation and brain tissue PO_2 as monitors of cerebral ischemia after head injury. Crit Care Med 1999;27: 2337–2345.
4. Kiening KL, Hartl R, Unterberg AW, et al. Brain tissue pO_2-monitoring in comatose patients: implications for therapy. Neurol Res 1997;19:233–240.
5. Manley GT, Pitts LH, Morabito D, et al. Brain tissue oxygenation during hemorrhagic shock, resuscitation, and alterations in ventilation. J Trauma 1999;46:261–267.
6. Erecinska M, Silver IA. Tissue oxygen tension and brain sensitivity to hypoxia. Respir Physiol 2001;128:263–276.
7. Imberti R, Bellinzona G, Langer M. Cerebral tissue PO_2 and $SjvO_2$ changes during moderate hyperventilation in patients with severe traumatic brain injury. J Neurosurg 2002;96:97–102.
8. Grohn OH, Kauppinen RA. Assessment of brain tissue viability in acute ischemic stroke by BOLD MRI. NMR Biomed 2001;14:432–440.
9. Sheinberg M, Kanter MJ, Robertson CS, et al. Continuous monitoring of jugular venous oxygen saturation in head-injured patients. J Neurosurg 1992;76:212–217.
10. van Santbrink H, Maas AI, Avezaat CJ. Continuous monitoring of partial pressure of brain tissue oxygen in patients with severe head injury. Neurosurgery 1996;38:21–31.
11. Fandino J, Stocker R, Prokop S, et al. Cerebral oxygenation and systemic trauma related factors determining neurological outcome after brain injury. J Clin Neurosci 2000;7:226–233.
12. Dearden NM, Midgley S. Technical considerations in continuous jugular venous oxygen saturation measurement. Acta Neurochir Suppl (Wien) 1993;59:91–97.
13. Kiening KL, Unterberg AW, Bardt TF, et al. Monitoring of cerebral oxygenation in patients with severe head injuries: brain tissue PO_2 versus jugular vein oxygen saturation. J Neurosurg 1996;85:751–757.
14. van den Brink WA, van Santbrink H, Steyerberg EW, et al. Brain oxygen tension in severe head injury. Neurosurgery 2000; 46:868–878.
15. Clark LC. Monitor and control of blood and tissue oxygen tension. Trans Am Soc Artif Int Organs 1956;2:41–48.
16. Valadka AB, Gopinath SP, Contant CF, et al. Relationship of brain tissue PO_2 to outcome after severe head injury. Crit Care Med 1998;26:1576–1581.
17. Meixensberger J, Kunze E, Barcsay E, et al. Clinical cerebral microdialysis: brain metabolism and brain tissue oxygenation after acute brain injury. Neurol Res 2001;23:801–806.
18. Doppenberg EM, Zauner A, Watson JC, et al. Determination of the ischemic threshold for brain oxygen tension. Acta Neurochir Suppl (Wien) 1998;71:166–169.
19. Sarrafzadeh AS, Kiening KL, Bardt TF, et al. Cerebral oxygenation in contusioned vs. nonlesioned brain tissue: monitoring of $PtiO_2$ with Licox and Paratrend. Acta Neurochir Suppl (Wien) 1998;71:186–189.
20. Farrar JK. Tissue PO_2 threshold of ischemic cell damage following MCA occlusion in cats. J Cereb Blood Flow Metab 1991;11:S553.
21. Bardt TF, Unterberg AW, Hartl R, et al. Monitoring of brain tissue PO_2 in traumatic brain injury: effect of cerebral hypoxia on outcome. Acta Neurochir Suppl (Wien) 1998;71:153–156.
22. Dings J, Jager A, Meixensberger J, et al. Brain tissue PO_2 and outcome after severe head injury. Neurol Res 1998; 20:S71–S75.
23. van den Brink WA, van Santbrink H, Avezaat CJ, et al. Monitoring brain oxygen tension in severe head injury: the Rotterdam experience. Acta Neurochir Suppl (Wien) 1998;71: 190–194.
24. Zhi DS, Zhang S, Zhou LG. Continuous monitoring of brain tissue oxygen pressure in patients with severe head injury during moderate hypothermia. Surg Neurol 1999;52:393–396.
25. Robertson CS, Gopinath SP, Uzura M, et al. Metabolic changes in the brain during transient ischemia measured with microdialysis. Neurol Res 1998;20:S91–S94.
26. Carmona Suazo JA, Maas AI, van den Brink WA, et al. CO_2 reactivity and brain oxygen pressure monitoring in severe head injury. Crit Care Med 2000;28:3268–3274.
27. Dings J, Meixensberger J, Amschler J, et al. Brain tissue PO_2 in relation to cerebral perfusion pressure, TCD findings and TCD-CO_2-reactivity after severe head injury. Acta Neurochir (Wien) 1996;138:425–434.
28. Dings J, Meixensberger J, Amschler J, et al. Continuous monitoring of brain tissue PO_2: a new tool to minimize the risk

of ischemia caused by hyperventilation therapy. Zentralbl Neurochir 1996;57:177–183.

29. Schneider GH, Sarrafzadeh AS, Kiening KL, et al. Influence of hyperventilation on brain tissue-PO_2, PCO_2, and pH in patients with intracranial hypertension. Acta Neurochir Suppl (Wien) 1998;71:62–65.

30. Unterberg AW, Kiening KL, Hartl R, et al. Multimodal monitoring in patients with head injury: evaluation of the effects of treatment on cerebral oxygenation. J Trauma 1997;42: S32–S37.

31. Bouma GJ, Muizelaar JP, Stringer WA, et al. Ultra-early evaluation of regional cerebral blood flow in severely head-injured patients using xenon-enhanced computerized tomography. J Neurosurg 1992;77:360–368.

32. Diringer MN, Videen TO, Yundt K, et al. Regional cerebrovascular and metabolic effects of hyperventilation after severe traumatic brain injury. J Neurosurg 2002;96:103–108.

33. Diringer MN, Yundt K, Videen TO, et al. No reduction in cerebral metabolism as a result of early moderate hyperventilation following severe traumatic brain injury. J Neurosurg 2000; 92:7–13.

34. Artru F, Jourdan C, Perret-Liaudet A, et al. Low brain tissue oxygen pressure: incidence and corrective therapies. Neurol Res 1998;20:S48–S51.

35. Filippi R, Reisch R, Mauer D, et al. Brain tissue PO_2 related to $SjvO_2$, ICP, and CPP in severe brain injury. Neurosurg Rev 2000;23:94–97.

36. Sarrafzadeh AS, Peltonen EE, Kaisers U, et al. Secondary insults in severe head injury: do multiply injured patients do worse? Crit Care Med 2001;29:1116–1123.

37. Goodman JC, Valadka AB, Gopinath SP, et al. Extracellular lactate and glucose alterations in the brain after head injury measured by microdialysis. Crit Care Med 1999; 27:1965–1973.

◆ 12 ◆

Should I Monitor Cerebral Blood Flow After Traumatic Brain Injury?

Paul M. Vespa

Brief Answer

The evidence from available studies supports monitoring cerebral blood flow (CBF) in traumatic brain injury (TBI) patients as a level III recommendation. Specifically, monitoring CBF to diagnose brain ischemia, posttraumatic vasospasm, and hyperemia in the setting of elevated intracranial pressure (ICP) may permit goal-directed management of the unstable TBI patient.

Background

The treatment of TBI patients centers on preventing secondary cell death in vulnerable brain tissue.[1] This concept is based on several studies that demonstrate that hypotension and hypoxia occur during the early phases of resuscitation and later in the intensive care unit (ICU) (class II data).[2,3] Pathologic postmortem series describe necrotic changes in brain regions remote from the primary insult (class III data).[4] These pathologic changes are nonspecific, but because many believe that they represent secondary ischemic injury, identification of ongoing ischemia and modification of treatment to avoid brain infarction are important goals. At the same time, treatment of elevated ICP is paramount after TBI. Elevated ICP may result from a variety of factors, including hemorrhagic mass lesions, brain edema, increased blood volume, and impaired cerebrospinal fluid outflow. In the acute postinjury period, treatment of ICP and prevention of brain ischemia are the main goals. It stands to reason that monitoring the effect of treatment would provide guidance and permit success at meeting these treatment goals. Such a model is used in coronary care units, where changes in cardiac performance and electrocardiograms identify ongoing ischemia and provide the basis of guiding treatment. A similar impetus has led to development of several modalities for assessing CBF. This chapter determines the strength of the evidence that assessing CBF makes a difference in patient care by guiding efforts to achieve the main treatment goals of lowering ICP and preventing secondary ischemic deficits.

Pearl

A model for the usefulness of monitoring CBF may be found in coronary care units, where changes in cardiac performance and electrocardiograms identify ongoing ischemia and provide the basis of guiding treatment.

There is a great deal of difference between believing that prevention of brain ischemia is important to outcome after TBI and demonstrating that monitoring CBF is necessary. To date, no randomized controlled trials demonstrate that monitoring CBF actually reduces the incidence of brain ischemia or improves outcome in TBI patients. A limited number of publications suggest that increasing cerebral perfusion pressure (CPP) >70 mmHg as promoted by Rosner and coworkers[5] leads to improved outcome (class II data). However, Robertson and coworkers[6] found no overall neurologic benefit of using a similar CPP-based therapy (class I data). Neither study actually modified treatment to reach a specific CBF goal, however, thus leaving the door open to the concept that measuring CBF and adjusting therapy to keep CBF in a normal range improves outcome. Thus, the large therapeutic question remains unanswered at present, and several questions remain to be addressed below.

This chapter outlines the evidence that monitoring CBF is useful and may lead to improved outcomes. This approach requires asking several questions about CBF measurements and considering the evidence for each question in turn. The questions are as follows: (1) Are methods of assessing CBF reliable enough to be clinically useful? (2) When should CBF testing be used? (3) Is CBF testing useful in determining prognosis of brain-injured patients? (4) Do the results of CBF testing and monitoring change patient management? Before discussion of these questions, the commonly used methods of measuring CBF in TBI patients are reviewed briefly.

Literature Review

Methods to Determine Cerebral Blood Flow

Several methods may be used to measure CBF: transcranial Doppler ultrasound (TCD), bedside Kety-Schmidt technique using nitrous oxide (N_2O) or radioactive xenon-133, cold xenon computed tomography (XeCT) of the brain, positron emission tomography, and laser Doppler flowmetry. Surrogate markers of CBF that are used to monitor the brain include brain tissue oxygen monitors, jugular venous oximetry, electroencephalography and other brain function monitors, and near-infrared spectroscopy. Although these techniques each have uniquely appealing qualities, some have proven not to be reliable, and others are not available for routine use and will not be outlined here.

The most frequently used modality of monitoring CBF is TCD, a noninvasive means of measuring blood flow velocity in the major extracranial and basal intracranial arteries. TCD is widely used for routine monitoring of patients with subarachnoid hemorrhage, but its use after TBI is less frequent. TCD is completely noninvasive, but it requires a high degree of operator expertise. TCD provides useful measures of changes in CBF, but they are not absolute measures per se. TCD is useful in determining the occurrence of posttraumatic vasospasm (class III and II data),[7,8] increases in ICP as reflected by increased pulsatility indices, and responses of CBF to clinical manipulations such as hyperventilation or to spontaneous changes in CPP (class II data).[9,10] TCD is usually performed as an intermittent diagnostic test rather than continuously. However, continuous monitoring applications have been used to accurately reflect changes in CBF if two conditions are present: (1) preserved angle of insonation, and (2) intact autoregulation.

The most commonly used way to measure CBF today is the XeCT technique involving computed tomography (CT) scanning after a bolus of inactive xenon. This technique has been used in several seminal contributions to the TBI literature.[11,12] It permits creation of a regional map of CBF in absolute units of cc/100 gm/min. In combination with CT scanning, it is useful for determining if mass effect is influencing CBF regionally (e.g., in the region of an intracerebral hematoma), and it can be useful in determining tissue viability (class III data).[13] However, XeCT cannot be used for continuous monitoring of the brain and entails some risk associated with travel to radiology.

Two bedside methods of measuring CBF may be used in the ICU: radioactive xenon-133 and N_2O techniques. The bedside radioactive xenon-133 technique entails the inhalation or intravenous infusion of a small bolus of the radioactive tracer and detection of the tracer by multiple detectors placed adjacent to the skull in well-defined spaces corresponding to major lobar divisions of the brain.[14] The detection of radioactivity is interpolated over a 15-minute time frame, yielding regional and global measures of CBF. This technique can be repeated in 2 to 4 hours, but the time required for the residual radioactivity to clear limits use of this technique on a continuous basis. This technique has been used in research protocols to evaluate the patterns of CBF early in the course of TBI.[14,15] In contrast, the N_2O technique compares known quantities of administered N_2O to continuously measured amounts of N_2O exiting the brain via the jugular bulb, as outlined by Kety and Schmidt.[16] This method enables serial measurements of CBF in the same patient. It has also been used to test questions of vasoreactivity and responsiveness of CBF to hemodynamic changes. Both the N_2O and xenon-133 techniques are somewhat labor-intensive, requiring quality control of the input and output functions of the test, thus limiting the duration of monitoring of CBF. Thus, like TCD, XeCT, xenon-133, and N_2O provide snapshots of CBF rather than truly continuous monitoring.

The advent of laser Doppler flowmetry (LDF) technology has enabled continuous monitoring of relative changes in CBF. This technique uses a small intraparenchymal probe that obtains a density measurement of moving blood and calibrates it to one of the flow measurement techniques outlined above. In several animal models of brain injury, LDF has had excellent reliability for detecting momentary percentage changes in CBF. Preliminary investigations in human TBI suggest that LDF may be accurately calibrated to XeCT measures of CBF and that clinical monitoring of CBF may be accomplished with this technology.[17]

Relevant Questions

Are Methods of Assessing Cerebral Blood Flow Reliable Enough to Be Clinically Useful?

As outlined above, measures of CBF have been tested in controlled settings[14] and compared with laboratory autoradiography studies to determine their validity. The XeCT and xenon-133 techniques have very low error rates in their absolute measurements of CBF. However, the heterogeneity of CBF across different brain regions is well documented, and extrapolation of global measures to specific regions of interest may not be valid. Thus, reliability and accuracy should be kept separate in the mind of the user. TCD has been validated as a monitor of relative changes in CBF, but it does not provide an accurate absolute measure of CBF (class II data).[18] Once TCD has been calibrated to a quantitative measure of CBF, it may be used to reliably describe the relationship between percent change in TCD velocities and corresponding changes in CBF.[18] An important question is whether these measures are reliable when used in multiple trauma patients, such as those with adult respiratory distress syndrome. Another issue is whether they are stable enough for continuous measurement or whether such an application will be hampered by potential problems with drift and accuracy that are inherent in clinical measurements. Continuous TCD measurements and automated vasoreactivity studies are labor-intensive and are used mostly as research tools,[10] but vasoreactivity indices may have some prognostic value and may be useful in guiding hemodynamic therapy.

Pearl

Once TCD has been calibrated to a quantitative measure of CBF, it may be used to reliably describe the relationship between percent change in TCD velocities and corresponding changes in CBF.

When Should Cerebral Blood Flow Testing Be Used?

Studies of the hyperacute phase of TBI demonstrate that brain ischemia may occur in up to 35% of patients within the initial 12 hours after injury (class II and class III data).[2,3,11,19,20] The early hemodynamic and surgical management of TBI strives to prevent this ischemia from occurring, but studies suggest that such management may not prevent ischemia if it is not guided by measurements of CBF. Ischemia may occur despite maintenance of mean arterial blood pressures >80 mmHg (class III data).[20] Thus, measuring the CBF directly or indirectly during the initial phase of management, such as the first 24 hours, seems to be a reasonable initial approach. No studies have determined which method should be used in the early period, but jugular venous oximetry and TCD facilitate continuous and repeated measures of the adequacy of CBF even during periods of rapid changes in hemodynamics. No outcome studies have demonstrated the efficacy of CBF monitoring during the hyperacute phase, but clinical reasoning suggests that CBF should be measured within the initial 24 hours or even the initial 12 hours, when the highest incidence of ischemia is thought to occur.

Pearl

Clinical reasoning suggests that CBF should be measured within the initial 24 hours or even the initial 12 hours, when the highest incidence of ischemia is thought to occur.

Beyond the initial 24 hours, the rationale for monitoring CBF during the initial week after injury stems from studies that demonstrate a correlation between intracranial hypertension and cerebral hyperemia (class II data).[21,22] Identifying hyperemia and adjusting hemodynamic management accordingly led to improved outcome in a case series that was compared with historical controls.[22] A second rationale for monitoring during the initial week is to detect cerebral ischemia associated with cerebral vasospasm.[7,8,23] The incidence of vasospasm after TBI may be as high as 40% (class II data), some of which results in secondary ischemic injuries. A third reason is that well-documented episodes of jugular venous oxygen desaturation occur during a similar time frame.[6] The desaturations may be due to intracranial hypertension, excessive ventilation, or cerebral vasospasm. Clearly, patients remain at risk for altered CBF for a long time after TBI, with apparent phasic changes of CBF over time after TBI. These phases occur in the following sequence: (1) hypoperfusion in the initial 24 hours, (2) hyperemia during postinjury days 1 to 3, (3) vasospasm during postinjury days 4 to 14, and (4) resolving reduced CBF for up to 3 weeks after TBI (class II data).[15] CBF may be measured during targeted clinical events to modify management that would increase or decrease CBF. These targeted clinical events may include elevated ICP, deterioration of neurologic exam, involuntary movements, or worsening of EEG or other monitors of brain function.

Is Cerebral Blood Flow Testing Useful in Determining Prognosis of Brain-Injured Patients?

CBF measurements are commonly performed in patients with severe TBI. They have correlated with outcome in a broad sense (class II data).[11,21] CBF reductions down to the range of cerebral ischemia have been seen in patients with progressive brain infarction that leads to brain death. Levels of CBF correlate well with score on the Glasgow Coma Scale (GCS). Furthermore, uncontrollable hyperemia has been demonstrated to occur in patients with intractable intracranial hypertension and to correlate with mortality. However, the lack of a phasic increase in CBF during the period from 24 to 72 hours after TBI may suggest a worsened outcome. Patients with persistence of very low CBF values have a poor prognosis. Similarly, low readings on indirect measures of CBF, namely jugular venous oximetry and brain parenchymal oxygen monitoring, correlate with increased mortality. Demonstration of absence of CBF may be very helpful in confirming brain death in the presence of sedating or paralyzing medications; for example, barbiturates. Thus, CBF values at the extremes of either ischemia or absolute hyperemia seem to correlate with a poor prognosis if combined with elevated ICP. However, the converse has not been demonstrated to be true; that is, midrange CBF values have been seen in patients with both good and poor outcomes (class II data).[21]

Pearl

CBF values at the extremes of either ischemia or absolute hyperemia seem to correlate with a poor prognosis when ICP is high, but midrange CBF values have been seen in patients with both good and poor outcomes.

Do the Results of Cerebral Blood Flow Testing and Monitoring Change Patient Management?

This question is difficult to answer because of the lack of prospective trials investigating treatment modification based on the results of CBF or TCD measurements. Nonetheless, observational studies suggest that detection of ischemia, hyperemia, and/or vasospasm occurs with great regularity across different reports. In the studies cited above, the frequency of one or more of these conditions ranges from 25 to 70%. Thus, many patients have CBF values that are abnormal and may be appropriate targets of therapy. Although not designed as an interventional trial, Kelly and coworkers[21] reported a trend toward increased mortality in patients with persistent hyperemia and intracranial hypertension (class II data). The Lund group reported improved survival when a standardized protocol to optimize CBF was used (class II data).[20] The knowledge that autoregulation is preserved may help guide treatment adjustments by allowing anticipation of the effects of proposed interventions on CBF measurements (class II data).[10] In the presence of oligemia or hyperemia, measures can be taken to increase or decrease CBF using manipulations of blood pressure, arterial pressure of carbon dioxide, and depth of sedation. In addition, the use of bedside autoregulation testing may have clinical utility in determining prognosis (class II data).[10]

Recommendations

The following level III recommendations suggest conditions and times under which CBF should be monitored:

1. TBI with GCS <9 during the initial 12 hours after trauma.
2. TBI with persistent GCS <9 during the initial 10 days after trauma.
3. TBI with intractable intracranial hypertension when conventional measures to reduce ICP fail.
4. TBI with neurologic deterioration during the initial two weeks after trauma.

Conclusions

The available studies suggest that CBF is altered in a phasic fashion after TBI, with reduced or increased CBF occurring at specific times after trauma. Moreover, these alterations of CBF may lead to brain ischemia from low flow during the initial 24 hours or from vasospasm several days later. In addition, increased CBF, or hyperemia, may contribute to elevated ICP and associated secondary injury. Thus, measuring CBF and adjusting treatment based on CBF values seem to be important. However, no clinical trials have measured the effect on outcome of directly adjusting CBF to keep it within a "normal" range after TBI. Consequently, any recommendations are based only on class III data. At the same time, however, if this were my brain, I would want you to monitor my CBF.

References

1. Jenkins LW, Moszynski K, Lyeth BG, et al. Increased vulnerability of the mildly traumatized rat brain to cerebral ischemia: the use if controlled secondary ischemia as a research tool to identify common or different mechanisms contributing to mechanical and ischemic brain injury. Brain Res 1989; 477:211–224.
2. Chesnut RM, Marshall LF, Klauber MR, et al. The role of secondary brain injury in determining outcome from severe head injury. J Trauma 1993;34:216–222.
3. Stocchetti N, Furlan A, Volta F. Hypoxemia and arterial hypotension at the accident scene in head injury. J Trauma 1996;40:764–767.
4. Graham DI, Lawrence AE, Adams JH, et al. Brain damage in non-missile head injury secondary to high intracranial pressure. Neuropathol Appl Neurobiol 1987;13:209–217.
5. Rosner MJ, Rosner SD, Johnson AH. Cerebral perfusion pressure: management protocol and clinical results. J Neurosurg 1995;83:949–962.

6. Robertson CS, Valadka AB, Hannay HJ, et al. Prevention of secondary ischemic results after severe head injury. Crit Care Med 1999;27:2086–2095.
7. Martin NA, Doberstein C, Zane C, et al. Posttraumatic cerebral arterial spasm: transcranial Doppler ultrasound, cerebral blood flow, and angiographic findings. J Neurosurg 1992;77: 575–583.
8. Lee JH, Martin NA, Alsina G, et al. Hemodynamically significant cerebral vasospasm and outcome after head injury: a prospective study. J Neurosurg 1997;87:221–233.
9. Czosnyka M, Smielewski P, Kirkpatrick P, et al. Continuous assessment of the cerebral vasomotor reactivity in head injury. Neurosurgery 1997;41:11–19.
10. Czosnyka M, Smielewski P, Kirkpatrick P, et al. Monitoring of cerebral autoregulation in head-injured patients. Stroke 1996; 27:1829–1834.
11. Bouma GJ, Muizelaar JP, Choi PG, et al. Cerebral circulation and metabolism after severe traumatic brain injury: the elusive role of ischemia. J Neurosurg 1991;75:685–693.
12. Marion DW, Darby J, Yonas H. Acute regional cerebral blood flow changes caused by severe head injuries. J Neurosurg 1991; 74:407–414.
13. Firlik AD, Kaufmann AM, Wechsler LR, et al. Quantitative cerebral blood flow determinations in acute ischemic stroke: relationship to computed tomography and angiography. Stroke 1997;28:2208–2213.
14. Obrist WD, Thompson HK Jr, Wang HS, et al. Regional cerebral blood flow estimated by 133-xenon inhalation. Stroke 1975; 6:245–256.
15. Martin NA, Patwardhan RV, Alexander MJ, et al. Characterization of cerebral hemodynamic phases following severe head trauma: hypoperfusion, hyperemia, and vasospasm. J Neurosurg 1997;87:9–19.
16. Kety SS, Schmidt CF. The nitrous oxide method for the quantitative determination of cerebral blood flow in man: theory, procedure, and normal values. J Clin Invest 1948;27:476–483.
17. Miller JI, Chou MW, Capocelli A, et al. Continuous intracranial multimodality monitoring comparing local cerebral blood flow, cerebral perfusion pressure, and microvascular resistance. Acta Neurochir Suppl (Wien) 1998;71:82–84.
18. Bishop CC, Powell S, Rutt D, et al. Transcranial Doppler measurement of middle cerebral artery blood flow velocity: a validation study. Stroke 1986;17:913–915.
19. Vigue B, Ract C, Benayed M, et al. Early $SjvO_2$ monitoring in patients with severe brain trauma. Intensive Care Med 1999; 25:445–451.
20. Eker C, Asgeirsson B, Grande PO, et al. Improved outcome after severe head injury with a new therapy based on principles for brain volume regulation and preserved microcirculation. Crit Care Med 1998;26:1881–1886.
21. Kelly DF, Kordestani RK, Martin NA, et al. Hyperemia following traumatic brain injury: relationship to intracranial hypertension and outcome. J Neurosurg 1996;85:762–771.
22. Asgeirsson B, Grande PO, Nordstrom CH. A new therapy of post-trauma brain oedema based on haemodynamic principles for brain volume regulation. Intensive Care Med 1994;20: 260–267.
23. Zurynski YA, Dorsch NW, Pearson I. Incidence and effects of increased cerebral blood flow velocity after head injury: a transcranial Doppler ultrasound study, I: Prediction of posttraumatic vasospasm and hyperemia. J Neurol Sci 1995;134: 33–40.

Brain Injury

General Management of Brain-Injured Patients

◆ 13 ◆

Does Raising Cerebral Perfusion Pressure Help Head-Injured Patients?

Roman Hlatky and Claudia S. Robertson

Brief Answer

Published recommendations for management of cerebral perfusion pressure (CPP) after traumatic brain injury (TBI) range from high values (>70–80 mmHg) intended to improve perfusion of the injured brain to reduced levels (50 mmHg) to minimize edema formation. No randomized trial has compared the results of these different management strategies in terms of neurologic outcome. Class II evidence from published clinical studies suggests that, based on measures of global cerebral blood flow (CBF) and global cerebral oxygenation, a CPP of 60 mmHg provides an adequate perfusion pressure for the majority of adult TBI patients. A single-institution randomized clinical trial (class I evidence) found that maintaining a CPP higher than that required to adequately perfuse the brain reduced the incidence of secondary ischemic insults associated with hypotension, but this management protocol did not result in superior long-term neurologic outcomes compared with simply treating hypotension promptly when it occurred. Moreover, this practice was associated with a fivefold higher risk of developing adult respiratory distress syndrome (ARDS).

Background

The traditional approach to the management of blood pressure and intracranial pressure (ICP) after TBI has been to direct all therapies at the ICP via a stair-step approach. Therapies were progressively added or subtracted as needed based on the response of the ICP, with the primary goal being control of ICP. Although avoidance of hypotension has been recognized as an important principle, the treatment of systemic hypertension, when present, was often one of the treatment modalities used to lower ICP. The outcome standard that is usually cited for this traditional treatment strategy is that from the Traumatic Coma Data Bank (TCDB) series that was published in 1991 (class II data).[1] Recently, several groups have advocated different overall strategies for the management of TBI, and each group has claimed improved neurologic outcome compared with the standard set by the TCDB series.

Literature Review

Cerebral Perfusion Pressure Management

Rosner et al[2] have advocated the management strategy that is widely known as "CPP management." This approach is based on the physiologic concept of the "vasodilatory cascade." According to this hypothesis, a reduction in CPP stimulates the cerebral vessels to dilate in an attempt to maintain CBF. The increase in cerebral blood volume that accompanies the vasodilation further reduces CPP by increasing ICP. This process sets up a cycle that leads to a progressively falling CPP. Based on observations that an increase in blood pressure will break the cycle and reduce ICP, Rosner et al emphasized maintaining CPP by raising mean arterial pressure (MAP) rather than by lowering ICP. Although it was never supported by a randomized trial, this approach became widely accepted. There was felt to be sufficient value in this practice that it was even included in the 1995 and 2000 versions of the Brain Trauma Foundation's head injury *Guidelines* as an option.[3] Several multicenter clinical trials of neuroprotective strategies have incorporated this approach to CPP management in their standard treatment regimen.

Lund Therapy

Another approach, called the "Lund therapy," emphasizes reduction in microvascular pressures to minimize formation of cerebral edema. This treatment strategy focuses on maintaining cerebral perfusion by treating the ICP side of the CPP equation (CPP = MAP – ICP). The goals of this approach are to preserve a normal colloid osmotic pressure, to reduce capillary hydrostatic pressures by reducing systemic blood pressures, and to reduce cerebral blood volume by vasoconstricting precapillary resistance vessels. Treatments that would promote transcapillary filtration of fluid, including targeting a high CPP, are avoided. Mortality has been reported to be 8% in a series of 53 patients managed by this approach, with 79% of patients described as achieving a Glasgow Outcome Scale score of good recovery or moderate disability by 6 months postinjury (class II data).[4]

Individualizing Treatment

Another approach has been to try to match the treatment to the underlying pathophysiology. This approach emphasizes that TBI is heterogeneous and that each individual patient has a predominant pathophysiologic pattern. In addition, it recognizes that the pathophysiology of TBI evolves over time. Treatment that is appropriate during the first few hours after injury may not necessarily be optimal several days after injury.[5]

Pearl

Different management strategies emphasize different parts of the overall equation that determines CBF: (MAP – ICP)/CVR = CBF where *CVR* represents cerebral vascular resistence. The CPP management strategy emphasizes increasing the MAP, whereas the Lund therapy emphasizes decreasing the ICP. Individualization of treatment emphasizes normalizing all parameters. The common goal is to improve perfusion of the injured brain.

What Is the Minimum Adequate Cerebral Perfusion Pressure After Traumatic Brain Injury?

The definition of what constitutes an adequate CPP varies with the management approach. Advocates of the Lund therapy consider the optimal CPP to be that which is sufficient for adequate perfusion of the brain. This group argues that a higher CPP does not improve cerebral perfusion and serves only to increase edema in the injured brain. In contrast, advocates of the CPP management approach argue that CPP should be kept above the lower limit of autoregulation. Below this level, the cerebral vasodilation that is induced as the brain compensates for a lower CPP can contribute to intracranial hypertension as long as pressure autoregulation remains intact.

To investigate the minimum safe threshold for CPP after TBI, many prospective clinical studies have examined the relationship between CPP and CBF or between CPP and a measure of cerebral oxygenation, such as jugular venous oxygen saturation ($SjvO_2$) or, more recently, partial pressure of oxygen in brain tissue. In these studies, an increase in CBF or in cerebral oxygenation as CPP increases is interpreted as indicating that further elevation of CPP would improve cerebral perfusion. Lack of change of CBF or of cerebral oxygenation in response to increases in CPP is interpreted as indicating that CBF is above the lower limit of autoregulation and is adequate for metabolic needs. As shown in Table 13-1, interpretation of the data in this manner yields a critical CPP threshold of 60 to 70 mmHg. One caution in accepting this result is that regional ischemia can occur despite seemingly adequate global oxygenation, and focal areas of the brain may be underperfused even at normal CPP levels (class II data).[6] In these circumstances, elevation of CPP beyond 60 to 70 mmHg can improve regional cerebral oxygenation.

Other prospective clinical studies have examined the relationship between different thresholds for CPP and outcome from TBI. These studies are limited in that a cause-and-effect relationship cannot be assumed even though an association with outcome can be demonstrated. Nevertheless, as shown in Table 13-1, these studies support the same general concept of a CPP threshold of 60 mmHg in adults.

The available information suggests that it is probably most correct to conclude that, after TBI, an adequate CPP is necessary but not sufficient to guarantee that CBF is adequate. Measurements of global CBF and global cerebral oxygenation in the available clinical studies suggest that a CPP of 60 mmHg provides

Pearl

A CPP of 60 mmHg seems to provide an adequate perfusion pressure for the majority of adult TBI patients. It must be emphasized, however, that regional ischemia may occur despite adequate global cerebral oxygenation.

Table 13-1 Brief Descriptions and Conclusions of Clinical Studies Addressing Various Aspects of Cerebral Perfusion Pressure Management

Type of Evidence	Reference	Description of Study	Conclusion
		What is an adequate CPP? Relationship between CPP and cerebral oxygenation	
Class II	Chan et al[12] 1992	This study used monitoring of $SjvO_2$ to study the relationship between CPP and cerebral oxygenation. $SjvO_2$ decreased with CPP below 70 mmHg, but was unrelated to CPP when above 70 mmHg	Cerebral oxygenation is dependent on CPP below 70 mmHg, but not when CPP is greater than 70 mmHg
Class II	Cruz et al[13] 1995	This study used monitoring of arteriojugular oxygen content difference to study the relationship between CPP and cerebral oxygenation; when CPP was maintained between 60 and 130 mmHg, there was no relationship between CPP and $SjvO_2$	Cerebral oxygenation is not dependent on CPP above a level of 60 mmHg
Class II	Kiening et al[14] 1997	This study used monitoring of $PbtO_2$ to investigate the effects of therapeutic interventions; when CPP was <40 mm Hg, raising CPP to 60 mmHg improved $PbtO_2$; mean values were: CPP: 32 ± 2 mmHg to 67 ± 4 mmHg $PbtO_2$: 13 ± 2 mmHg to 21 ± 1 mmHg $SjvO_2$: $54 \pm 3\%$ to $65 \pm 3\%$ Further elevation of CPP above 60 mmHg did not improve oxygenation	A CPP of at least 60 mmHg provides adequate cerebral oxygenation
Class II	Bruzzone et al[15] 1998	This study used monitoring of $PbtO_2$ to study the relationship between CPP and cerebral oxygenation; below a CPP of 60 mmHg, there was a significant relationship between CPP and $PbtO_2$	Cerebral oxygenation is dependent on CPP below a level of 60 mmHg
		What is an adequate CPP? Relationship between CPP and outcome	
Class II	Marmarou et al[16] 1991	This study examined the prospectively collected TCDB data for the relationship between various thresholds for ICP and MAP and outcome; the most important determinants of outcome were the proportion of time that ICP and MAP were beyond the thresholds of 20 and 80 mmHg, respectively	The proportion of time ICP is above 20 mmHg and the proportion of time MAP is below 80 mmHg are associated with a poor outcome
Class III	Downard et al[17] 2000	This retrospective study investigated the relationship between physiologic parameters and outcome in 118 children with ICP monitors placed within 24 hours of injury; no patient survived with a mean CPP (for the first 48 hour) <40 mmHg; there was no relationship to outcome when mean CPP was >40 mmHg	In children, the threshold for CPP may be lower; a mean CPP below 40 mmHg is associated with a high mortality
Class II	Struchen et al[18] 2001	This study examined prospectively collected data from 184 patients for a relationship between outcome and adverse physiologic events after severe head injury; the length of time that ICP, MAP, and CPP were beyond the thresholds of 25, 80, and 60 mmHg, respectively, were significantly associated with GOS and DRS	The length of time CPP is below 60 mmHg is associated with a poor outcome
Class II	Chambers et al[19] 2001	This study examined prospectively collected data from 291 patients (207 adults and 84 children) and analyzed the relationship between physiologic parameters and outcome after severe head injury; the maximum value of a 2-minute rolling average of ICP readings and the minimum value of the CPP readings were used to calculate the sensitivity and specificity of receiver-operating characteristic curves over a range of values	A threshold value of 55 mmHg for minimum CPP and 35 mmHg for maximum ICP were the best predictors of outcome in adults; for children the levels appear to be 43 to 45 mmHg for minimum CPP and 35 mmHg for maximum ICP; higher levels of minimum CPP seemed important in adults with mass lesions

(*continued*)

Table 13-1 *(continued)*

Type of Evidence	Reference	Description of Study	Conclusion
		Does a higher CPP prevent secondary ischemic insults due to hypotension?	
Class I	Robertson et al[10] 1999	This clinical trial randomized 189 patients to either a CBF-targeted or ICP-targeted management protocol to test the hypothesis that a treatment strategy targeted at preventing hypotension and hypocarbia would reduce the incidence of secondary ischemic insults after a severe head injury; the CBF-targeted protocol was designed to prevent hypotension by setting goals for MAP and CPP of >90 mmHg and >70 mmHg, respectively, and to prevent hypocarbia by not using hyperventilation in the treatment algorithm for intracranial hypertension; the ICP-targeted (control) protocol used traditional ICP management strategies, with normal goals for MAP (>70 mmHg) and for CPP (>50 mmHg), and used moderate hyperventilation not as a routine, but rather as one of the modalities used to treat intracranial hypertension	The CBF-targeted group had a significantly higher MAP, CPP, $ETCO_2$, and CBF than the ICP-targeted group; there was also a significant reduction in the incidence of jugular venous desaturation, from 50.6% with the ICP-targeted protocol to 30% with the CBF-targeted protocol
		Does a higher CPP reduce ICP?	
Class II	Bouma et al[11] 1992	This prospective study examined the acute ICP effects of raising CPP in 47 patients with severe head injury. ICP, MAP, and CBF were measured before and after increasing MAP by infusion of phenylephrine; the patients were divided into two groups depending on the changes in CBF that were induced by the blood pressure change	In patients with intact pressure autoregulation, ICP did not change as the blood pressure was raised, but ICP increased with blood pressure in the patients with impaired pressure autoregulation
Class I	Robertson et al[10] 1999	This randomized clinical trial studied 189 patients assigned to either a CBF-targeted or ICP-targeted management protocol as described above; the goal for MAP was >70 mmHg in the ICP-targeted group and >90 mmHg in the CBF-targeted group	Maintaining an elevated MAP had no adverse effects on ICP; the average ICP, the length of time that ICP was above 25 mmHg, and the incidence of refractory intracranial hypertension were similar in the two treatment groups

CBF, cerebral blood flow; CPP, cerebral perfusion pressure; DRS, Disability Rating Scale; $ETCO_2$, end-tidal CO_2; GCS, Glasgow Coma Scale; GOS, Glasgow Outcome Scale; ICP, intracranial pressure; MAP, mean arterial pressure; $PbtO_2$, partial pressure of oxygen in brain tissue; $SjvO_2$, jugular venous oxygen saturation; TCDB, Traumatic Coma Data Bank.

an adequate perfusion pressure for the majority of adult TBI patients. It must be emphasized, however, that regional ischemia may occur despite adequate global cerebral oxygenation.

Does Increasing Cerebral Perfusion Pressure Above 60 mmHg Have a Beneficial Therapeutic Effect?

There exists general agreement that CPP should be kept at a level that provides adequate perfusion of the injured brain; that is, at least 60 mmHg. The practice of raising CPP to even higher levels could have both beneficial effects and detrimental consequences. The risk:benefit ratio of this practice, and therefore its overall effect on outcome, is controversial. No multicenter randomized clinical trials have compared these different management strategies in terms of neurologic outcome. One single-site randomized clinical trial and numerous prospective clinical studies do address potential benefits of elevating CPP, including fewer secondary ischemic insults and lower ICP. In addition, these studies give some information on outcome effect. They are summarized in Tables 13-1 and 13-2.

Does a Higher Cerebral Perfusion Pressure Prevent Secondary Ischemic Insults Due to Hypotension?

Several investigators have linked secondary ischemic insults to poor neurologic outcome (class II data).[7–9] Thus, one might reasonably expect that a potential benefit of keeping CPP at an elevated level might be a reduction in the incidence of secondary ischemic insults.

One randomized clinical trial has addressed this question directly. Robertson et al[10] randomly assigned 189 patients to either a CBF-targeted or an ICP-targeted

Table 13-2 Glasgow Outcome Scale Scores After Traumatic Brain Injury in Selected Prospective Studies

	Glasgow Outcome Scale (at 6 Months Unless Otherwise Specified)			Parameter					
Author	**Good Outcome, %**	**Poor Outcome, %**	**Dead, %**	**Age (Yrs)**	**GCS Score**	**% with Masses**	**CPP**	**ICP**	**Goal for CPP**
				Traditional ICP-based management					
Marshall et al[1] 1991 (TCDB) (outcomes at median of 674 days)	43	57	36	30	6**	42			
Robertson et al[10] 1999 (ICP-targeted group)	49	51	24	30	7**	35	73	18	>50
				CPP-based management					
Rosner et al[2] 1995 (outcomes at 10.5 months?)	59	41	29	28	5**	27	83	27	>70
Robertson et al[10] 1999 (CBF-targeted group)	40	60	25	30	7**	36	77	17	>70
				CPP-based management in clinical trials of other therapeutic agents					
Clifton et al[20] 1993 (normothermia control group) (outcomes at 3 months)	36	64		30†	41% GCS 4–5; 59% GCS 6–7	32	81†	17†	>70†
Marion et al[21] 1997 (normothermia control group)	33	67	24	35	38% GCS 3–4; 62% GCS 5–7	48	81†	19†	>70
Morris et al[22] 1999 (Selfotel control group)	58	42	21	31	6.1*	31			>60
Clifton et al[23] 2001 (hypothermia control group)	43	57	27	32	5.8*	36	77	18	>70

*Mean value; **median value; †estimated value.

CBF, cerebral blood flow; CPP, cerebral perfusion pressure; DRS, Disability Rating Scale; $ETCO_2$, end-tidal CO_2; GCS, Glasgow Coma Scale; GOS, Glasgow Outcome Scale; ICP, intracranial pressure; MAP, mean arterial pressure; $PbtO_2$, partial pressure of oxygen in brain tissue; $SjvO_2$, jugular venous oxygen saturation; TCDB, Traumatic Coma Data Bank.

Good outcome: moderate disability or good recovery; poor outcome: severe disability, persisent vegetative state, or death.

management protocol to test the hypothesis that a treatment strategy targeted at preventing hypotension and hypocarbia would reduce the incidence of secondary ischemic insults after severe TBI (class I data). The CBF-targeted protocol was designed to prevent hypotension by setting goals for MAP and CPP at >90 mmHg and >70 mmHg, respectively, and to prevent hypocarbia by eliminating hyperventilation from the treatment algorithm for intracranial hypertension. The ICP-targeted protocol consisted of a traditional ICP management protocol with goals for MAP and CPP of >70 mmHg and >50 mmHg, respectively, and allowed moderate hyperventilation not as a routine, but rather as one of the modalities used to treat persistent intracranial hypertension. Because of the differences in the management protocols, the CBF-targeted group had a significantly higher MAP, CPP, end-tidal CO_2, and CBF than the ICP-targeted group. The outcome of the study demonstrated a significant reduction in the incidence of jugular venous oxygen desaturation, from 50.6% in the ICP-targeted group to 30% with the CBF-targeted protocol.[10]

One criticism of this study has been that, although the difference in CPP between the two treatment groups was statistically significant, the absolute difference in the median values for CPP in the two groups was not large (77 and 73 mmHg in the CBF and ICP-targeted groups, respectively; $p = .004$). However, the purpose of the CBF-targeted protocol was to prevent hypotensive episodes, and summary values such as mean or median are very insensitive measures for detecting transient, but still important, differences. The length of time that CPP was <60 mmHg was much longer in the ICP-targeted group: a median of 13 hours, compared with 4 hours in the CBF-targeted group ($p = .008$). Perhaps even more importantly, the length of time that $SjvO_2$ was low because of hypotension totaled 58.9 hours for the entire ICP-targeted group but only 7.8 hours in the CBF-targeted group. Finally, to achieve the desired difference in MAPs, significant differences in treatment were required; e.g., higher fluid intake and more frequent use of pressors.

Another criticism of the study has been that two physiologic parameters (blood pressure and $PaCO_2$)

were varied in the same trial, potentially making it impossible to state conclusively that the reduction in ischemic insults was due to targeting a higher CPP. To put this point in perspective, it is important to remember that avoiding hyperventilation has always been a part of the CPP management strategy as described by Rosner et al.[2] Also, the physiologic effects of manipulation of blood pressure and $PaCO_2$ are different, and the end point of jugular venous desaturation can be further categorized according to the underlying cause of the desaturation. The incidence of hypotension-induced jugular venous desaturation was significantly lower in the CBF-targeted group. Nevertheless, it is probably more correct to interpret the data as showing that a management strategy designed to minimize both hypotension and hypocarbia significantly reduced the incidence of secondary ischemic insults.

Does a Higher Cerebral Perfusion Pressure Reduce Intracranial Pressure?

Manipulation of blood pressure in TBI patients has a variable effect on ICP. Both initial and delayed effects must be considered. The initial ICP response to increased MAP depends on the status of pressure autoregulation. Bouma et al[11] published the results of 58 tests of autoregulation in 47 patients in whom phenylephrine was used to elevate mean arterial blood pressure (class II data). The CBF response to elevation of MAP was used to divide patients into two groups: those with intact pressure autoregulation and those with defective pressure autoregulation. In the group with intact autoregulation, MAP increased from 93 ± 11 mmHg to 119 ± 11 mmHg, but ICP and CBF did not change significantly. In the group with defective autoregulation, MAP increased from 99 ± 12 mmHg to 126 ± 9 mmHg, ICP increased from 16 ± 7 mmHg to 20 ± 9 mmHg ($p < .01$), and CBF increased from 35 ± 10 mL/100 g/min to 50 ± 14 mL/100 g/min (not statistically significant).

Raising CPP, however, could theoretically increase cerebral edema, with the long-term effect of actually increasing ICP and prolonging the need for treatment. Evidence to support such a possibility may be found in Rosner et al's own series. As shown in Table 13-2, although the average CPP in Rosner et al's patients was higher than that in any other listed series, the average ICP was also 8 to 10 mmHg higher than in the other reports. In addition, the average duration of "acute monitoring" in the Rosner et al series was 17.7 days. If this parameter represents the length of time that ICP monitoring was required, then it far exceeds the median of 4 to 5 days reported in the other studies.

The randomized clinical trial by Robertson et al[10] described above also examined the effect of the CBF-targeted protocol on ICP control as a secondary outcome measure. In this study, no significant differences existed between the two treatment groups in duration of ICP monitoring, in any measure of ICP severity (mean ICP, length of time ICP was greater than 25 mmHg, or number of patients who died of refractory intracranial hypertension), or in any measure of ICP treatment.

Does a Higher Cerebral Perfusion Pressure Improve Neurologic Outcome?

The TCDB study published by Marshall et al[1] describes outcomes in a multicenter prospective study of 746 TBI patients with Glasgow Coma Scale scores <9. No prescribed treatment protocol was used in the study, but the investigators all followed traditional ICP treatment strategies. The overall mortality rate at 6 months postinjury was 36.3%. At 6 months, 42.9% of the patients had a favorable outcome (good recovery or moderate disability), and 57.1% of the patients had a poor outcome (severe disability, vegetative state, or death).

Rosner et al[2] reported a prospective series of 158 patients managed with a protocol based on his CPP management strategy. The average CPP in this clinical series was 83 ± 14 mmHg (ICP 27 ± 12 mmHg and MAP 109 ± 14 mmHg). Mortality was 29%, and 59% of the patients achieved good recovery or moderate disability by 10.5 months postinjury (class II data).[2] These outcomes appear to be improvements over the results of the TCDB series. However, different demographic characteristics in the two groups of patients might also explain the better outcome in Rosner et al's series, including the lower age (28 vs. 30 years) and the lower incidence of mass lesions (27% vs. 42%) in the Rosner et al series.

Several recent clinical studies provide additional prospectively collected information on outcomes of head-injured patients managed with protocols that include maintaining CPP >70 mmHg. Table 13-2 lists selected parameters from several studies, including the CPP management paper by Rosner et al, the control groups from some recent multicenter clinical trials that followed a CPP management strategy, and the CBF-targeted group from the Robertson study. Although most of these groups of patients share the management goal of keeping CPP >70 mmHg, the studies cannot be directly compared because of differences in patient demographics, in entry/exclusion criteria, and in other aspects of treatment. Despite these potentially confounding factors, however, none of these prospectively collected clinical series, either alone or collectively, demonstrates convincingly a beneficial effect on outcome from maintaining CPP >70 mmHg.

The randomized trial by Robertson et al[10] examined long-term neurologic outcome as a secondary outcome measure. The results, which are also summarized in Table 13-2, did not show a significant improvement in outcome in the CBF-targeted group. The sample size for this study was powered to enable detection of a 20% improvement in favorable outcome, which is probably too large an effect to expect from the difference in management practice that was studied. Nevertheless, the investigators could not find even a suggestion that outcome was improved by the CBF-targeted management strategy. When potential complications of maintaining an elevated CPP were explored, the investigators found a fivefold increase in the incidence of ARDS. This complication may have offset any potential beneficial effects.

Because the only randomized trial that has compared the consequences of targeting different levels of CPP failed to demonstrate a long-term benefit and, in fact, demonstrated a clearly detrimental effect (increased incidence of ARDS) associated with a CPP target of >70 mmHg, there exists no compelling reason to raise CPP in all patients beyond that required to adequately perfuse the brain.[10] It seems likely that a CPP of 60 mmHg provides adequate perfusion for most cases. Higher levels of CPP should probably be reserved for those TBI patients who demonstrate a specific indication for induced hypertension, for example, regional cerebral ischemia.

Pearl

Maintenance of a CPP target of >70 mmHg has been shown to prevent secondary ischemic insults from hypotension, but with no reduction in intracranial pressure and no improvement in neurologic outcome.

Conclusions

A CPP of at least 60 mmHg seems adequate for most patients with severe head injury. Because an adverse effect on pulmonary function has been associated with induced hypertension, CPP levels higher than 70 mmHg should be reserved for patients who demonstrate a specific indication for induced hypertension, such as regional cerebral ischemia.

Recommendations

Level I

As a part of an overall management strategy to minimize cerebral ischemic insults after TBI, the practice of raising CPP above the level required for adequate perfusion of the brain significantly reduces the incidence of hypotension-induced secondary ischemic insults. However, preventing secondary ischemic insults in this manner does not significantly improve neurologic outcome compared with promptly treating insults when they occur. In addition, maintaining an elevated CPP is associated with an increased incidence of ARDS.

Level II

The short-term ICP effect of raising CPP is dependent on the status of pressure autoregulation in the individual patient. If autoregulation is intact, then ICP may acutely decrease as blood pressure is increased. If autoregulation is impaired, then ICP may increase as blood pressure is increased. Raising CPP above the level required for adequate perfusion of the brain has not been demonstrated to have a long-term beneficial or detrimental effect on ICP.

Acknowledgment

This work is supported by National Institutes of Health grant P01-NS38660.

References

1. Marshall LF, Gautille T, Klauber MR, et al. The outcome of severe closed head injury. J Neurosurg 1991;75:S28–S36.
2. Rosner MJ, Rosner SD, Johnson AH. Cerebral perfusion pressure: management protocol and clinical results. J Neurosurg 1995;83:949–962.
3. The Brain Trauma Foundation, the American Association of Neurological Surgeons, and the Joint Section on Neurotrauma and Critical Care. Management and prognosis of severe traumatic brain injury: guidelines for cerebral perfusion pressure. J Neurotrauma 2000;17:507–511.
4. Eker C, Asgeirsson B, Grande PO, et al. Improved outcome after severe head injury with a new therapy based on principles for brain volume regulation and preserved microcirculation. Crit Care Med 1998;26:1881–1886.
5. Miller JD, Piper IR, Dearden NM. Management of intracranial hypertension in head injury: matching treatment with cause. Acta Neurochir Suppl (Wien) 1993;57:152–159.
6. Stocchetti N, Chieregato A, De Marchi M, et al. High cerebral perfusion pressure improves low values of local brain tissue O2 tension (PtiO2) in focal lesions. Acta Neurochir Suppl (Wien) 1998;71:162–165.
7. Chesnut RM, Marshall LF, Klauber MR, et al. The role of secondary brain injury in determining outcome from severe head injury. J Trauma 1993;34:216–222.
8. Gopinath SP, Robertson CS, Contant CF, et al. Jugular venous desaturation and outcome after head injury. J Neurol Neurosurg Psychiatry 1994;57:717–723.
9. Signorini DF, Andrews PJ, Jones PA, et al. Adding insult to injury: the prognostic value of early secondary insults for survival after traumatic brain injury. J Neurol Neurosurg Psychiatry 1999;66:26–31.
10. Robertson CS, Valadka AB, Hannay HJ, et al. Prevention of secondary ischemic insults after severe head injury. Crit Care Med 1999;27:2086–2095.
11. Bouma GJ, Muizelaar JP, Bandoh K, et al. Blood pressure and intracranial pressure-volume dynamics in severe head injury: relationship with cerebral blood flow. J Neurosurg 1992;77:15–19.
12. Chan KH, Miller JD, Dearden NM, et al. The effect of changes in cerebral perfusion pressure upon middle cerebral artery blood flow velocity and jugular bulb venous oxygen saturation after severe brain injury. J Neurosurg 1992;77:55–61.

13. Cruz J, Jaggi JL, Hoffstad OJ. Cerebral blood flow, vascular resistance, and oxygen metabolism in acute brain trauma: redefining the role of cerebral perfusion pressure? Crit Care Med 1995;23: 1412–1417.
14. Kiening KL, Hartl R, Unterberg AW, et al. Brain tissue pO2-monitoring in comatose patients: implications for therapy. Neurol Res 1997;19:233–240.
15. Bruzzone P, Dionigi R, Bellinzona G, et al. Effects of cerebral perfusion pressure on brain tissue pO2 in patients with a severe head injury. Acta Neurochir Suppl (Wien) 1998;71: 111–113.
16. Marmarou A, Anderson RL, Ward JD, et al. Impact of ICP instability and hypotension on outcome in patients with severe head injury. J Neurosurg 1991;75:S59–S66.
17. Downard C, Hulka F, Mullins RJ, et al. Relation of cerebral perfusion pressure and survival in pediatric brain-injured patients. J Trauma 2000;49:654–658.
18. Struchen MA, Hannay HJ, Contant CF, et al. The relation between acute physiological variables and outcome on the Glasgow Outcome Scale and the Disability Rating Scale following severe traumatic brain injury. J Neurotrauma 2001;18: 115–125.
19. Chambers IR, Treadwell L, Mendelow AD. Determination of threshold levels of cerebral perfusion pressure and intracranial pressure in severe head injury by using receiver-operating characteristic curves: an observational study in 291 patients. J Neurosurg 2001;94:412–416.
20. Clifton GL, Allen S, Barrodale P, et al. A phase II study of moderate hypothermia in severe brain injury. J Neurotrauma 1993; 10:263–271.
21. Marion DW, Penrod LE, Kelsey SF, et al. Treatment of traumatic brain injury with moderate hypothermia. N Engl J Med 1997;336:540–546.
22. Morris GF, Bullock R, Marshall SB, et al. Failure of the competitive *N*-methyl-D-aspartate antagonist Selfotel (CGS 19755) in the treatment of severe head injury: results of two phase III clinical trials. J Neurosurg 1999;91:737–743.
23. Clifton GL, Miller ER, Choi SC, et al. Lack of effect of induction of hypothermia after acute brain injury. N Engl J Med 2001;344: 556–563.

◆ 14 ◆

What Are the Best Ventilator Settings for Head-Injured Patients? What Is the Role of Hyperventilation?

Christopher Mendello, William M. Coplin, and J. Kraus

Brief Answer

1. There is no support for the use of hyperventilation to treat elevated intracranial pressure (ICP) except as a short-term temporizing measure while other diagnostic and therapeutic interventions are initiated (class II and III evidence).
2. There is no role for prophylactic hyperventilation to prevent intracranial hypertension (class II and III evidence).
3. Chronic hyperventilation may worsen cerebral ischemia (class II and III evidence).
4. There is inadequate evidence to either support or refute the use of positive end-expiratory pressure (PEEP) at the end of each breath for brain-injured patients (class III evidence).
5. There may be a role for the use of normobaric supranormal concentrations of inspired oxygen (class III evidence).
6. Optimal ventilator settings and the use of hyperventilation for brain-injured patients should be individually assessed at the bedside by a practitioner experienced in both ventilatory and neurological issues.

Background

The three major components of the intracranial cavity are brain parenchyma, cerebral blood volume (CBV), and cerebrospinal fluid (CSF). A reduced volume of any one of these components, such as redistribution of CSF to external drainage, may decrease elevated ICP and prevent herniation of an edematous brain. Since the middle of the last century, we have known that hyperventilation dramatically decreases ICP due to cerebral arterial constriction secondary to reduced arterial carbon dioxide tension ($PaCO_2$). However, the desired vasoconstriction may also decrease cerebral blood flow (CBF), resulting in hypoperfusion and subsequent global or focal ischemic injury. Because of these concerns, the dogma of "therapeutic hyperventilation" for the treatment of prolonged elevations in ICP has been challenged in recent years. Class II and class III data currently support a management strategy of hyperventilation for acutely elevated ICP to reverse signs and symptoms of brain herniation. Conversely, analyses of patient outcomes, both long- and short-term, do not support the use of prophylactic or continuous hyperventilation in patients at risk of developing elevated ICP or in those who already have chronic elevations of ICP.

Pearl

By decreasing CBV, hyperventilation-induced vasoconstriction may be helpful to lower acutely elevated ICP while diagnostic and other therapeutic maneuvers are initiated.

Pearl

Hyperventilation-induced vasoconstriction may also decrease CBF, resulting in hypoperfusion and subsequent ischemic injury.

Ventilator Basics

Adjustment of ventilator settings allows a caregiver to control a patient's ventilation and oxygenation. Tidal volume (V_T), or the volume of air delivered in each breath, and respiratory rate (RR), or number of breaths per minute, affect the $PaCO_2$; that is, ventilation. Inspired oxygen concentration (FiO_2) and positive pressure at the end of each breath (PEEP) affect the PaO_2 or oxygenation. The recent literature supports the use of a smaller V_T, ~5 to 7 mL/kg of body mass, to reduce barotrauma to the pulmonary parenchyma, especially when lung compliance is decreased (class I data).[1] Minute ventilation (V_E), which is the RR multiplied by the V_T, need not exceed 10 to 12 L per minute to achieve adequate ventilation in most patients. FiO_2 has the most influence over PaO_2, and PEEP has a supporting role through alveolar recruitment, which allows a greater surface area for oxygen exchange. A balance between FiO_2 and PEEP must be established to provide an optimal PaO_2 with minimal risks of O_2 toxicity and barotrauma.

Review of Cerebral Hemodynamics and Oxidative Metabolism after Brain Injury

Cerebral physiology and metabolism differ greatly between injured and healthy brain. Glucose and oxygen, delivered by the cerebral circulation, are the primary fuels on which the brain functions. Under normal conditions, oxidative metabolism and CBF are coupled, a concept known as "metabolic autoregulation."[2] Cerebral metabolism is quantified primarily by the difference between oxygen delivery and oxygen extraction by the brain parenchyma, a concept referred to as the cerebral metabolic rate of oxygen consumption ($CMRO_2$). In the normal brain, CBF is maintained at a relatively constant rate, proportional to the cerebral perfusion pressure (CPP) and inversely proportional to cerebral vascular resistance (CVR). This "pressure autoregulation" allows for relatively unaltered levels of CBF despite a wide range of perfusion pressures, from as low as 50 to as high as 150 mmHg.[2] In the healthy state, ~30 to 40% of oxygen in arterial blood is extracted and utilized, as demonstrated by the cerebral oxygen extraction fraction (CEO_2) or the difference between the partial pressures of oxygen in arterial and venous blood ($AVDO_2$). Mathematically, the Fick principle relates O_2 metabolism, CBF, O_2 extraction (arteriovenous difference of oxygen, or $AVDO_2$), and O_2 uptake, such that CBF is proportional to O_2 metabolism divided by $AVDO_2$ (O_2 metabolism = CBF $\times$ $AVDO_2$).

Pearl

When the relationship between $CMRO_2$ and CBF becomes uncoupled, either a hyperemic state (blood flow exceeding metabolic need) or an oligemic state (inadequate blood flow in relation to metabolic demand) may develop.

Under normal circumstances, O_2 delivery exceeds the brain's demand for oxygen. In settings characterized by decreased cerebral oxygen delivery, an increase in oxygen extraction by the brain parenchyma leads to a widened $AVDO_2$ and a constant $CMRO_2$.[3] Failure of autoregulatory mechanisms to meet increased oxygen demand leads to insufficient oxygen delivery, metabolic failure, neuronal dysfunction, and cell death.[4,5] When the relationship between $CMRO_2$ and CBF becomes uncoupled, either a hyperemic state (blood flow exceeding metabolic need) or an oligemic state (inadequate blood flow in relation to metabolic demand) may develop.[6] As predicted by the Fick principle, extreme oligemia (<18 mLO_2/100 g brain tissue/minute) results in ischemic injury, with the threshold largely dependent on the rate of oxygen consumption. A decreased $CMRO_2$ lowers the ischemic injury threshold.[5–7] For the clinician, this means cerebral ischemia can be identified only after measurements of $CMRO_2$ and $AVDO_2$ in relation to CBF are obtained. There exists class II and III evidence that $CMRO_2$ is markedly decreased after brain injury and that uncoupling exists between CBF and $CMRO_2$.[8–10] As many as 30% of patients with severe traumatic brain injury (TBI) demonstrate reduced CBF; in contrast, others have reported that 20% of patients may have elevated CBF when compared with healthy subjects (class II and III data).[9–11] This uncoupling makes it very difficult for clinicians to predict from CBF analysis alone which patients are suffering from secondary ischemia because reduced CBF with an even greater reduction in $CMRO_2$ could mean a relatively hyperemic state, with adequate O_2 delivery. Some investigators have reported that elevated ICP measurements correlate well with the hyperemic state (class III data)[10] and predict a worse outcome when not managed appropriately. What remains unclear is whether further reductions of an already reduced CBF, despite the existence of a relatively hyperemic state, can lead to worsening cerebral ischemia.

Pearl

It is very difficult to predict from CBF studies alone which patients are suffering from secondary ischemia because reduced CBF with an even greater reduction in $CMRO_2$ could produce a relatively hyperemic state, with adequate O_2 delivery.

Monitoring Techniques

Several reports have documented early cerebral ischemia in TBI patients, with severity of ischemia predictive of worsened patient outcomes (class II data).[12] Within the medical community there is tremendous debate regarding optimal management of patients with TBI, much of which stems from modern medicine's inability to assess cerebral ischemia with technical precision. Most measurements of cerebral $AVDO_2$ represent average determinations of global cerebral oxidative metabolism and do not assess focal ischemic areas that may exist within the brain parenchyma.[13] Conversely, more modern techniques that measure intracranial PO_2, pH, lactate, and PCO_2 within small anatomic areas may not adequately measure or reflect overall cerebral perfusion.[14] There is class II evidence pointing to regional differences in parenchymal oxygen tension ($PbtO_2$) between normal and damaged tissue without histologic evidence of ischemia due to hypocapneic vasoconstriction, possibly because of locally disrupted autoregulation after brain injury.[15] Whether the differences in $PbtO_2$ are due to altered vasoreactivity or altered metabolism is not clear, but more work in monitoring cerebral tissue metabolism needs to occur before a consensus is reached.

The role of monitoring CPP to determine cerebral oxygenation status is even less clear. Earlier studies linked elevated CPP with increased cerebral oxygenation and assumed a direct relationship between CPP and CBF.[16,17] As discussed above, the mechanism of "pressure autoregulation" in healthy brain maintains constant CBF and oxygen delivery over a wide range of perfusion pressures. Investigators examined the link between CPP and oxygen metabolism in brain-injured patients and could not document a relationship between $CMRO_2$ and CPP or between $AVDO_2$ and CPP over a wide range of CPP values (60 mmHg to 130 mmHg) (class II data).[18] However, positive correlations were seen between $CMRO_2$ versus CBF, $AVDO_2$ versus CVR, and $CMRO_2$ versus $AVDO_2$, confirming earlier data on the relationship among O_2 metabolism, CBF, and O_2 extraction. Interestingly, negative correlations were noted between $AVDO_2$ and CVR with CBF. The authors concluded that, in the presence of normal or high CPP, cerebral hemodynamics and metabolic patterns are more closely associated with CVR than with CPP.[18] It is important to note that the study did not examine the relationships of $CMRO_2$, CBF, and $AVDO_2$ versus CPP in association with CPP <60 mmHg. These data suggest that CPP may or may not be the optimal parameter for drawing conclusions at the bedside about the status of CBF in brain-injured patients.

Literature Review

Hyperventilation

In the 1970s, investigators discovered that CBF and CBV could be manipulated using hyperventilation, allowing indirect adjustment of ICP.[19] These and other data were used to justify the use of hyperventilation in brain-injured patients to manage acute elevations of ICP. It is now recognized, however, that such a practice may be quite deleterious.

The mechanism behind the manipulation of ICP and CBF is adjustment of CSF pH via arteriolar vasoconstriction. This pH-driven vasoconstriction is transitory to the extent that carbonic anhydrase metabolism in the choroid plexus is able to correct CSF pH. Normally, within 4 to 6 hours, there is either normalization of cerebral arteriolar caliber, ICP, and CBF or a rebound effect of hyperemia with increased ICP. Carmona-Suazo et al[20] showed that the cerebral arteriolar response to CSF pH was dampened in patients with decreased CBF (class II data).

Pearl

Normally, within 4 to 6 hours of initiating hyperventilation, there is either normalization of cerebral arteriolar caliber, ICP, and CBF or a rebound hyperemia with increased ICP.

Managing brain injury with endotracheal intubation and mechanical ventilation permits a physician to control a potentially unstable airway and to adjust $PaCO_2$ and PaO_2 according to a patient's needs. However, ventilation, oxygenation, and airway management are completely separate processes, and the decisions to intubate a patient and to initiate ventilatory support must be based on an individual patient's needs. It has been suggested that delaying extubation of comatose patients who have a cough and who are free of copious secretions or respiratory infection (regardless of mental status or gag reflex) does not confer benefit and may actually increase undesirable consequences, such as higher rates of pneumonia, longer hospital stays, and increased costs (class II data).[21]

A 1991 survey of 261 randomly selected trauma centers found that 83% used hyperventilation as a means of managing brain-injured patients.[22] However, the 2000 update of the *Guidelines for the Management of Severe Traumatic Brain Injury* found only a limited number of meaningful studies that investigated hyperventilation in brain-injured patients.[23] Follow-up of patient outcomes after TBI is difficult because of the extended time course and diversity of end points. Our literature review located no class I evidence addressing patient outcome. Class II and III studies looking at the effects of hyperventilation on surrogate markers such as CBF, $PbtO_2$, and $AVDO_2$ have not provided conclusive evidence that hyperventilation improves clinical outcome.

There is but one prospective, randomized, controlled study (class II evidence) regarding hyperventilation after brain injury, reported by Muizelaar et al[24] in 1991. This study evaluated the use of hyperventilation with respect to patient outcomes. Investigators monitored ICP, $PaCO_2$, $AVDO_2$, CBF, $CMRO_2$, and CSF and blood pH and lactate levels in three groups of brain-injured patients and assessed the Glasgow Outcome Scale at 3, 6, and 12 months. The groups were divided into eucapneic ventilation ($PaCO_2$ 35 ± 2 mmHg), hyperventilation ($PaCO_2$ 25 ± 2 mmHg), and hyperventilation with administration of tromethamine, a weak base with the ability to cross the blood–brain barrier and alkalinize the CSF. This study showed that 5 days of prophylactic hyperventilation resulted in worse outcomes at 3 and 6 months for patients with otherwise good prognostic indicators on admission; that is, Glasgow motor score of 4 or 5. At 12 months postinjury, there was a trend toward worse outcomes among the hyperventilated patients, but this did not reach statistical significance. Of interest, the eucapneic (control) group tended to have a higher mortality compared with the hyperventilation group, but this also did not meet statistical significance. Patients with poor prognostic indicators on admission had poor outcomes in all three treatment groups.

Augmenting Arterial Oxygenation

Several investigators have looked at the effects of delivering normobaric supranormal FiO_2 on cerebral metabolism. In two separate studies (both class III), one on patients undergoing anesthesia for neurosurgical procedures[25] and one on head-injured patients,[26] investigators found that increasing FiO_2 improved PaO_2, cerebral O_2 delivery, and $AVDO_2$. Similar findings were reported by Menzel et al[27] (class III evidence), who noted decreased levels of lactate in cerebral microdialysate during periods of hyperoxygenation to PaO_2 levels of 200 to 400 mmHg. An important caveat, however, is that no study to date has correlated decreased cerebral lactate or increased $PbtO_2$ with improved patient outcomes.

Pearl

Increasing FiO_2 improved $PbtO_2$, cerebral O_2 delivery, $AVDO_2$, and cerebral lactate levels.

Class II data regarding the use of PEEP to improve PaO_2 indicate that PEEP may increase lung barotrauma and ICP (albeit with no clinical consequences).[28] Additionally, increased PEEP may impede cerebral venous outflow from the cranium to the thorax and lead to elevated ICP. However, increased PEEP routinely alters several hemodynamic variables, including cardiac output and blood pressure, which may offset effects of PEEP on ICP. It is therefore recommended that the use of PEEP and its effects on ICP and hemodynamics be evaluated at the patient's bedside.

Pearl

The use of PEEP and its effects on ICP and hemodynamics should be individualized by careful assessment at the patient's bedside.

Conclusions

Given the lack of evidence specifically addressing the use of hyperventilation in brain-injured patients vis-à-vis patient outcome, we cannot make any level I recommendations regarding the "optimal" ventilator settings for these patients. We agree with statements from the Brain Trauma Foundation that there remains a tremendous need for data from well-designed randomized trials addressing these issues and that hypoxemia and routine excessive hyperventilation should be avoided. The safest ventilatory management goals for brain-injured patients at this time remain the maintenance of eucapneic ventilation (by delivering individualized tidal volumes and delivery pressures) with oxygen delivery sufficient to avoid hypoxemia or tissue hypoxia. Clearly, prophylactic hyperventilation has no role in the routine ventilatory management of brain-injured patients. Judicious use of hyperventilation (never to a $PaCO_2$ <26 mmHg) should be reserved as a temporizing measure to treat clinically important ICP elevations and brain herniation while the underlying causes and definitive therapies are otherwise assessed and instituted. Furthermore, we recommend that future investigations address and clarify a multitude of other ventilatory management issues for brain-injured patients, including the safety of PEEP and the potential role of normobaric hyperoxia therapy.

Recommendations

The available evidence does not support the existence of uniformly applicable "optimal" ventilator settings for head-injured patients. Rather, we recommend that individual ventilation needs be assessed and managed on a case-by-case basis at the bedside. It is our opinion that a specialist experienced in managing both mechanical ventilation and brain-injured patients may best perform ventilatory management for these patients. In reviewing the existing literature, we found no evidence to support the use of prophylactic hyperventilation or the use of long-term hyperventilation for chronically elevated ICP, and we recommend avoidance of these unsubstantiated practices (level II recommendations). In contrast, based on the available class II data, we strongly recommend short-term moderate ($PaCO_2$ >25 mmHg) hyperventilation as a temporizing measure for cases of acutely elevated ICP and suspected brain herniation (level II recommendation). There is some evidence in support of using normobaric supranormal alveolar oxygenation to attempt to augment cerebral O_2 delivery and thereby increase the cerebral aerobic/anaerobic metabolism ratio (level III recommendation); however, one must weigh concerns regarding an increased risk of oxygen toxicity against attempts to increase oxygen delivery. The clinical importance of such interventions and their associated potential for adverse effects remain largely unknown.

References

1. Acute Respiratory Distress Syndrome Network. Ventilation with lower tidal volumes as compared with traditional tidal volumes for acute lung injury and the acute respiratory distress syndrome. N Engl J Med 2000;342:1301–1308.
2. Lassen NA, Christensen MS. Physiology of cerebral blood flow. Br J Anaesth 1976;48:719–734.
3. Sutton LN, McLaughlin AC, Dante S, et al. Cerebral venous oxygen content as a measure of brain energy metabolism with increased intracranial pressure and hyperventilation. J Neurosurg 1990;73:927–932.
4. Powers WJ. Hemodynamics and metabolism in ischemic cerebrovascular disease. Neurol Clin 1992;10:31–48.
5. Powers WJ, Grubb RL Jr, Darriet D, et al. Cerebral blood flow and cerebral metabolic rate of oxygen requirements for cerebral function and viability in humans. J Cereb Blood Flow Metab 1985;5:600–608.
6. Obrist WD, Langfitt TW, Jaggi JL, et al. Cerebral blood flow and metabolism in comatose patients with acute head injury: relationship to intracranial hypertension. J Neurosurg 1984;61: 241–253.
7. Astrup J, Siesjo BK, Symon L. Thresholds in cerebral ischemia: the ischemic penumbra. Stroke 1981;12:723–725.
8. Muizelaar JP, Marmarou A, DeSalles AA, et al. Cerebral blood flow and metabolism in severely head-injured children, I: relationship with GCS score, outcome, ICP, and PVI. J Neurosurg 1989;71:63–71.
9. Skippen P, Seearr M, Poskitt K, et al. Effect of hyperventilation on regional cerebral blood flow in head-injured children. Crit Care Med 1997;25:1402–1409.
10. Obrist WD, Langfitt TW, Jaggi JL, et al. Cerebral blood flow and metabolism in comatose patients with acute head injury: relationship to intracranial hypertension. J Neurosurg 1984; 61:241–253.
11. Bouma GJ, Muizelaar JP, Choi SC, et al. Cerebral circulation and metabolism after severe traumatic brain injury: the elusive role of ischemia. J Neurosurg 1991;75:685–693.
12. Robertson CS, Contant CF, Gokaslan ZL, et al. Cerebral blood flow, arteriovenous oxygen difference, and outcome in head injured patients. J Neurol Neurosurg Psychiatry 1992;55: 594–603.
13. Bouma GJ, Muizelaar JP, Stringer WA, et al. Ultra-early evaluation of regional cerebral blood flow in severely head-injured patients using xenon-enhanced computerized tomography. J Neurosurg 1992;77:360–368.
14. Doppenberg EM, Zauner A, Bullock R, et al. Correlations between brain tissue oxygen tension, carbon dioxide tension, pH, and cerebral blood flow—a better way of monitoring the severely injured brain? Surg Neurol 1998;49:650–654.
15. Gupta AK, Hutchinson PJ, Al-Rawi P, et al. Measuring brain tissue oxygenation compared with jugular venous oxygen saturation for monitoring cerebral oxygenation after traumatic brain injury. Anesth Analg 1999;88:549–553.
16. Cruz J, Miner ME, Allen SJ, et al. Continuous monitoring of cerebral oxygenation in acute brain injury: injection of mannitol during hyperventilation. J Neurosurg 1990;73:725–730.
17. Rosner MJ, Daughton S. Cerebral perfusion pressure management in head injury. J Trauma 1990;30:933–941.
18. Cruz J, Jaggi JL, Hoffstad OJ. Cerebral blood flow, vascular resistance, and oxygen metabolism in acute brain trauma: redefining the role of cerebral profusion pressure? Crit Care Med 1995;23:1412–1417.
19. Raichle ME, Posner JB, Plum F. Cerebral blood flow during and after hyperventilation. Arch Neurol 1970;23:394–402.
20. Carmona-Suazo JA, Maas AI, van den Brink WA, et al. CO_2 reactivity and brain oxygen pressure monitoring in severe head injury. Crit Care Med 2000;28:3268–3274.
21. Coplin WM, Pierson DJ, Cooley KD, et al. Implications of extubation delay in brain-injured patients meeting standard weaning criteria. Am J Respir Crit Care Med 2000;161:1530–1536.
22. Ghajar J, Hariri RJ, Narayan RK, et al. Survey of critical care management of comatose, head-injured patients in the United States. Crit Care Med 1995;23:560–567.
23. Brain Trauma Foundation, American Association of Neurological Surgeons, Joint Section on Neurotrauma and Critical Care. Guidelines for the management of severe traumatic brain injury. Hyperventilation. J Neurotrauma 2000; 17:513–520.
24. Muizelaar JP, Marmarou A, Ward JD. Adverse effects of prolonged hyperventilation in patients with severe head injury: a randomized clinical trial. J Neurosurg 1991;75: 731–739.
25. Matta BF, Lam AM, Mayberg TS, et al. The influence of arterial oxygenation on cerebral oxygen saturation during hyperventilation. Can J Anaesth 1994;41:1041–1046.
26. Thiagarajan A, Goverdhan PD, Chari P, et al. The effect of hyperventilation and hyperoxia on cerebral venous oxygen saturation in patients with traumatic brain injury. Anesth Analg 1998;87:850–853.
27. Menzel M, Doppenberg EM, Zauner A, et al. Increased inspired oxygen concentration as a factor in improved brain tissue oxygenation and tissue lactate levels after severe human head injury. J Neurosurg 1999;91:1–10.
28. Cooper KR, Boswell PA, Choi SC. Safe use of PEEP in patients with severe head injury. J Neurosurg 1985;63:552–555.

◆ 15 ◆

What Is the Optimal Hematocrit and Hemoglobin for Head-Injured Patients?

Harel Deutsch and Jamie S. Ullman

Brief Answer

A hematocrit between 30 and 35% is widely believed to be optimal for head-injured patients. This number has been derived from experimental studies of blood viscosity and oxygen-carrying capacity. When cerebral autoregulation is intact, viscosity has little effect on cerebral blood flow (CBF), which is determined primarily by vessel diameter. With loss of autoregulation, vessels are maximally dilated, and viscosity becomes an important determinant of CBF. Halving the blood viscosity by reducing the hematocrit from 45–50% to 30–35% results in a doubling of CBF. Reducing the hematocrit to less than 30% is generally believed to result in only a slight decrease in viscosity at the expense of a greater decrease in oxygen-carrying capacity. However, no direct clinical studies exist to support this practice.

Background

The optimal hematocrit for head-injured patients has been the subject of intense study by physiologists and neurosurgeons for several decades. Initial theories involved the classical description of fluid dynamics as expressed by the Hagen-Poiseuille equation:

$$Q = \frac{P\pi r^4}{8L\eta}$$

where Q is blood flow, P is the pressure gradient, r is the vessel radius, L is the vessel length, and η is the viscosity. Under normal conditions, vessel radius is the most important determinant of blood flow. Autoregulation of CBF functions by adjusting blood vessel radius to compensate for changes in pressure gradients and blood viscosity. In situations where autoregulation is lost and vessel radius is maximal, viscosity becomes an important determinant of CBF. According to the Hagen-Poiseuille equation, halving the blood viscosity doubles the CBF.

Pearl

When autoregulation is lost and vessel radius is maximal, viscosity becomes an important determinant of CBF.

The hematocrit is a major determinant of blood viscosity. The viscosity of plasma is 1.2 times that of water, whereas blood with a normal hematocrit of 45% has an apparent viscosity 2.4 times that of plasma. Reducing the hematocrit from 45 to 30% will halve the measured viscosity and therefore theoretically double the CBF. A linear relationship exists between hematocrit and the logarithm of blood viscosity at a given shear rate.[1] Further hematocrit reduction will increase CBF, but at a substantial cost in terms of diminished oxygen delivery capacity. The oxygen delivery capacity is a function of hemoglobin and is calculated as:

$$C = (1.39\,\text{mLO}_2/\text{gm of hemoglobin}) \times (\text{g of hemoglobin/dL})$$

This equation assumes 100% hemoglobin saturation and disregards the very small amount of O_2 dissolved in plasma. Based on these calculations, the optimal hematocrit for head-injured patients has been classically quoted to be between 30 and 35%.[2]

Pearl

Reducing the hematocrit from 45 to 30% will halve the measured viscosity and therefore theoretically double the CBF while decreasing oxygen-carrying capacity by only a third.

Further research has revealed that these calculations may not be accurate because the cerebral microcirculation has been found to be more complex than initially believed.[3] Poiseuille's equation only applies to ideal, or Newtonian, fluids. Blood is a non-Newtonian fluid, the viscosity of which changes with vessel diameter. Most suspensions of rigid particles display increasing viscosity as they flow through progressively narrower tubes. Fahraeus discovered that blood viscosity, however, actually decreases when the tube diameter becomes less than 0.3 mm. The Fahraeus effect is attributed to accumulation of red blood cells in the faster axial stream, whereas plasma tends to flow in the slower marginal layers. By contributing to shear thinning, that is, the decreased tendency for erythrocytes to aggregate as flow velocity increases, faster axial flow rates act to reduce viscosity. As the capillary size decreases to less than 7 μm, viscosity greatly increases because the vessel diameter is close to the erythrocyte size, an effect known as the inversion phenomenon. The erythrocytes travel through the capillaries faster than the plasma, resulting in a decreased apparent hematocrit in the capillaries. In a 300 μm or larger tube, the hematocrit is close to the hematocrit in larger vessels, but below 300 μm, the hematocrit steadily decreases. At 30 μm, the hematocrit is 40% less than in the larger blood vessels. The effects of the microcirculation on the optimal hematocrit are uncertain, but they do cast doubt on the validity of previous calculations based on Poiseuille's equation.

Literature Review

Many animal studies have demonstrated increased CBF and decreased ischemia as a result of hemodilution and reduced hematocrit.[4–6] When autoregulation is intact, lowered viscosity results in cerebral vessel narrowing and constant CBF. With loss of autoregulation in ischemic conditions, a reduction in blood viscosity results in an increase in CBF.[7]

Administration of whole blood to induce nondilutional hypervolemia has been shown not to improve collateral perfusion to ischemic regions or to reduce infarct size in experimental models of focal cerebral ischemia, despite significant augmentation of cardiac output.[8] Analogous observations have been made in patients with idiopathic erythrocytosis (class III data). The strokes are attributed to elevated blood viscosity.[9]

Recent animal experiments have tried to address the role of the microcirculation in defining an optimal hematocrit. Experiments using in vivo red blood cell fluorescence videomicroscopy in intracortical capillaries have demonstrated an increasing red blood cell supply as hematocrit is lowered from 44 to 15%.[10] Theoretically, hematocrits below 30% may be desirable in head trauma patients, but convincing experimental data are lacking.

Clinical studies examining optimal hematocrit after head trauma do not exist. Clinical data concerning the relationship between hematocrit and CBF are sparse. Class III data include a study by Harrison et al[11] that found a correlation between elevated hematocrit and size of cerebral infarction after occlusive carotid disease. Thomas et al[12] (class II data) measured CBF with an intravenous ^{133}Xe isotopic clearance technique in two groups of patients, one with hematocrits between 47 and 53% and another in whom those values ranged from 36 to 46%. The group with the higher values had an average CBF of 46.1 mL/100 g/min, whereas the group with the lower hematocrits had an average CBF of 65.0 mL/100 g/min ($p > .001$). Venesection was performed on 19 patients, reducing their hematocrit from 49.3 to 42.6%, with a resulting 50% increase in CBF from 41.4 mL/100 g/min to 62.1 mL/100 g/min. Oxygen-carrying capacity was calculated to fall by 13% in the venesection group but was accompanied by a 50% increase in CBF.[12]

Pearl

In clinical studies, elevated hematocrit has been associated with lower CBF and larger infarct volumes.

Muhling et al[13] (class II data) measured CBF velocity using transcranial Doppler in 11 healthy volunteers undergoing isovolemic hemodilution using venesection and transfusion with hydroxyethyl starch. The subjects' hematocrits decreased from 41.8 to 29.6%, whereas blood flow velocity in the middle cerebral artery increased from 61.2 cm/sec to 77.3 cm/sec ($p < .01$). These investigations demonstrating an association between increased CBF and lowered hematocrit support the use of mild hemodilution to increase CBF in head trauma patients.

Recommendations

The available clinical evidence does not support level I or II recommendations about the optimal hematocrit in head trauma. Level III recommendations may be formulated by generalizing experimental and clinical data involving ischemia and hematocrit. Hemodilution should be used to obtain a hematocrit of ~30 to 35% and a hemoglobin of 10 mg/dL. This reduction of viscosity results in a doubling of CBF with a less dramatic decrease in oxygen-carrying capacity. Further clinical studies are necessary to determine the effect of this practice on clinical outcome and other important measures.

References

1. Pearson TC. Hemorheology in the erythrocytoses. Mt Sinai J Med 2001;68:182–191.
2. Muizelaar JP. CBF and management of the head-injured patient. In: Narayan RK, Wilberger JE, Povlishock JT, eds. Neurotrauma. New York: McGraw-Hill, 1996:553–561.
3. Kee DB, Wood JH. Rheology of the cerebral circulation. Neurosurgery 1984;15:125–131.
4. Korosue K, Heros RC. Mechanism of cerebral blood flow augmentation by hemodilution in rabbits. Stroke 1992;23:1487–1492.
5. Cole DJ, Drummond JC, Osborne TN, Matsumura J. Hypertension and hemodilution during cerebral ischemia reduce brain injury and edema. Am J Physiol 1990;259:H211–217.
6. Tomiyama Y, Brian JE Jr, Todd MM. Plasma viscosity and cerebral blood flow. Am J Physiol Heart Circ Physiol 2000;279:1949–1954.
7. Muizelaar JP, Wei EP, Kontos HA, et al. Cerebral blood flow is regulated by changes in blood pressure and in blood viscosity alike. Stroke 1986;17:44–48.
8. Wood JH, Snyder LL, Simeone FA. Failure of intravascular volume expansion without hemodilution to elevate cortical blood flow in region of experimental focal ischemia. J Neurosurg 1982;56:80–91.
9. Pearson TC, Wetherley-Mein G. Vascular occlusive episodes and venous haematocrit in primary proliferative polycythaemia. Lancet 1978;2:1219–1222.
10. Hudetz AG, Wood JD, Biswal BB, et al. Effect of hemodilution on RBC velocity, supply rate, and hematocrit in the cerebral capillary network. J Appl Physiol 1999;87:505–509.
11. Harrison MJ, Pollock S, Kendall BE, et al. Effect of haematocrit on carotid stenosis and cerebral infarction. Lancet 1981;2:114–115.
12. Thomas DJ, Marshall J, Russell RW, et al. Effect of haematocrit on cerebral blood-flow in man. Lancet 1977;2:941–943.
13. Muhling J, Dehne MG, Sablotzki A, et al. Cerebral blood flow velocity during isovolemic hemodilution and subsequent autologous blood retransfusion. Can J Anaesth 1999;46:550–557.

◆ 16 ◆

How Soon Should Patients Receive Nutrition? How Much, Which Formulation, and by Which Route?

Shelly D. Timmons

Brief Answer

Nutritional management of patients with traumatic brain injury (TBI) may be important in determining overall outcome by minimizing mortality and morbidity from infectious complications, thereby allowing earlier and potentially greater neurologic improvement. As long as adequate early caloric and nitrogen intake can be achieved via enteral nutrition (EN), this is the preferred route of administration. In some patients who are unable to tolerate EN, parenteral nutrition (PN) is an acceptable means of providing support in the early postinjury phase.

Pearl

Patients with severe brain injuries exhibit metabolic responses similar to those of patients with 20 to 40% of body surface area burns.

Background

In considering appropriate nutrition for patients with TBI, one must address the timing of initiation of nutritional therapy, the route of delivery, and the formulation to be given. For brain-injured patients who are unable to eat due to depressed level of consciousness, endotracheal intubation, or alimentary tract dysfunction (depressed gag reflex, delayed gastric emptying, ileus, dysphagia), EN and PN nutrition provide excellent opportunities for temporary nutritional support. Indeed, alternative means of nutrition are necessary adjuncts to the treatment of severely brain-injured patients who experience prolonged coma and mechanical ventilation. This patient population often has concurrent major injuries of other body systems, putting them at further risk of nutritional depletion and infectious complications in the acute postinjury period.

It has long been recognized that injured patients enter hypermetabolic hypercatabolic states, suffer derangements in glucose metabolism, and experience other metabolic changes such as increased catecholamine release. However, it has only been in the past two decades that specific attention has been given to the study of nutritional and metabolic considerations in brain-injured patients. Relatively few randomized prospective studies have been done to address the optimal timing and route of nutritional support, especially with regard to neurologic outcome.

Pearl

Resting metabolic expenditure has been shown to be as high as 168% ± 53% of expected levels in the most severely brain-injured patients [Glasgow Coma Scale (GCS) of 4–5].[1]

There has been some controversy about the ideal route of administration of nutritional formulations.

Studies from the 1980s focused on differences between PN and EN with regard to their respective abilities to provide adequate caloric and nitrogen intake and positive nitrogen balance. Somewhat concurrently, techniques were evolving for various means of providing EN and for assessing nutritional status. Early investigators were also confronted with the variable use of steroid therapy in brain-injured patients. Accepted forms of treatment for elevations in intracranial pressure (ICP) have also changed over this time period. Finally, published studies on nutritional supplementation differed significantly in their design and goals. For these reasons, the results described in the existing literature can seem conflicting.

The enteral route is thought to be preferable because EN preserves mucosal integrity, minimizes bacterial translocation, and better preserves intestinal immunocompetence. However, in this patient population, gastrointestinal problems can lead to intolerance of enteral feedings, putting the patient at risk for aspiration-related pulmonary complications.[2–4]

Literature Review

Timing of Administration of Nutrition

Seven prospective randomized trials have specifically addressed the issue of timing of administration of nutrition in TBI patients (Table 16-1). The majority of these studies were designed to compare routes of administration, but because of the time period necessary to achieve adequate calorie and protein intake in the enteral groups, differences in timing may be at the root of differences in results. Rapp et al[5] investigated the differences between traditional delayed EN and early PN in 38 TBI patients with GCS scores of 3 to 10 (class I data).

Table 16-1 Class I Studies Examining Timing of Initiation of Nutritional Support

Date of Publication	Authors	Study Groups	Number of Patients	Conclusions
1983[5]	Rapp et al.*	EN versus PN	38 (18 EN/20 TPN)	Increased mortality was seen in EN group. PN patients had more + nitrogen balance and improved indices of nutritional status. PN patients had more improvement in GOS from discharge to 1 year, possibly related to greater no. of deaths in EN group. Time to optimal nutrition was longer in EN group, suggesting that results were possibly due to the degree of nutritional replacement in the acute phase rather than the route.
1986[6]	Hadley et al.	EN versus PN	45 (21 EN/24 PN)	No differences were identified in safety between the two groups. Higher calorie and nitrogen intake were achieved somewhat sooner in the PN group than the EN group. Early provision of nutrition overall (both groups) resulted in improved indices of nutritional status.
1987[2]	Young et al.*	EN versus PN	51 (28 EN/23 PN)	Neurologic recovery occurred more rapidly in patients with better nutritional support (the PN group in this case). Overall outcomes (GOS at 1 year) were not different. Optimal nutrition was supplied earlier in the PN group.
1987[8]	Young et al.	EN versus PN	96 (#s not noted)	PN and EN had similar effects on intracranial pressure (ICP) and ICP therapy. PN was noted to be safely given without causing serum hyperosmolality.
1995[10]	Sacks et al.	PN (early) versus PN (late)	9 (4 early/5 late)	Early PN modified immunologic function by increasing CD4 cells, CD4-CD8 ratios, and T-lymphocyte responsiveness.
1999[9]	Taylor et al.*	Enhanced EN versus standard EN	82 (41 enhanced/ 41 standard)	Enhanced EN (feeding started at rate that met estimated energy and nitrogen requirements) resulted in accelerated neurologic recovery (GOS) compared with standard EN. No differences remained by 6 months. Enhanced EN reduced incidence of infectious complications and inflammatory responses. No cost differences were seen.
2000[11]	Minard et al.	EN (early) versus EN (very early)	27 (15 early/ 12 very early)	The authors defined the groups as early and delayed, but in comparison to other studies and vis-à-vis metabolic requirements, could be categorized as very early and early. No differences were seen between the two groups with respect to LOS or infectious complications.

PR, prospective, randomized trial; PN, parenteral nutrition; EN, enteral nutrition; GOS, Glasgow Outcome Scale; LOS, length of stay; TPN, total parenteral nutrition.

*These studies specifically addressed outcome.

EN was begun when resumption of gastrointestinal tract function was identified. They found significant differences in peak temperature during the first 24 hours of hospitalization (higher in PN), in-hospital deaths (higher in EN), nitrogen and caloric intake (both greater in PN), and loss of triceps skinfold thickness (greater in EN). Importantly, there was notable improvement in Glasgow Outcome Scale (GOS) score at 1 year compared with discharge for the PN group, suggesting that, by diminishing early deaths, PN provided the opportunity for improved long-term neurologic outcome. [The EN group had fewer long-term survivors (eight out of 18 patients compared with 16 out of 19 PN patients), but their outcomes as a group also improved between discharge and 1-year follow-up.] Both PN and EN groups experienced negative nitrogen balance through day 16, providing confirmation of the profound catabolic state of brain-injured patients. Other authors have reported the same finding (in class I studies).[3,6,7]

Young and coworkers[2] (the same group of investigators) studied 51 TBI patients with GCS scores of 4 to 10 (class I data). They again demonstrated higher cumulative caloric and protein intake in a PN group compared with an EN group. EN feedings were administered via nasogastric or nasoduodenal routes. They noted no significant differences in infections or traditional tests of nutritional status in the first 2 weeks after injury. In this study, neurologic recovery occurred more rapidly in the PN group, though 1-year GOS scores were not significantly different from those of the EN group.

When these investigators looked at ICP data in 96 patients in the two treatment groups, they noted no significant differences in ICP, treatment for elevated ICP, or serum osmolality measurements (class I data).[8] The latter finding is important because some have suggested that the fluid composition of PN formulas may exacerbate cerebral edema to a greater degree than EN formulas and thereby lead to ICP elevations, with resultant negative effects on outcome.

Taylor et al[9] examined the effects of standard EN versus "enhanced" EN, in which the feedings were started at rates that approximated estimated caloric and nitrogen requirements (class I data). The standard treatment arm consisted of gradually increased enteral feedings. Each group consisted of 41 patients with severe TBI. They demonstrated fewer infectious complications, fewer overall complications, and a reduced inflammatory response (as shown by the ratio of concentrations of serum C-reactive protein to albumin) in the enhanced EN group. They also showed faster neurologic recovery in the enhanced EN group. These results lend further credence to the idea that the route of nutrition administration is not as important as the time until adequate intake is achieved, as suggested by the Rapp and Young papers.

This idea is further supported by the work of Hadley et al,[6] who compared PN to EN in 45 TBI patients (mean admission GCS = 5.8) (class I data). Both routes were used early (nutritional support initiated within 48 hours), and treatment was tailored to individual needs as estimated by resting energy expenditure and indirect calorimetry measurements. No differences were discovered with respect to maintenance of serum albumin, weight loss, incidence of infection, nitrogen balance, or final outcome as assessed by GCS.

The decrease in bacterial infections seen when caloric and protein needs are met earlier in the course of treatment supports the concept that adequate nutrition promotes immunocompetence. Sacks et al[10] noted that early aggressive nutritional support of TBI patients (GCS 3–12) resulted in increased CD4 cell counts, CD4/CD8 ratios, and T-lymphocyte responsiveness to certain stimuli (class I data). Their experimental groups consisted of patients given early PN at day 1 or delayed PN at day 5, and though sample sizes were small ($n = 4$ and 5, respectively), statistical significance was achieved for the above findings.

Minard et al[11] investigated the timing of EN in two groups of TBI patients (GCS 3–11; $n = 27$) (class I data). Both groups were given an immune-enhancing formula via endoscopically placed nasoenteric tubes (early) or nasogastric tube after resolution of ileus (delayed). The early group had feedings initiated within 33 ± 15 hours, and the delayed group within 84 ± 41 hours. In view of the rapidity with which support was provided overall, these treatment arms could easily be considered as "very early" versus "early" groups, rather than "early" and "delayed" groups. For this reason, it is not surprising that no differences were seen in infectious complication rates or hospital lengths of stay between the two groups.

In summary, patients appear to have fewer infectious complications and improved outcomes when feedings are begun early in the therapeutic course. The actual route of administration may play a less important role.

Route of Nutrition

In addition to the four studies cited above, which involved differences between EN and PN, three other prospective, randomized studies of this question have been published (Table 16-2).

Thirty-two head-injured patients with GCS <10 were studied by Grahm and coworkers[4] (class I data). They were able to achieve early EN via nasojejunal tubes placed with fluoroscopic guidance. Their EN patient group was able to receive support equal to measured resting energy expenditures within 36 hours of injury. A control group underwent gastric feeding when bowel sounds returned. Although no significant differences were seen in standard nutritional indices, the early jejunally fed group had improved daily caloric and nitrogen intake and nitrogen balance, a lower incidence of bacterial infections, and shorter intensive care unit stay.

Table 16-2 Class I Studies Examining Route of Nutritional Support

Date of Publication	Authors	Study Groups	Number of Patients	Conclusions
1983[5]	Rapp et al.*	EN versus PN	38 (18 EN/20 PN)	See Table 16-1. Critical to interpreting results is the fact that the EN group took much longer to reach nutritional goals, thereby probably affecting results.
1989[4]	Grahm et al.	EN (jejunal) versus EN (gastric)	32 (17J/15G)	Jejunal feedings resulted in higher caloric and nitrogen intake and improved nitrogen balance. Jejunal feedings also resulted in decreased bacterial infections and days of intensive care.
1985[12]	Hausmann et al.	EN + PN versus PN	20 (10 EN + PN/ 10 PN)	No differences were seen in mortality, nitrogen balance, or other metabolic markers studied.
1986[6]	Hadley et al.	EN versus PN	45 (21 EN/24 PN)	See Table 16-1.
1987[2]	Young et al.	EN versus PN	58 51(28 EN/23 PN)	See Table 16-1. Critical to interpreting results is the fact that the EN group took much longer to reach nutritional goals, thereby probably affecting results.
1987[8]	Young et al.	EN versus PN	96 (#s not noted)	See Table 16-1. Critical to interpreting results is the fact that the EN group took much longer to reach nutritional goals, thereby probably affecting results.
1994[3]	Borzotta et al.	EN versus PN	48 (27 EN/21 PN)	EN and PN had comparable infectious complication rates and nutritional markers when prescriptions were based on individual measured energy expenditure and nitrogen excretion. PN resulted in higher patient charges, but hospital costs were similar for EN and PN.

PR, prospective, randomized trial; PN, parenteral nutrition; EN, enteral nutrition.
*This study specifically addressed outcome.

Pearl

Jejunal feedings were tolerated despite the absence of detectable bowel sounds and the presence of gastric dysfunction.[4]

Borzotta and his group[3] found that early PN ($n = 21$) and early EN ($n = 27$) were equally effective at meeting nutritional goals for severe TBI (GCS 3–7) patients (class I data). There was no difference in the frequency of infectious complications. They asserted that the key to their findings was that both types of support were tailored to the individual patient's nutritional needs as estimated by measured energy expenditure and urinary nitrogen excretion, and both types were begun early. They utilized jejunal feeding with simultaneous gastric decompression when possible to facilitate early tube feedings. Furthermore, they did note similar hospital costs for both regimens, although patient charges were higher for PN. This study and Hadley et al's study, discussed above, are the most accurate comparisons of the two types of feeding routes. The earlier study by Rapp and colleagues did not achieve adequate nutritional intake via the enteral route and could thus be more properly viewed as a study comparing PN to relative starvation, as the authors acknowledged in a later report.[2]

Hausmann and coinvestigators[12] sought to detect differences between PN and a combined PN-EN regimen ($n = 10$ for each treatment arm) given to patients with TBI (GCS 5–7) (class I data). They did not observe any differences among mortality, nitrogen balance, or other markers of nutritional status. They also suggested that testing regurgitated gastric fluid for elevated protein concentration could direct management by identifying patients who would tolerate the combined protocol less well.

Research presented by Suchner and colleagues[13] suggested that PN and EN were equally effective in 34 patients who had undergone neurosurgical procedures (class II data). EN was thought to preserve several gastrointestinal physiologic functions better than PN, but this was a fairly heterogeneous patient population not limited to head trauma patients. The authors confirmed the findings of others[2–4,6,7,14] that nitrogen balance per se is probably insufficient to predict efficacy of nutritional replacement.

Formulation of Nutrition

Several formulations of PN and EN are available, and individualized formulations can be produced in many institutions. Insofar as hyperglycemia has been associated with poor neurologic outcome after TBI (class II data),[15,16] its occurrence should be prevented, whatever formulation is used.

Clifton et al[7] investigated enteral feedings in 20 brain-injured patients (GCS 3–7) (class I data). They demonstrated that high-calorie and high-protein formulations could be delivered via the enteral route and suggested that increasing nitrogen content from 14 to 22% may improve nitrogen retention. Investigations into metabolic expenditure have reported increases over the expected amounts ranging from 101 to 175%, with a mean around 140%.[4,14] No significant differences in resting metabolic expenditure have been identified in steroid versus non–steroid-treated patients. Energy needs have been shown to be increased in patients with agitation, infections, or persistent hypertonicity.[3]

Complications

Complications associated with PN include line sepsis, pneumothorax, hyperlipidemia, hyperglycemia, electrolyte imbalance, and volume overload. Complications associated with EN include aspiration (causing aspiration pneumonitis and/or pneumonia) and general infectious complications related to delay in achieving adequate caloric and protein intake. In hemodynamically unstable patients, enteral feedings may produce intestinal ischemia. Both types of nutritional supplementation can be associated with diarrhea. Tube dislodgment is a common problem in enteral feeding, particularly with nasally placed tubes in agitated patients.

Conclusions

Early initiation of nutritional support benefits brain-injured patients by decreasing the likelihood of infectious complications, decreasing mortality, and enhancing speed of recovery from neurologic deficits.

EN provides advantages over PN, including decreased risk of line-related and other complications and improved immunocompetence.

The hypermetabolism and hypercatabolism associated with severe TBI suggest that feedings should consist of ~140% of expected caloric requirements with ≥15% of calories supplied as protein.

Recommendations

Timing of Nutrition Administration

Evidence suggests that earlier feeding results in a trend toward fewer infectious complications and lower mortality. Some evidence suggests improved and more rapid neurologic outcome when nutrition is initiated earlier. Initiation of some form of nutritional support within 48 to 72 hours of injury is recommended (level I). Adequate replacement should be in place by postinjury day 7 to achieve sufficient intake to prevent major nitrogen losses (level II).

Route of Nutrition

PN may be associated with more complications. EN must often be delayed secondary to gastrointestinal dysmotility; however, jejunal feeding catheters provide an option for early enteral administration of adequate calories and protein without the complications sometimes associated with gastric feeding. The enteral route is recommended if adequate calorie and protein intake can be achieved within the first few days after injury. The jejunal route is preferable as a means of minimizing complications and optimizing nutrition, with or without simultaneous gastric decompression. Recommendations regarding route of therapy (PN versus EN) are level II. Various EN techniques can only currently be presented as level III recommendations but merit further study.

Formulation of Nutrition

Good evidence suggests that nutritional requirements vary widely among patients. It is therefore recommended that the composition of feedings be tailored to individual nutritional needs. This requires the creation of a routine for estimating caloric and protein needs and for monitoring the adequacy of nutritional support. At least 140% of resting metabolic expenditure should be provided, with at least 15% of calories being provided as protein (level III).

References

1. Robertson CS, Clifton GL, Grossman RG. Oxygen utilization and cardiovascular function in head-injured patients. Neurosurgery 1984;15:307–314.
2. Young B, Ott L, Twyman D, et al. The effect of nutritional support on outcome from severe head injury. J Neurosurg 1987;67: 668–676.
3. Borzotta AP, Pennings J, Papasadero B, et al. Enteral versus parenteral nutrition after severe closed head injury. J Trauma 1994;37:459–468.
4. Grahm TW, Zadrozny DB, Harrington T. The benefits of early jejunal hyperalimentation in the head-injured patient. Neurosurgery 1989;25:729–735.
5. Rapp RP, Young B, Twyman D, et al. The favorable effect of early parenteral feeding on survival in head-injured patients. J Neurosurg 1983;58:906–912.
6. Hadley MN, Grahm TW, Harrington T, et al. Nutritional support and neurotrauma: a critical review of early nutrition in forty-five acute head injury patients. Neurosurgery 1986;19: 367–373.

7. Clifton GL, Robertson CS, Contant CF. Enteral hyperalimentation in head injury. J Neurosurg 1985;62:186–193.
8. Young B, Ott L, Haack D, et al. Effect of total parenteral nutrition upon intracranial pressure in severe head injury. J Neurosurg 1987;67:76–80.
9. Taylor SJ, Fettes SB, Jewkes C, et al. Prospective, randomized, controlled trial to determine the effect of early enhanced enteral nutrition on clinical outcome in mechanically ventilated patients suffering head injury. Crit Care Med 1999;27:2525–2531.
10. Sacks GS, Brown RO, Teague D, et al. Early nutrition support modifies immune function in patients sustaining severe head injury. JPEN J Parenter Enteral Nutr 1995;19:387–392.
11. Minard G, Kudsk KA, Melton S, et al. Early versus delayed feeding with an immune-enhancing diet in patients with severe head injuries. JPEN J Parenter Enteral Nutr 2000;24: 145–149.
12. Hausmann D, Mosebach KO, Caspari R, et al. Combined enteral-parenteral nutrition versus total parenteral nutrition in brain-injured patients: a comparative study. Intensive Care Med 1985;11:80–84.
13. Suchner U, Senftleben U, Eckart T, et al. Enteral versus parenteral nutrition: effects on gastrointestinal function and metabolism. Nutrition 1996;12:13–22.
14. Clifton GL, Robertson CS, Grossman RG, et al. The metabolic response to severe head injury. J Neurosurg 1984;60:687–696.
15. Lam AM, Winn HR, Cullen BF, et al. Hyperglycemia and neurological outcome in patients with head injury. J Neurosurg 1991;75:545–551.
16. Young B, Ott L, Dempsey R, et al. Relationship between admission hyperglycemia and neurologic outcome of severely brain-injured patients. Ann Surg 1989;210:466–473.

17

Are There Safe Upper and Lower Limits for Serum Sodium and Serum Osmolality in Head-Injured Patients? Should I Use Hypertonic Saline or Fluid Restriction to Treat Hyponatremia?

Shon W. Cook, Pejman Cohan, and Daniel F. Kelly

Brief Answer

Safe Upper and Lower Limits for Serum Sodium and Serum Osmolality in Head-Injured Patients

Little solid evidence is available for identifying a safe absolute lower limit for serum sodium and serum osmolality in acutely head-injured patients. However, acute and progressive hyponatremia and hypo-osmolality are known to be associated with worsening brain swelling, intracranial hypertension, and seizure activity. Therefore, the suggestion that every effort be made to avoid hyponatremia, for example, serum sodium <135 mEq/L, may be offered as a level III recommendation.

Evidence that defines an absolute safe upper limit for serum sodium and serum osmolality in acutely head-injured patients is also sparse. Induced hypernatremia with hypertonic saline is being used increasingly as a treatment for refractory intracranial hypertension in head-injured patients. Although rapid elevations of serum sodium may cause central myelinolysis, a relatively large increase in serum sodium is needed to induce myelinolysis if a patient is normonatremic at baseline.[1] On the other hand, subsequent excessively rapid correction of iatrogenic hypernatremia may cause or aggravate cerebral edema. Therefore, as a level III recommendation, excessive hypernatremia (e.g., serum sodium >150 mEq/L) should be avoided, especially when it develops rapidly.

Use of Hypertonic Saline or Fluid Restriction to Treat Hyponatremia

The most effective treatment for hyponatremia in acutely head-injured patients is often difficult to identify because the treatment of posttraumatic hyponatremia depends in large part on its etiology. The preponderance of recent data seems to indicate that hyponatremia in the neurosurgical setting is caused by a combination of early inappropriate release of antidiuretic hormone and a later period of salt wasting. Because many head-injured patients with hyponatremia already appear to have an element of cerebral salt wasting (CSW) with relative volume depletion when they are diagnosed, therapies that raise serum sodium without restricting free water, such as hypertonic saline, intravenous urea, or fludrocortisone acetate, are probably the safest and most effective initial treatments. Regardless of the method used, the rate of sodium correction should not exceed 15 mEq/L per day to avoid central myelinolysis (class III data) (although myelinolysis seems to be uncommon after correction of acute, as opposed to chronic, hyponatremia).[1] An attempt should also be made to differentiate between CSW and the syndrome of inappropriate secretion of antidiuretic hormone (SIADH) because inappropriate treatment may exacerbate a patient's hyper- or hyponatremia or systemic volume disturbance.

Treatment of Hypernatremia

Hypernatremia is best treated by careful administration of more free water, by restriction of the amount of sodium administered to a patient, and, in severe cases, by administration of deamino-8-D-arginine vasopressin (DDAVP) (desmopressin) to decrease renal excretion of water.

Background and Literature Review: Safe Upper and Lower Limits for Serum Sodium and Serum Osmolality in Head-Injured Patients

No class I studies have addressed the safe range of serum sodium and serum osmolality in head-injured patients. For ethical reasons, it is unlikely that a prospective, randomized, controlled study will be done to determine definitively a safe upper or lower limit for serum sodium in head-injured patients. Currently available evidence is primarily class III, but some class II studies (not limited to head-injured patients) are available.

Significance of Hyponatremia

Acute hyponatremia is relatively common following head injury, occurring in 8% of moderately or severely injured patients in one retrospective series (class III data).[2] A review of the literature since 1935 reveals multiple cases of symptomatic hyponatremia following neurologic surgery, sometimes accompanied by coma and seizures (class III data).[3] Hyponatremia is often delayed in onset and may not appear for several days after an intracranial insult (class III data).[4]

Class III evidence suggests that hyponatremia may lower the seizure threshold,[5] exacerbate cerebral edema,[2] and cause or contribute to delayed elevations in intracranial pressure.[4] Conscious patients may initially develop such nonspecific symptoms as headache, nausea, emesis, and weakness. Worsening hyponatremia may lead to progressive neurologic deterioration and convulsions (class III data).[6] Class II data in subarachnoid hemorrhage patients indicate that those with hyponatremia have a significantly higher risk of cerebral ischemia than those without hyponatremia, but this predisposition is apparently not associated with an increase in mortality.[7]

Predicting the serum sodium concentration at which an individual will develop symptoms is difficult, but the degree of hypo-osmolality and especially the rate of decrease seem to correlate in general terms with severity of symptoms (class II data).[8] Many patients seem to become symptomatic or deteriorate neurologically when serum sodium levels fall below 130 mEq/L. In one series, all patients with a serum sodium level below 125 mEq/L had some degree of symptomatology (class II data).[8] Major neurologic manifestations, including seizures and coma, are common when sodium concentrations fall below this level (class III data).[5,9] Class II and III evidence suggests that female gender (menstruant women), hypoxia, and young age may worsen the prognosis of hyponatremic encephalopathy.[1]

Pearl

Hyponatremia may lower the seizure threshold, exacerbate cerebral edema, and cause or contribute to delayed elevations in intracranial pressure.

Etiology of Hyponatremia

In the early 1950s, renal salt wasting was first reported in patients with intracranial disease. Because the pituitary-adrenal axis was intact, the excessive natriuresis was thought to be due to disruption of direct neural regulation of renal tubular activity and therefore was named CSW (class III data).[10–12] In 1957, however, SIADH was described (class III data),[13] and it soon became the favored explanation for hyponatremia in neurosurgical patients (class III data).[2,14–16] The popularity of SIADH as a diagnosis in hyponatremic patients fueled recommendations to restrict fluid intake during the acute management of neurosurgical patients (class III data),[17] including those with head injuries (class III data).[18]

In recent years it has become evident that many hyponatremic patients with acute brain disease are in fact relatively hypovolemic (class II and III data),[19–21] compatible with the original diagnosis of CSW. There has also been an increase in the number of reports describing such instances as hyponatremia with normal ADH (class III data)[22,23] and high plasma atrial natriuretic peptide (class III data)[22]; delay or failure of correction with fluid restriction (class III data)[24,25]; successful treatment with mineralocorticoids (class III data)[25,26] or with administration of fluids and salt (class II data)[27]; and clinical biochemical results being

Pearl

Mounting evidence favors CSW over SIADH as the primary cause of hyponatremia in acutely ill neurological patients.

more consistent with CSW than SIADH (class III data).[28] Overall, these studies support the concept that CSW is a common cause of hyponatremia in patients with cerebral pathologies. Several articles nicely summarize the mounting evidence in favor of CSW over SIADH as the primary cause of hyponatremia in acutely ill neurologic patients.[6,21,29–34]

Differentiation Between Cerebral Salt Wasting and the Syndrome of Inappropriate Secretion of Antidiuretic Hormone

The differentiation between CSW and SIADH is critical because not only are the treatments different, but the incorrect choice of treatment may exacerbate conditions associated with hyponatremia. For example, a retrospective review of subarachnoid hemorrhage patients revealed that fluid restriction in patients with hyponatremia was associated with a higher risk of cerebral infarction (class III data).[35]

The physiologic changes in these two entities can be differentiated based on the mechanism of each disorder. Simplistically, CSW is a renal loss of sodium, and with it water. Conversely, SIADH is retention of free water, with a compensatory attempt at volume reduction by excretion of sodium. See Table 17-1 for a summary of clinical and laboratory findings used to differentiate CSW from SIADH.

The key factor distinguishing CSW from SIADH is hypovolemia (class II).[21,27] Clinically, patients with CSW show signs of dehydration such as poor skin turgor, lack of hand vein distention when in a dependent position, and dry mucous membranes. Orthostatic hypotension develops if dehydration is severe. A rapid weight loss with a negative fluid balance also suggests hypovolemia. If invasive monitoring is available, it will show that patients with CSW have a low central venous pressure, a low pulmonary capillary wedge pressure (in the absence of cardiac or pulmonary disease), and a low plasma volume.

Laboratory values consistent with CSW include markedly increased urinary sodium, mildly increased or normal urinary potassium, and increased or normal urine osmolality. The hematocrit and blood urea nitrogen (BUN) are elevated due to dehydration, and uric acid should be normal.

Table 17-1 Comparison of Findings in CSW and SIADH

Clinical Findings	CSW	SIADH
Dehydration symptoms	Present	Absent
Weight	Decreased	Increased
Fluid balance	Negative	Positive
Orthostatic hypotension	Likely	Possible
Central venous pressure	Decreased	Increased
Pulmonary capillary wedge pressure	Decreased	Increased
Plasma volume	Decreased	Increased
Laboratory Findings	**CSW**	**SIADH**
Urine sodium	Increased	Increased
Serum potassium	Increased or normal	Decreased or normal
Serum osmolality	Increased or normal	Decreased
Urine osmolality	Increased	Increased
Hematocrit	Increased	Decreased or normal
Urea nitrogen (BUN)	Increased	Normal
Uric acid	Normal	Decreased

Pearl

The key factor distinguishing CSW from SIADH is hypovolemia.

In SIADH, water is not excreted appropriately, so unlike CSW, the extracellular volume increases. Consequently, the glomerular filtration rate increases, the renin-angiotensin-aldosterone axis is suppressed, and atrial natriuretic peptide is secreted. Each of these responses leads to a paradoxical *increase* in urinary sodium excretion. The diagnosis is based on the findings of hypervolemic hyponatremia, serum hypo-osmolality, and an inappropriately high urine osmolality. A definitive diagnosis of SIADH can be made by observing an abnormal response to a water load test. However, because this test may exacerbate hyponatremia in patients who may already be volume-overloaded, it should be used judiciously in critically ill patients.

In a retrospective series of postoperative female neurosurgical patients in whom the average plasma sodium level reached 108 mEq/L, all 15 patients developed grand mal seizures, followed by respiratory arrest requiring intubation (class III data).[5] At that time, the urinary sodium concentration and osmolality averaged 68 mEq/L and 501 mOsm per kilogram, respectively, suggesting inappropriate secretion of antidiuretic hormone. Net postoperative fluid retention averaged 7.5 L.

Hypernatremia

It is likely that hypernatremia in head-injured patients is most commonly iatrogenic, although unrecognized diabetes insipidus (DI) can also result in rapid loss of free water and hypernatremia. DI may be caused by cranial base fractures and resultant hypothalamic and/or pituitary stalk injuries. In one retrospective military series, posttraumatic hypernatremia was seen in 8% of head-injured patients; one third of the hypernatremic patients died within 30 days of injury (class III data).[36] A retrospective review of neurosurgical patients who developed DI (most of whom suffered from subarachnoid hemorrhage or severe head injury) reported a mortality rate of 72% (class III data).[37] The diagnosis of DI is typically made after polyuria of over 200 mL/h for 3 hours accompanied by a urine specific gravity of 1.005 or less and a rising serum sodium concentration.

Background and Literature Review: Treatment of Hyper- and Hyponatremia

Class I studies aimed at defining the optimal treatment modality for hyponatremia in head-injured patients are not currently available. This problem is due, at least in part, to the continued controversy about the underlying etiology of hyponatremia in this patient population. Class II and III studies are reviewed below.

Treatment of Cerebral Salt Wasting (Table 17-2)

The treatment of CSW should be dictated by the magnitude of the hyponatremia, by the presence and severity of clinical symptoms, and by the degree to which the patient is at risk for complications of hyponatremia. For head-injured patients with brain swelling and/or hemorrhagic lesions on computed tomography scan, hyponatremia of any degree should be aggressively treated because of the potential for worsening brain swelling. In addition, hyponatremia may lower the seizure threshold in patients who are already predisposed to seizures because of traumatic brain injury. If hyponatremia develops in the acute postinjury period in such patients, rapid correction to mild hyponatremia or to a normal serum sodium level is generally well tolerated.

Pearl

If hyponatremia develops in the acute postinjury period in such patients, rapid correction to mild hyponatremia or to a normal serum sodium level is generally well tolerated.

Oral Salt

Administration of oral salt is the least intrusive method of sodium replacement. Its use is most reasonable when hyponatremia is mild; for example, serum sodium 130 to 134 mEq/L. Because patients must be capable of taking oral medication, this route is used most frequently with mild head injury patients (Glasgow Coma Scale score 13–15). The dose is typically 3 to 4 g three times a day. Administration with meals may minimize the development of resultant nausea (class III data).[27] Dehydrated patients must be rehydrated if this treatment is to be used, and normovolemic patients must be carefully monitored so they do not become dehydrated.

Hypertonic Saline

If the hyponatremia is more severe (serum sodium <130 mEq/L), or if the oral route is not available, intravenous hypertonic saline (usually 3% or 5%) can be administered. In a study of 58 patients with subarachnoid hemorrhage or head injury, hypertonic saline shortened the duration of hyponatremia by more than 60% compared with that in untreated patients, and hypertonic saline also appeared to reduce the duration of hyponatremia more than phenytoin, glucose/insulin/potassium therapy, or water restriction (class II data).[38]

Adequate sodium replacement can usually be achieved with 25 to 75 mL per hour of 3% NaCl. Typically, an infusion of 3% NaCl will initially raise serum sodium by 1 mEq/L/h if given at 1 mL/kg/h. Thus, in a 70-kg patient, a 70 mL/h infusion of 3% NaCl will initially raise serum sodium by ~1 mEq/L/h, whereas a 35 mL/h infusion will initially raise it by 0.5 mEq/L/h (class III data).[39] To monitor sodium repletion, serum sodium should be checked every 4 to 6 hours, and appropriate adjustments in the rate should be made to prevent hypernatremia or continued hyponatremia.

Sodium chloride solutions become more irritating and sclerosing to veins as they increase in tonicity, so central venous access may be necessary for 5% NaCl or high rates of 3% NaCl, though 25 to 30 mL/hour of 3% NaCl can be used for a few days in patients with good peripheral venous access.

The following is a useful formula for calculating the effect of treatment on serum sodium:

$$\text{Change in serum Na (mEq/L)} = \frac{\text{(Infusate Na} - \text{serum Na) (mEq/L)} \times \text{Volume of infusate (L)}}{\text{Total body water (L)}}$$

Table 17-2 Treatment Options for CSW and SIADH

CSW		
Treatment	**Dose or Amount**	**Recommendation Level**
Salt tablets or high dietary sodium	Up to 3–4 g orally three times a day with meals	Level III
Hypertonic saline	3% NaCl intravenously at 25–75 mL/h; check serum sodium every 4–6 hours	Level II
Fludrocortisone acetate	0.1–0.3 mg po daily (though doses up to 0.6 mg/day are supported in the literature, and 1 mg/day is used in patients with postural hypotension)	Level II
Urea	40 g urea in 100 to 150 mL normal saline intravenously q 8 hour	Level III
SIADH: Acute		
Treatment	**Dose or Amount**	**Recommendation Level**
Fluid restriction	Free water intake 500 mL less than daily urine output	Level III
Hypertonic saline	3% NaCl intravenously at 25–75 mL/h; check serum sodium every 6 hours; monitor fluid balance carefully to prevent fluid overload	Level III
Mannitol with furosemide	No standard dosing	Animal studies
SIADH: Chronic		
Treatment	**Dose or Amount**	**Data Class**
Fluid restriction	1200–1800 mL/d	Level III
Furosemide with oral sodium	20–40 mg furosemide daily + 3 g NaCl po three times a day	Level III
Urea	30–60 g po daily	Level III
Demeclocycline	300 mg po two to four times a day	Level III

Infusate Na in mEq/L can be calculated by %NaCl × 171, for example, 3% NaCl contains 513 mEq/L. Total body water in liters is a fraction of body mass in kilograms, which ranges from 0.6 in children and nonelderly men to 0.5 in nonelderly women and elderly men to 0.45 in elderly women (class III data).[40] These formulas do not consider sodium loss, so the difference between the calculated expected response to therapy and the actual response can give a rough estimate of how much sodium is being lost.

Fludrocortisone Acetate

Use of fludrocortisone acetate has become well established as an effective and safe alternative or additional treatment if the serum sodium concentration remains low despite maximal rates of sodium replacement (class III data).[25,26] Fludrocortisone is a potent mineralocorticoid with direct renal inhibition of natriuresis. Typical doses used to treat hyponatremia range from 0.1 to 0.3 mg/day, but doses as high as 0.6 mg/day have been used successfully without side effects[41] (class II data), and doses as high as 1 mg/day have been used in the treatment of chronic orthostatic hypotension (class III data).[42] Nevertheless, patients should be closely monitored for potential side effects (particularly the elderly), which include hypokalemia, hypertension, edema, and congestive heart failure.

Urea

Another option when maximum sodium replacement is still not able to offset sodium loss is urea. Urea is an osmotic diuretic that also inhibits natriuresis in the kidney. Urea allows a rapid reduction of brain edema and intracranial pressure, which is followed by subsequent correction of hyponatremia (class III data).[1] Experimental data also suggest that treatment of hyponatremia with urea is associated with a lower incidence of myelinolysis.[1]

Various treatment regimens have been described for both oral and intravenous forms of urea. Decaux et al[43] reported seven patients with hyponatremia treated by oral intake of two to three doses of 30 g of urea over 24 hours or infusion of 80 g of urea as a 30% solution over 6 hours, along with water restriction and sodium supplementation (class III data). In another report they described an additional patient treated similarly (class III data).[44] The regimen described by Reeder and Harbaugh[24] in 48 neurosurgical patients with hyponatremia from various causes consisted of 40 g urea dissolved in 100 to 150 mL normal saline as an intravenous drip every 8 hours (class III data). An average of 2.5 treatments was necessary to correct hyponatremia in a series of patients with delayed hyponatremia after transsphenoidal surgery (class III).[45] No treatment complications were reported in these series, though urea is contraindicated in patients with renal failure or advanced liver disease because of the potential for hyperammonemia and hepatic encephalopathy, respectively.

Treatment of Syndrome of Inappropriate Secretion of Antidiuretic Hormone (Table 17-2)

As with CSW, aggressiveness of treatment depends on the severity of hyponatremia, presence of symptoms, and risks of hyponatremia. If hyponatremia is known to have developed acutely, then rapid normalization is generally well tolerated.

Fluid Restriction

A conservative goal of fluid restriction in the asymptomatic or minimally symptomatic patient is to limit daily water intake to 500 mL less than daily urine output.

Hypertonic Saline

Intravenous 3% NaCl administered at 25 to 75 mL/h may be considered for the correction of symptomatic, severe hyponatremia. Frequent checks of serum sodium every 6 hours or at similarly frequent intervals should be considered, and fluid balance should be monitored carefully to prevent fluid overload.

Furosemide

Fluid restriction limits can be eased by using furosemide to increase excretion of water. Furosemide generally induces a diuresis equivalent to half-normal saline by inhibiting reabsorption of Na^+ and Cl^- predominantly in the ascending limb of the loop of Henle. An initial dose of 20 to 40 mg/day can be used, depending on how positive the fluid balance is. Patients can then be taught to monitor their daily weight as an indicator of their volume status and to adjust the medication dose up or down as needed without significantly restricting fluids (class III data).[46] It is important to maintain a high-salt diet and to monitor potassium levels to compensate for the increased urinary excretion of sodium and potassium.

Urea

As discussed above for CSW, urea is an osmotic diuretic that inhibits natriuresis in the kidney and can be given both intravenously and orally. Urea may be used as an adjunctive outpatient treatment, allowing patients to be less strict with water restriction (class III data).[47] Oral doses of 30 to 60 g/day are usually sufficient to aid in increasing water excretion and decreasing sodium excretion while minimizing the development of azotemia. The most common complaint regarding oral urea is poor palatability.

Mannitol

This osmotic diuretic is very effective in causing excretion of free water. Rats that were administered hypotonic saline, a loop diuretic, vasopressin, and labeled mannitol by the intraperitoneal route excreted a predictable volume of free water because the urine was iso-osmotic to plasma and contained *all* of the administered mannitol within 210 minutes.[48] If mannitol happens to be retained, the measured serum osmolality will be much higher than the serum osmolality calculated on the basis of the hyponatremia because mannitol contributes to oncotic pressure; therefore, the risk of cerebral edema is greatly reduced (class III data).[49]

Demeclocycline

Demeclocycline is known to produce a reversible nephrogenic DI. Patients lose weight, and biochemical features of SIADH are rapidly corrected despite an unchanged fluid intake and persistence of high plasma levels of ADH. The typical oral dose is 300 mg two to four times daily.[50] The effect of treatment may not be seen for several days,[51] so 3 to 4 days should be allowed to pass between dosage increases. Acute renal failure was observed in one patient treated with 2400 mg/24 hours, possibly because of a nephrotoxic effect of high circulating levels of demeclocycline (class III data).[52] Renal function returned to normal after the demeclocycline was stopped.

Vasopressin Antagonists

In the near future, vasopressin antagonists will become available for clinical use. In 1992, an oral nonpeptide antagonist to the V2 receptor in the kidney was described.[53] Since then, several comparable agents with similar effects have been developed. All increase urinary volume and decrease urinary osmolality.[54] Preliminary experience has already demonstrated their efficacy in inducing a sustained water diuresis and a correction of hyponatremia in human patients with SIADH (class II data).[55,56]

Treatment of Hypernatremia

Mild hypernatremia is easily treated by administering more free water; for example, by changing to a less concentrated saline solution for intravenous infusions and/or by administering repeated small boluses of water through enteral feeding tubes.

In patients who are awake and alert, mild DI can be adequately treated by ensuring that patients have unlimited access to water because most patients will drink enough to compensate for mild impairments in ability to concentrate urine. Hypernatremia from more severe forms of DI can be treated with 0.5 to 2 μg of DDAVP subcutaneously or intravenously every 8 to 12 hours. Alternatively, the shorter-acting aqueous form of vasopressin can be given in a dose of 5 to 10 units intramuscularly[57] or subcutaneously two to four times a day or as a continuous infusion at a rate of 1 to 3 units per hour (carefully titrated to urine output). Finally, DDAVP may be administered intranasally.[58] The recommended intranasal dose is 10 to 40 μg daily, administered as a single dose or divided into as many as three separate doses.

Recommendations

Upper and Lower Limits for Serum Sodium in Head-Injured Patients

Currently available data suggest that both hyponatremia and hypernatremia may result in secondary cerebral insults and increased morbidity in head-injured patients. In one sense, marked hyponatremia may be more deleterious (because of potential exacerbation of cerebral edema) than hypernatremia. As a level III recommendation, every attempt should be made to maintain normonatremia in head-injured patients. A reasonable target for serum sodium concentration is 135 to 150 mEq/L.

Treatment

Attempts should be made to identify the etiology of sodium abnormalities in head-injured patients so that treatment can be tailored to the specific cause. Until such an etiology is identified, or in the absence of a clear etiology, it is most prudent to treat hyponatremia with therapies that raise serum sodium without restricting free water, such as hypertonic saline (level II for CSW), fludrocortisone acetate (level II for CSW), or intravenous urea (level III for CSW and SIADH). Care should be taken to avoid rates of sodium correction in excess of 15 mEq/L per day to avoid the risk of central myelinolysis (level III).

Hypernatremia is best treated by careful administration of more free water, by restricting the amount of sodium administered to a patient, and, in severe cases, by administration of DDAVP to decrease renal excretion of water (level III).

References

1. Soupart A, Decaux G. Therapeutic recommendations for management of severe hyponatremia: current concepts on pathogenesis and prevention of neurologic complications. Clin Nephrol 1996;46:149–169.
2. Dóczi T, Tarjányi J, Huszka E, et al. Syndrome of inappropriate secretion of antidiuretic hormone (SIADH) after head injury. Neurosurgery 1982;10:685–688.
3. DeFronzo RA, Arieff AI. Hyponatremia: pathophysiology and treatment. In: Arieff AI, DeFronzo RA, eds. Fluid, Electrolyte and Acid-Base Disorders, 2nd ed. New York: Churchill Livingstone, 1995:255–303.
4. Unterberg A, Kiening K, Schmiedek P, et al. Long-term observations of intracranial pressure after severe head injury: the phenomenon of secondary rise of intracranial pressure. Neurosurgery 1993;32:17–24.
5. Arieff AI. Hyponatremia, convulsions, respiratory arrest, and permanent brain damage after elective surgery in healthy women. N Engl J Med 1986;314:1529–1535.
6. Bracco D, Favre JB, Ravussin P. Hyponatremia in neurologic intensive care: cerebral salt wasting syndrome and inappropriate antidiuretic hormone secretion. Ann Fr Anesth Reanim 2001;20:203–212.
7. Hasan D, Wijdicks EF, Vermeulen M. Hyponatremia is associated with cerebral ischemia in patients with aneurysmal subarachnoid hemorrhage. Ann Neurol 1990;27:106–108.
8. Arieff AI, Llach F, Massry SG. Neurological manifestations and morbidity of hyponatremia: correlation with brain water and electrolytes. Medicine (Baltimore) 1976;55:121–129.
9. De Troyer A, Demanet JC. Clinical, biological and pathogenic features of the syndrome of inappropriate secretion of antidiuretic hormone. A review of 26 cases with marked hyponatraemia. Q J Med 1976;45:521–531.
10. Peters JP, Welt LG, Sims EAH, et al. A salt wasting syndrome associated with cerebral disease. Trans Assoc Am Physicians 1950;63:57–64.
11. Welt LG, Selden DW, Nelson WI, et al. Role of the central nervous system in metabolism of electrolytes and water. Arch Intern Med 1952;90:355–378.
12. Cort JH. Cerebral salt wasting. Lancet 1954;1:752–754.
13. Schwartz WB, Bennet W, Curelop S, et al. A syndrome of renal sodium loss and hyponatremia probably resulting from inappropriate secretion of antidiuretic hormone. Am J Med 1957;23: 529–542.
14. Hald T, Holm HH, Nielsen B. Head injury followed by transient hyponatremia, probably caused by inappropriate antidiuresis. Acta Neurol Scand 1967;43:530–534.
15. Davis BP, Matukas VJ. Inappropriate secretion of antidiuretic hormone after cerebral injury. J Oral Surg 1976;34:609–615.
16. Imbert Y, Peroua JJ, Coomans D, et al. Inappropriate secretion of antidiuretic hormone (ISADH) after head injury. Sem Hop 1982;58:1151–1154.
17. Shenkin HA, Bezier HS, Bouzarth WF. Restricted fluid intake: rational management of the neurosurgical patient. J Neurosurg 1976;45:432–436.
18. Steinbok P, Thompson GB. Metabolic disturbances after head injury: abnormalities of sodium and water balance with special reference to the effects of alcohol intoxication. Neurosurgery 1978;3:9–15.
19. Nelson PB, Seif SM, Maroon JC, et al. Hyponatremia in intracranial disease: perhaps not the syndrome of inappropriate secretion of antidiuretic hormone (SIADH). J Neurosurg 1981;55:938–941.
20. Wijdicks EF, Vermeulen M, ten Haaf JA, et al. Volume depletion and natriuresis in patients with a ruptured intracranial aneurysm. Ann Neurol 1985;18:211–216.
21. Sivakumar V, Rajshekhar V, Chandy MJ. Management of neurosurgical patients with hyponatremia and natriuresis. Neurosurgery 1994;34:269–274.
22. Yamamoto N, Miyamoto N, Seo H, et al. Hyponatremia with high plasma ANP level—report of two cases with emphasis on the pathophysiology of cerebral salt wasting. No Shinkei Geka 1987;15:1019–1023.
23. Zerbe R, Stropes L, Robertson G. Vasopressin function in the syndrome of inappropriate antidiuresis. Annu Rev Med 1980; 31:315–327.
24. Reeder RF, Harbaugh RE. Administration of intravenous urea and normal saline for the treatment of hyponatremia in neurosurgical patients. J Neurosurg 1989;70:201–206.
25. Kawajiri K, Matsuoka Y, Kan M. Cerebral salt wasting syndrome secondary to head injury: a case report. No Shinkei Geka 1992;20:1003–1007.
26. Ishikawa SE, Saito T, Kaneko K, et al. Hyponatremia responsive to fludrocortisone acetate in elderly patients after head injury. Ann Intern Med 1987;106:187–191.
27. Damaraju SC, Rajshekhar V, Chandy MJ. Validation study of a central venous pressure-based protocol for the management of

neurosurgical patients with hyponatremia and natriuresis. Neurosurgery 1997;40:312–317.
28. Lolin Y, Jackowski A. Hyponatraemia in neurosurgical patients: diagnosis using derived parameters of sodium and water homeostasis. Br J Neurosurg 1992;6:457–466.
29. Betjes MG, Koopmans RP. Hyponatremia in acute intracranial disorders: cerebral salt wasting. Ned Tijdschr Geneeskd 2000; 144:553–556.
30. Harrigan MR. Cerebral salt wasting syndrome: a review. Neurosurgery 1996;38:152–160.
31. Harrigan MR. Cerebral salt wasting syndrome. Crit Care Clin 2001;17:125–138.
32. Maesaka JK, Gupta S, Fishbane S. Cerebral salt-wasting syndrome: does it exist? Nephron 1999;82:100–109.
33. Uygun MA, Ozkal E, Acar O, et al. Cerebral salt wasting syndrome. Neurosurg Rev 1996;19:193–196.
34. Zafonte RD, Mann NR. Cerebral salt wasting syndrome in brain injury patients: a potential cause of hyponatremia. Arch Phys Med Rehabil 1997;78:540–542.
35. Wijdicks EF, Vermeulen M, Hijdra A, et al. Hyponatremia and cerebral infarction in patients with ruptured intracranial aneurysms: is fluid restriction harmful? Ann Neurol 1985;17:137–140.
36. Bacic A, Gluncic I, Gluncic V. Disturbances in plasma sodium in patients with war head injuries. Mil Med 1999;164:214–217.
37. Wong MF, Chin NM, Lew TW. Diabetes insipidus in neurosurgical patients. Ann Acad Med Singapore 1998;27:340–343.
38. Morinaga K, Tabuse H, Ohkawara S. Mechanism and therapy of hyponatremia with central origin. No Shinkei Geka 1989;17: 539–544.
39. Verbalis JG. Adaptation to acute and chronic hyponatremia: implications for symptomatology, diagnosis, and therapy. Semin Nephrol 1998;18:3–19.
40. Adrogué HJ, Madias NE. Hyponatremia. N Engl J Med 2000; 342:1493–1499.
41. Morinaga K, Hayashi S, Matsumoto Y, et al. Therapeutic effect of a mineralocorticoid in patients with hyponatremia of central origin. No To Shinkei 1995;47:671–674.
42. Kochar MS. Management of postural hypotension. Curr Hypertens Rep 2000;2:457–462.
43. Decaux G, Unger J, Brimioulle S, et al. Hyponatremia in the syndrome of inappropriate secretion of antidiuretic hormone: rapid correction with urea, sodium chloride, and water restriction therapy. JAMA 1982;247:471–474.
44. Decaux G, Unger J, Mockel J. Urea therapy for inappropriate antidiuretic hormone secretion from tuberculous meningitis. JAMA 1980;244:589–590.
45. Kelly DF, Laws ER Jr, Fossett D. Delayed hyponatremia after transsphenoidal surgery for pituitary adenoma: report of nine cases. J Neurosurg 1995;83:363–367.
46. Decaux G, Waterlot Y, Genette F, et al. Treatment of the syndrome of inappropriate secretion of antidiuretic hormone with furosemide. N Engl J Med 1981;304:329–330.
47. Decaux G, Genette F. Urea for long-term treatment of syndrome of inappropriate secretion of antidiuretic hormone. Br Med J (Clin Res Ed) 1981;283:1081–1083.
48. Porzio P, Halberthal M, Bohn D, et al. Treatment of acute hyponatremia: ensuring the excretion of a predictable amount of electrolyte-free water. Crit Care Med 2000;28:1905–1910.
49. Oster JR, Singer I. Hyponatremia, hyposmolality, and hypotonicity: tables and fables. Arch Intern Med 1999;159:333–336.
50. Perks WH, Walters EH, Tams IP, et al. Demeclocycline in the treatment of the syndrome of inappropriate secretion of antidiuretic hormone. Thorax 1979;34:324–327.
51. Miyagawa CI. The pharmacologic management of the syndrome of inappropriate secretion of antidiuretic hormone. Drug Intell Clin Pharm 1986;20:527–531.
52. Padfield PL, Hodsman GP, Morton JJ. Demeclocycline in the treatment of the syndrome of inappropriate antidiuretic hormone release: with measurement of plasma ADH. Postgrad Med J 1978;54:623–627.
53. Yamamura Y, Ogawa H, Yamashita H, et al. Characterization of a novel aquaretic agent, OPC-31260, as an orally effective, nonpeptide vasopressin V2 receptor antagonist. Br J Pharmacol 1992;105:787–791.
54. Palm C, Reimann D, Gross P. The role of V2 vasopressin antagonists in hyponatremia. Cardiovasc Res 2001;51: 403–408.
55. Kuhn K, Reimann D, Gross P. Beneficial effects of V_2-vasopressin-antagonist (ANTAG) in the hyponatremia (HYPO) of clinical cardiac failure (CHF), SIADH, and liver cirrhosis (CI). Kidney Blood Press Res 1998;21:183.
56. Saito T, Ishikawa S, Abe K, et al. Acute aquaresis by the nonpeptide arginine vasopressin (AVP) antagonist OPC-31260 improves hyponatremia in patients with syndrome of inappropriate secretion of antidiuretic hormone (SIADH). J Clin Endocrinol Metab 1997;82:1054–1057.
57. Shucart WA, Jackson I. Management of diabetes insipidus in neurosurgical patients. J Neurosurg 1976;44:65–71.
58. Coculescu M, Antipa C, Cucu C. Effects of DDAVP in cranial diabetes insipidus as compared to other antidiuretic drugs. Endocrinologie 1977;15:275–281.

◆ 18 ◆

When Should Follow-Up Computed Tomography Scans Be Obtained?

John A. Lopez and J. Paul Elliott

BRIEF ANSWER

The evidence supports a level III recommendation for use of serial computed tomography (CT) for clinical management and determination of prognosis following severe traumatic brain injury (TBI). However, use of serial CT scans to improve patient outcome can be supported only as a level III recommendation.

Background

Clearly, CT scans have improved our understanding of the evolution of TBI. In their 1977 seminal study on the value of head CT, French and Dublin[1] reported a 52% incidence of new lesions or progression of known lesions in their patients who had two or more CT scans following TBI (class III data). However, no prospective randomized controlled trials have evaluated serial head CT scanning in TBI patients. Identification of the optimal number and timing of follow-up head CT scans in these patients requires further evaluation with respect to outcome-based measures.

Pearl

Although entry criteria and patient populations vary, several studies have documented that more than half of head-injured patients demonstrate new findings on repeat head CT scans.

Literature Review

Determining Prognosis with Serial Computed Tomography Scans

Several studies have provided evidence that serial CT scanning may be helpful in predicting outcome. Kobayashi et al[2] (class III data) performed serial CT scanning on 138 patients with severe head injuries [Glasgow Coma Scale (GCS) score ≤8). Scans were obtained upon admission (within hours of the injury) and after 1, 3, and 7 days, and after 1 month. New findings (not visualized on the initial CT scan) were seen in 91 of the 138 patients, and significant new lesions were found in 60 of the 91 patients. A significant correlation existed between the development of new lesions and poor outcome at the time of discharge. The authors concluded that serial CT scanning can help to predict outcome in severe TBI patients and that serial scans are especially useful when clinical symptoms may be masked by therapy.

Cooper et al[3] (class III data) also found that serial CT scanning was useful in prognostic assessments and that it may also be of value in improving the accuracy of clinical assessment. Their study found that follow-up CT scans demonstrated new lesions in 30 of 58 patients (52%) and that the development of new lesions was strongly associated with a bad outcome. The authors could not find any evidence that operation or reoperation indicated by the results of repeat CT scanning actually improved outcome.

Lobato et al[4] found that 51% of 587 severely head-injured patients demonstrated CT changes that were significant enough to change their initially assigned category (either worse or better) on the Marshall CT classification scale (class III data). Of the 587 patients, 97% had their first repeat scan within 3 days after injury, with the average interval between the first and second scan being 37 hours. Final outcomes were more closely correlated with the repeat scans than with the initial CT diagnoses. Thus, a pathologic categorization made by using an early repeat scan rather than the initial scan might be most useful for prognostic purposes. The authors recommended follow-up CT scanning within the first 2 days after injury.

Pearl

The appearance of new lesions has been associated with a poor prognosis after TBI, but it has been difficult to show that prompt detection and evacuation of these new lesions improves outcome.

Serial Computed Tomography Scans in Clinical Management

It is well known that lesions accompanying TBI evolve over time. However, even though the literature suggests that sequential CT scanning can help in the diagnosis of new lesions, and even though sequential CT scanning following TBI is a common practice, it is not clear that more expeditious detection of new lesions necessarily improves outcome. To complicate this issue further, the proliferation of CT scanners in general hospitals and improvements in trauma systems and in patient transport practices have reduced the interval between head injury and initial CT scan in many regions. As a result, it has become more likely that an admission scan may demonstrate a lesion very early in its course, before it has reached its most dramatic appearance. Since appropriate timing of follow-up CT scans remains poorly defined except for a few specific lesions, and since different lesions appear to have different propensities to progress, the safest strategy may be to tailor serial scanning to the type of lesions found on the initial CT scan and to the postinjury time at which the initial scan was obtained.

Based on an analysis of the European Brain Injury Consortium database, Servadei et al[5] recommended a follow-up CT scan whenever the initial scan reveals evidence of diffuse injury (level III recommendation). They found that one in six such patients demonstrates significant CT evolution of the lesions. When the initial scan revealed Marshall-type II, III, and IV diffuse injuries,[6] subsequent scans had high rates of progression to mass lesions (13–14% for types II and III and 20% for type IV). The authors suggested that a CT scan be repeated within 12 hours whenever the initial scan was obtained within 3 hours of injury and within 24 hours in all other instances (level III recommendation). A third scan was recommended on the third day after trauma, although the authors acknowledged that this recommendation was empiric.

Compared with other types of brain injuries, traumatic intracerebral hematomas and epidural hematomas probably have the greatest propensity to expand. Yamaki et al[7] (class III data) performed a retrospective review of 48 patients who developed a traumatic intracerebral hemorrhage $\geqslant$3 cm in diameter at some point during their acute hospitalization. The initial scan was performed between 0.5 and 6 hours after the head injury. Traumatic intracerebral hematomas $>$3 cm in diameter developed in 56% of patients within 6 hours, in 81% of patients within 12 hours, and in 100% of patients within 24 hours of the initial trauma. Servadei et al[8] (class III data) also found that the lesions that are most prone to enlarge are epidural hematomas and intracerebral hemorrhages. Performance of the initial CT scan within 3 hours of the initial trauma did not exclude rapid evolution of a new mass lesion or expansion of a lesion identified initially. They recommended that a follow-up CT scan be obtained within 12 hours in patients in whom the first scan was obtained within 3 hours of the initial injury.

Pearl

Lesions seen on CT scans that have been performed within 3 to 6 hours of injury may not yet have reached their ultimate size.

Knuckey et al[9] (class III data) studied "asymptomatic" epidural hematomas and found 6 hours to be the critical time for evaluation. Deterioration was seen in 43% of those with an initial CT scan performed within 6 hours of injury and in 55% of patients with a skull fracture traversing the middle meningeal artery or a major venous sinus. Furthermore, 71% of patients with both risk factors required evacuation of the epidural hematoma. Interestingly, only 13% of patients with a small epidural hematoma that was diagnosed on a scan obtained more than 6 hours after injury subsequently required surgical evacuation of the hematoma.

Pearl

Consideration should be given to reevaluating a nonoperative acute epidural hematoma by follow-up CT scanning at 6 hours after injury.

Specific clinical factors may suggest a propensity for a lesion to expand. Follow-up CT scanning may be more appropriate when such factors are present. Stein et al[10] (class III data) found that the appearance of delayed cerebral insults on follow-up CT scans was significantly associated with the severity of the initial brain injury and with the presence of coagulopathy on admission. They found serial CT scanning to be useful in defining and monitoring the development of delayed brain injury. They recommended a follow-up scan immediately in all patients who deteriorate or at 12 to 24 hours after admission in patients with coagulopathy or incomplete recovery.

Although most studies of serial CT scanning have focused on severely injured patients, serial CT scanning has also been reported to be useful in minor and moderate head injury. The Study Group on Head Injury of the Italian Society for Neurosurgery[11] (class III data) recognized the relationship between coagulopathy and the propensity for new lesions to develop in patients with minor head injury. They recommended that coagulopathic patients with minor head injury undergo repeat CT scanning prior to discharge even when the initial scan did not demonstrate an intracranial lesion. In a retrospective analysis of 341 patients with moderate head injury (GCS score 9 to 12), Stein et al[12] (class III data) noted that most patients with normal or near-normal scans improve within hours. They recommended a second CT scan 12 hours after admission for any patient who deteriorates or who fails to achieve a GCS score of 14 or 15 by that time. Almost 50% of their patients required a follow-up scan because of clinical deterioration or failure to improve, and 32% of those demonstrated radiologic deterioration.

Although it seems reasonable that better diagnosis would improve outcome, there exists little direct evidence linking follow-up CT scanning to an improved clinical outcome. Turazzi et al,[13] however, argued that the systematic repetition of CT scans could be a major factor in preventing the worsening of a patient's clinical status (class III data). Patients in their study were treated with initial CT scans on admission and then daily thereafter regardless of their clinical status (every patient was scanned at least three times). They compared this series to a historical control group from the era immediately preceding the advent of CT scanning. They found that serial CT scanning made it easier to operate on patients with new or expanding lesions before they deteriorated to a GCS score of 8 or less. To establish cause and effect, however, a study of this type would require more clearly defined end points.

Follow-Up Scans May Not Always Be Useful

Although the majority of studies argue that scheduled repeat scans are of some use in prognosis and clinical management, other studies have found them to be of limited value. In their early study of serial CT scanning, Roberson et al[14] (class III data) investigated the value of prearranged routine sequential CT scanning of patients with severe head injury. They performed serial CT scans prospectively on 107 comatose patients on days 1 (the day of admission), 3, 5, and 7, and at 2 weeks and 3 months postinjury and, in some patients, at 1 year. They found that repeat CT scans were unproductive if the initial scan was normal and the patient showed clinical improvement. Although 18% of patients in this category developed some new CT abnormality, none required surgical treatment or a change in their clinical management. In no instances did prearranged CT scanning reveal unsuspected surgical mass lesions when neurologic status and intracranial pressure (ICP) were being monitored. The study's final recommendations were to repeat CT scans at 24 hours after craniotomy; in patients not improving by day 3 postinjury; and after 2 to 3 weeks, after 3 months, and, if the patient's condition remained abnormal, at 1 year postinjury. Of course, a repeat CT scan should be performed immediately for clinical deterioration.

Another important issue is the complication rate associated with transport of critically ill patients for a CT scan when the scan may be of low yield. The risk of secondary injury, such as hypotension or hypoxia, may be significant during prolonged "road trips," especially in the multiply injured patient. In a retrospective review of the medical records of 117 patients with moderate or severe head injury, Lee et al[15] (class III data) concluded that follow-up CT scans should be obtained only for clinical deterioration unexplained by ICP changes alone. They found a positive correlation between change in CT scan and change in GCS score; that is, when patients had an unchanged or improved GCS score, 73.1% had an improved or unchanged CT scan appearance, but when patients had a decreased GCS score, the CT scan was worse in 77.9%. Importantly, there was a 16.9% complication rate, including hemodynamic instability and increased ICP, during follow-up scanning. This rate was higher in severe TBI patients than in those with moderate TBI.

Pearl

Transport of severely injured patients to the radiology department may be associated with a high complication rate.

Few studies have specifically investigated the utility of follow-up CT scans in patients with nonoperative lesions on their initial head CT scans. Muszynski et al[16] (class III data) retrospectively studied the role of serial CT scans in the nonoperative management of 41 patients with extraaxial intracranial hematomas and a midline shift of less than 0.5 cm. They found that the follow-up CT examinations did not specifically alter the decisions to manage the patients nonoperatively because the patients remained clinically stable. They concluded that the clinical examination remains the most important factor in determining management. In 11% of patients, however, follow-up CT scanning did alert the physician to an increase in the size of the hematomas, which may have prompted closer observation in this group.

Recommendations

The current literature supports a level III recommendation for follow-up CT scanning in head-injured patients in the first 24 hours after the initial traumatic event.

Several additional level III recommendations can be made. Several of these were not explicitly discussed in this chapter, but we feel that they are reasonable based on a careful review of the literature and on our personal experience. An initial head CT should be performed when TBI is suspected or known to have occurred. When an acute, nonoperative small epidural hematoma is present, a repeat scan should be obtained in 6 hours. For the remainder of nonoperative lesions, a repeat CT scan should be obtained at 12 to 24 hours, or sooner if neurologic deterioration or increased ICP occurs. We believe that all patients should receive an immediate head CT scan following surgery for TBI to serve as a baseline in the event of subsequent decline in neurologic status or increase in ICP. The ordering of subsequent CT scans is tailored to the individual case, guided principally by clinical examination and ICP. Finally, we recommend a head CT scan in patients with significant neurologic abnormality just prior to their transfer to a subacute care facility.

References

1. French BN, Dublin AB. The value of computerized tomography in the management of 1000 consecutive head injuries. Surg Neurol 1977;7:171–183.
2. Kobayashi S, Nakazawa S, Otsuka T. Clinical value of serial computed tomography with severe head injury. Surg Neurol 1983;20:25–29.
3. Cooper PR, Maravilla K, Moody S, et al. Serial computerized tomographic scanning and the prognosis of severe head injury. Neurosurgery 1979;5:566–569.
4. Lobato RD, Gomez PA, Alday R, et al. Sequential computerized tomography changes and related final outcome in severe head injury patients. Acta Neurochir (Wien) 1997;139:385–391.
5. Servadei F, Murray GD, Penny K, et al. The value of the "worst" computed tomographic scan in clinical studies of moderate and severe head injury. Neurosurgery 2000;46:70–77.
6. Marshall LF, Marshall SB, Klauber MR, et al. A new classification of head injury based on computerized tomography. J Neurosurg 1991;75:S14–S20.
7. Yamaki T, Hirakawa K, Ueguchi T, et al. Chronological evaluation of acute traumatic intracerebral haematoma. Acta Neurochir (Wien) 1990;103:112–115.
8. Servadei F, Nanni A, Nasi MT, et al. Evolving brain lesions in the first 12 hours after head injury: analysis of 37 comatose patients. Neurosurgery 1995;37:899–907.
9. Knuckey NW, Gelbard S, Epstein MH. The management of "asymptomatic" epidural hematomas: a prospective study. J Neurosurg 1989;70:392–396.
10. Stein SC, Spettell C, Young G, et al. Delayed and progressive brain injury in closed-head trauma: radiological demonstration. Neurosurgery 1993;32:25–31.
11. The Study Group on Head Injury of the Italian Society for Neurosurgery. Guidelines for minor head injured patients' management in adult age. J Neurosurg Sci 1996;40:11–15.
12. Stein SC, Ross SE. Moderate head injury: a guide to initial management. J Neurosurg 1992;77:562–564.
13. Turazzi S, Bricolo A, Pasut ML, et al. Changes produced by CT scanning in the outlook of severe head injury. Acta Neurochir (Wien) 1987;85:87–95.
14. Roberson FC, Kishore PR, Miller JD, et al. The value of serial computerized tomography in the management of severe head injury. Surg Neurol 1979;12:161–167.
15. Lee TT, Aldana PR, Kirton OC, et al. Follow-up computerized tomography (CT) scans in moderate and severe head injuries: correlation with Glasgow Coma Scores (GCS), and complication rate. Acta Neurochir (Wien) 1997;139:1042–1048.
16. Muszynski CA, Hayman LA, Weingarten K, et al. Conservative management of extra-axial hematomas diagnosed by CT. Neuroradiology 1999;41:875–881.

Do Patients with Intracranial Pressure Monitors Need Prophylactic Antibiotics?

Daniel B. Michael

Brief Answer

The literature contains conflicting evidence about the benefits and risks of prophylactic antibiotics for preventing infection of intracranial pressure (ICP) monitors. Several studies supporting prophylactic antibiotic use also demonstrate increased incidence of infection due to unusual or resistant microorganisms. The currently available evidence supports a recommendation (level III) that patients with ICP monitors do not need prophylactic antibiotics other than a single dose of cefazolin 30 minutes prior to the start of the procedure.

Background

The modern era of ICP monitoring began with the report of the use of intraventricular catheters by Guillaume and Janny in 1951.[1] Despite subsequent advances in technology, the ventriculostomy catheter remains the "gold standard" among ICP monitoring devices. Its widespread use is often considered to be a factor in the improved outcome of neurotrauma patients when compared with earlier outcomes (despite lack of class I evidence to support this assumption).[2]

The most common complications of ventriculostomy catheters are hemorrhage, overdrainage, and infection.[3] The first two may be minimized by meticulous surgical technique, by careful regulation of the amount of cerebrospinal fluid (CSF) drained, and by monitoring of the patient's clinical condition while ventricular drainage is being used.

ICP monitor infection has been the subject of investigation, speculation, and controversy for over 30 years. The following factors have been thought to affect the risk of infection: experience and technique of the surgeon; setting of procedure; type of monitor placed; duration of monitoring; patient's underlying pathology; leakage or flushing of the drainage system; use of steroids; other concurrent infection; and use of prophylactic antibiotics. The infection rates of ICP monitors in selected publications range from zero to 26.8%, with an overall rate of ~7.7% (Table 19-1).

The vast majority of published studies examining risk factors for infection of ICP monitors have been retrospective (class III or, at best, class II). Caution must be used in interpreting such data. Early series showed increased infection in devices that had been in place for a long time, leading some authors to suggest that ventriculostomies should be routinely changed at certain intervals to reduce the chance of infection (class II and class III data).[4,5] At least one early study, however, did not support duration of use as a significant risk factor.[6]

Pearl

Although early series suggested that ventriculostomies should be routinely changed at certain intervals to reduce the chance of infection, subsequent studies have suggested that such a practice may not be necessary.

Table 19-1 Antibiotic Prophylaxis for Intracranial Pressure Monitors

First Author	Year	Class	Total Patients	Infections (%)	Comment Conclusion
Rebuck[13] (included nonventricul-ostomies)	2000	III	215	16 (7.4%)	Risk of infection same with or without antibiotics (given before or at time of insertion)
Alleyne[12]	2000	III	308	12 (3.9%)	Risk of infection same with or without antibiotics (given after insertion procedure)
Zingale[16]	1999	III	143	15 (10.5%)	Recommended prophylactic antibiotics
Jacobs[11] (nonventricul-ostomies only)	1998	III	14	0	Long-term antibiotic prophylaxis is potentially harmful (more sepsis and pneumonia)
Poon[10]	1998	I	228	15 (6.6%)	Prophylaxis (beyond time of insertion) decreased infection but selected resistant organisms
Guyot[3]	1998	III	274	20 (7.3%)	Increased infection rate in ventriculostomy vs. intraparenchymal devices
Kahn[17]	1998	III	104	5 (4.8%)	Trend toward increased infection rate in ventriculostomy vs. intraparenchymal devices
Holloway[7]	1996	II	584	61 (10.4%)	Routine replacement of venticulostomy does not reduce infection
Bader[15]	1995	III	75	0	All patients received long-term prophylaxis
Paramore[18]	1994	III	135	9 (6.7%)	Calls for prospective study
Bogdahn[19]	1992	III	94	1/63 (1.6%) without CSF leak; 4/31 (12.9%) with CSF leak	Drainage system was flushed three times a day with gentamicin; higher infection rate associated with CSF leakage beside bedside catheter
Clark[5] (included nonventricul-ostomies)	1989	III	140	12 (8.6%)	Risk of infection same with or without antibiotics
Sundbarg[20]	1988	III	648	25 (3.9%)	Duration of monitoring is "of subordinate importance for the development of infection"
Aucoin[21]	1986	III	41	11(26.8%)	Risk of infection same with or without prophylactic antibiotics
Kanter[6] (included nonventricul-ostomies)	1985	III	65	9 (13.8%)	All patients received antibiotic prophylaxis
Mayhall[4]	1984	II	172	19 (11.0%)	Risk of infection same with or without antibiotics (given at time of insertion and for one day following)
Rosner[9] (included nonventricul-ostomies)	1976	III	112	20 (17.9%)	Risk of infection same with or without antibiotics
Smith[22]	1976	III	56	3 (5.4%)	Recommended antibiotic prophylaxis for duration of monitoring
Wyler[8]	1972	III	70	11 (15.7%)	Antibiotic prophylaxis for duration of monitoring decreases infection
TOTAL			3478	268 (7.7%)	

Later, a well-designed class II study failed to support the hypothesis that the risk:benefit ratio of routine catheter replacement was favorable.[7]

As used in this chapter, "prophylactic" use of antibiotics refers to intravenous administration at the time of insertion of an ICP monitor, with continued scheduled dosing until the device has been removed. Only one class I study examining this question has been published to date. The remainder of the studies report class II or class III data.

Literature Review

Table 19-1 summarizes selected studies pertinent to the question of prophylactic use of antibiotics in patients with ICP monitors. The classes of evidence provided by these studies may be summarized as follows: 16 studies report class III data, two studies describe class II evidence, and one study contains class I data.

In 1972 Wyler and Kelly[8] reported a series of 102 ventriculostomies in 70 patients. In this class III review, prophylactic ampicillin reduced the infection rate from 27 to 9%. Three of the four infections in the prophylactic group were due to coagulase-positive *Staphylococcus* spp., whereas the fourth was due to *Serratia* sp. The authors concluded that prophylactic antibiotics should be used, and they recommended a more aggressive regimen of either intravenous methicillin or oral cloxacillin to provide better coverage against the gram-positive cocci that caused most of their infections; these organisms were usually coagulase-positive in patients who developed infections despite antibiotic prophylaxis.

Rosner and Becker[9] performed another retrospective, multivariate analysis of complications of ICP monitors. They identified monitoring duration but not antibiotic prophylaxis as a significant risk factor for infection in this class III study.

Mayhall et al[4] published a prospective series of ventriculostomies that was not randomized with respect to antibiotic use. This class II study reported on two groups: a group receiving no antibiotic prophylaxis, and a group receiving no more than four doses of nafcillin within the first 24 hours of the procedure. The overall infection rate was 11%: 12.9% in the prophylactic group and 6.1% in the group receiving no antibiotics. However, the difference between the groups was not significant, and the authors did not identify antibiotic use as a significant determinant of ventriculostomy infection.

Poon et al[10] have reported the only class I study specifically designed to examine antibiotic prophylaxis in ventriculostomy. This study from the Prince of Wales Hospital in Hong Kong randomized ventriculostomy patients to one of two groups: those receiving only perioperative Unasyn (ampicillin/sulbactam) and those receiving Unasyn and aztreonam for the duration of monitoring with a ventriculostomy catheter. Prolonged antibiotic use reduced the CSF infection rate from 11 to 3% ($p = .01$). The infections in the prophylactic group were caused by methicillin-resistant *Staphylococcus aureus* and *Candida albicans*, as opposed to *Staphylococcus* spp., *Bacillus* sp., *Escherichia coli*, *Klebsiella* sp., *Acinetobacter* sp., *Aeromonas hydrophilia*, and *Xanthomonas maltophilia* in the perioperative group. This finding is similar to the results of Wyler and Kelly[8] in that use of prophylactic antibiotics seems to select for resistant or opportunistic organisms. The authors also reported a lower incidence of extracranial infections in the prophylaxis group, but such results have been challenged by others.[11]

Pearl

A class I study suggested that use of prophylactic antibiotics reduces ventriculostomy infection rates but seems to select for resistant or opportunistic organisms.

Alleyne et al[12] published a class III study that compared ventriculostomy infection rates and incremental cost in cohorts of patients receiving either three or fewer doses of perioperative cefuroxime or prophylactic continuation of the same antibiotic for the duration of external ventricular drainage. The infection rate was 4.0% in the perioperative group and 3.8% in the prophylaxis group. This difference was not significant. The authors calculated that discontinuing the use of prophylactic antibiotics would save their institution approximately $80,000 per year in direct drug costs.

Pearl

The authors of one study calculated that discontinuing the use of prophylactic antibiotics at their institution would save approximately $80,000 per year in direct drug costs.

Rebuck et al[13] reported the results of a class III study comparing infection rates between patients receiving no antibiotics (6/87, 6.9%) and those receiving any antibiotic prophylaxis (10/128, 7.8%). Duration of antibiotic use and time of administration relative to ICP monitor placement were not identified as significant risk factors.

The Medical Letter on Drugs and Therapeutics acknowledges the sparse and often conflicting evidence in the literature regarding antibiotic prophylaxis for cranial, spinal, and CSF shunt surgery. This publication makes a level III recommendation to use a single dose of 1 to 2 g of intravenous cefazolin (or 1 g of vancomycin if patients are allergic to penicillins or cephalosporins) just prior to a craniotomy.[14]

The discrepancy in results between the single class I study showing benefit from antibiotic prophylaxis and several class II and III studies that failed to demonstrate a significant effect of antibiotic prophylaxis may be explained by study design and by differences in other known risk factors, including patients' underlying pathologies and concurrent infections. Also, the importance of careful surgical technique during insertion of ICP monitors should not be forgotten.[15]

The potential benefits of antibiotic prophylaxis in preventing ventriculitis must be weighed against the reported risks of selection of resistant organisms, more frequent systemic infections, and increased institutional costs, as well as concerns over increased mortality rate, significant morbidity, and prolongation of length of stay from nosocomial ventriculitis. Of note, the studies reviewed did not report a single death from ventriculitis despite an overall infection rate of 7.7% in 3478 patients (Table 19-1). A well-designed, prospective, multicenter study of the risk:benefit ratio of prophylactic antibiotic administration during ICP monitoring appears to be justified, but the numbers of patients that might be needed to make such a trial worthwhile could also prevent it from being economically feasible.

Conclusions and Recommendations

Multiple factors contribute to the risk of developing an ICP monitor–related infection. Conflicting reports emphasize either the benefits or the risks of antibiotic prophylaxis. Some studies report a reduction in infection with long-term prophylaxis, whereas others fail to document any such benefit (Table 19-1). Even studies that support the use of prophylaxis report that this practice promotes antimicrobial drug resistance, which threatens current and future neurosurgical patients. In the author's opinion, use of a single dose of cefazolin administered prior to insertion balances the risks and benefits identified in the published literature, but this advice is offered only as a level III recommendation because of the conflicting nature of the published evidence.

References

1. Guillaume J, Janny P. Manometric intracranienne continue: interet de la methode aux premiers resultats. Rev Neurol (Paris) 1951;84:131–142.
2. Brain Trauma Foundation, American Association of Neurological Surgeons, Joint Section on Neurotrauma and Critical Care. Management and prognosis of severe traumatic brain injury: indications for intracranial pressure monitoring. J Neurotrauma 2000;17:479–491.
3. Guyot LL, Dowling C, Diaz FG, et al. Cerebral monitoring devices: analysis of complications. Acta Neurochir Suppl (Wien) 1998;71:47–49.
4. Mayhall CG, Archer NH, Lamb VA, et al. Ventriculostomy-related infections: a prospective epidemiologic study. N Engl J Med 1984;310:553–559.
5. Clark WC, Muhlbauer MS, Lowrey R, et al. Complications of intracranial pressure monitoring in trauma patients. Neurosurgery 1989;25:20–24.
6. Kanter RK, Weiner LB, Patti AM, et al. Infectious complications and duration of intracranial pressure monitoring. Crit Care Med 1985;13:837–839.
7. Holloway KL, Barnes T, Choi S, et al. Ventriculostomy infections: the effect of monitoring duration and catheter exchange in 584 patients. J Neurosurg 1996;85:419–424.
8. Wyler AR, Kelly WA. Use of antibiotics with external ventriculostomies. J Neurosurg 1972;37:185–187.
9. Rosner MJ, Becker DP. ICP monitoring: complications and associated factors. Clin Neurosurg 1976;23:494–519.
10. Poon WS, Ng S, Wai S. CSF antibiotic prophylaxis for neurosurgical patients with ventriculostomy: a randomised study. Acta Neurochir Suppl (Wien) 1998;71:146–148.
11. Jacobs DG, Westerband A. Antibiotic prophylaxis for intracranial pressure monitors. J Natl Med Assoc 1998;90:417–423.
12. Alleyne CH Jr, Hassan M, Zabramski JM. The efficacy and cost of prophylactic and perioprocedural antibiotics in patients with external ventricular drains. Neurosurgery 2000;47:1124–1129.
13. Rebuck JA, Murry KR, Rhoney DH, et al. Infection related to intracranial pressure monitors in adults: analysis of risk factors and antibiotic prophylaxis. J Neurol Neurosurg Psychiatry 2000;69:381–384.
14. Antimicrobial prophylaxis in surgery. Med Lett Drugs Ther 2001;43:92–97.
15. Bader MK, Littlejohns L, Palmer S. Ventriculostomy and intracranial pressure monitoring: in search of a 0% infection rate. Heart Lung 1995;24:166–172.
16. Zingale A, Ippolito S, Pappalardo P, et al. Infections and re-infections in long-term external ventricular drainage: a variation upon a theme. J Neurosurg Sci 1999;43:125–133.
17. Khan SH, Kureshi IU, Mulgrew T, et al. Comparison of percutaneous ventriculostomies and intraparenchymal monitor: a retrospective evaluation of 156 patients. Acta Neurochir Suppl (Wien) 1998;71:50–52.
18. Paramore CG, Turner DA. Relative risks of ventriculostomy infection and morbidity. Acta Neurochir (Wien) 1994;127:79–84.
19. Bogdahn U, Lau W, Hassel W, et al. Continuous-pressure controlled, external ventricular drainage for treatment of acute hydrocephalus—evaluation of risk factors. Neurosurgery 1992;31:898–904.
20. Sundbarg G, Nordstrom CH, Soderstrom S. Complications due to prolonged ventricular fluid pressure recording. Br J Neurosurg 1988;2:485–495.
21. Aucoin PJ, Kotilainen HR, Gantz NM, et al. Intracranial pressure monitors: epidemiologic study of risk factors and infections. Am J Med 1986;80:369–376.
22. Smith RW, Alksne JF. Infections complicating the use of external ventriculostomy. J Neurosurg 1976;44:567–570.

◆ 20 ◆

Do Head-Injured Patients Need Prophylactic Anticonvulsants? For How Long?

José A. Menéndez, Nancy R. Temkin, and David W. Newell

Brief Answer

The literature contains reasonable evidence that the frequency of early seizures after brain injury is reduced by administration of antiepileptic drugs (AEDs). The drug that has been most studied for this indication is phenytoin. It is therefore reasonable to treat patients for 1 week with phenytoin if they are at high risk for developing early posttraumatic seizures (PTSs) (level I recommendation for prevention of early PTS). Continuation of such treatment for only 1 week reduces the incidence of early PTS while maintaining an acceptably low risk of adverse effects. The studies done to date, however, have not been designed to investigate the effect of prevention of early PTS on secondary brain injury and neurobehavioral outcome. For this reason, there is no evidence that prevention of early seizures reduces mortality, morbidity, or the development of late posttraumatic epilepsy. Thus, anticonvulsant prophylaxis is only a level III recommendation in terms of improving outcome. Treatment of patients after 1 week for late PTS prophylaxis is not recommended (level I recommendation).

Background

Each year more than 422,000 people in the United States are hospitalized for head injury (class III data).[1] As a result, tens of thousands of Americans are affected by PTS (class III data).[2] The estimated number of new occurrences per year ranges from 5,000 to 30,000. According to some reports (some of which predate the use of the Glasgow Coma Scale classification of head injury), ~20 to 25% of all patients who suffer a serious head injury might be expected to experience at least one PTS (class III data)[3] (the use of prophylactic AEDs in these reports was variable).

Pearl

Approximately 20 to 25% of patients who sustain serious head injuries can be expected to have at least one PTS.

PTSs have been classified into three groups according to the time of their occurrence: (1) immediate seizures, which occur during the first few hours of injury (most occur during the first hour); (2) early seizures, which occur during the first week; and (3) late seizures, which occur more than 1 week after the initial insult (class III data).[3,4]

Retrospective analyses by Annegers and collaborators[5] show that the overall standardized incidence ratio for development of new unprovoked seizures after head trauma is 3.1 (95% confidence interval, 2.5 to 3.8); that is, that those with head trauma have a risk of developing unprovoked seizures that is 3.1 times higher than that of the general population (class III data). This analysis also investigated the relationship between the severity of the injury and the development of posttraumatic seizures. Injuries were classified as mild when accompanied by a loss of consciousness or amnesia lasting less than 30 minutes; as moderate when associated with a skull fracture or with a loss of consciousness or amnesia lasting 30 minutes to 24 hours; and as severe when accompanied by an intracranial hematoma, by a brain contusion, or by a loss of consciousness or amnesia lasting more than 24 hours. The authors found that the standardized incidence ratio was 1.5 after mild injuries, but with no increase over the expected number after 5 years. The standardized incidence ratio was 2.9 after moderate injuries and 17.0 after severe injuries.

The highest seizure rates occur after penetrating injuries. In cohort studies of veterans who sustained penetrating brain injuries in Vietnam, over 53% developed a seizure during the 15 years following injury (class II data).[6,7] Approximately 40% of those who developed seizures within 15 years of injury had their first seizure within 4 months after the trauma, 50% within 8 months, and 75% within ~30 months. Despite the relatively high seizure rate after penetrating trauma, patients have a 95% chance of not developing PTS if they remain seizure-free for 3 years after injury (class II data).[4,7]

Pearl

Over half of the veterans who sustained penetrating brain injuries in Vietnam had a seizure during the subsequent 15 years.

Literature Review

Early Posttraumatic Seizures

The risk of early posttraumatic seizures is related to the severity of the head injury. Jennett[8] found that the main risk factors are brain contusions and subdural hematomas, which are associated with an incidence of early seizures of greater than 25% (class III data). Annegers et al[9] described a 19% incidence of early seizures in patients with brain contusions or hematomas (class III data). Epidural hematomas, amnesia that lasts more than 24 hours, or focal neurologic deficits are associated with an increase in the incidence of early seizures of 4 to 10%.[8]

The development of PTS also seems to be influenced by several factors. In terms of patient age, Jennett[3] described an early seizure rate of 9% in children under the age of 5 years, as opposed to 4% in older children and adults (class III data). Hahn et al[10] reported a seizure rate of 32% in children with subdural hematomas, but no increase in rate associated with epidural or intraparenchymal hematomas (class III data). They also found that diffuse cerebral edema and a Glasgow Coma Scale score of 12 or less were other important risk factors.

The significance of early PTS is their association with—and predisposition of patients to—late seizures. Even when they follow mild trauma, early seizures are associated with development of late posttraumatic epilepsy in 25% of cases (class III data).[3] This rate contrasts dramatically with a late seizure incidence of ~1% for mild head injuries unaccompanied by early seizures, acute hematomas, or depressed fractures (class III data).[3] The development of late seizures is not determined by the number or type of early seizures, and late seizures are seen less often in children than in adults (class III data).[3] PTSs may occasionally lead to complications, including aspiration pneumonia and status epilepticus. Patients may also suffer major psychosocial sequelae after experiencing a seizure. For example, a temporary loss of driving privileges is mandated in some states.

Pearl

Early seizures are associated with development of late posttraumatic epilepsy in 25% of cases.

Late Posttraumatic Epilepsy

The mechanisms responsible for late posttraumatic epilepsy are not yet well understood. Multiple elements have been proposed as factors for the development of a seizure focus, including biochemical, electrical, and structural changes; development of pacemaker neurons; decreased inhibitory control mechanisms; disturbances of acetylcholine, glutamic acid, and potassium metabolism; postsynaptic hypersensitivity; impairment of acid-base balance; deposition of iron salts from hemorrhage; lipid peroxidation; and genetic influences.[2]

The severity and type of injury play an important role in the development of late seizures. According to Jennett's[3] studies, almost half of patients with subdural or intracerebral hematomas develop late PTS, as compared with ~20% of patients with epidural hematomas (class III data). Early seizures (28%), dural tears (24%), depressed skull fractures (14%), signs of focal dysfunction of a cerebral hemisphere (29%), or amnesia that persists more than 24 hours (34%) are all associated with a significantly increased risk of late seizures (class III data).[3]

Prevention

Prophylaxis is distinguished from treatment or suppression of an epileptogenic focus in that, when successful, it prevents the formation of an epileptogenic focus and consequent seizures. This concept implies that after completion of a predetermined course of a prophylactic agent, the risk of seizure occurrence is significantly less.

Many neurosurgeons routinely treat head-injured patients with prophylactic AEDs. In a survey of neurosurgeons in 1973, Rapport and Penry[11] reported that 60% of respondents prescribed prophylactic anticonvulsants for trauma patients (class III data), but under a variety of conditions. Several reasons are given as justification for this practice. One is the belief that seizures beget seizures and cause damage to brain tissue, with corresponding deterioration of neurologic function. Concern over the acute consequences of seizures is another reason given to support prophylactic use of AEDs. A third justification is the fact that PTSs reduce quality of life, create socioeconomic problems, and often require lifelong treatment. Finally, failure to use PTS prophylaxis may also have medicolegal implications because of a widespread (but not substantiated) belief that PTS or posttraumatic epilepsy may be preventable with proper treatment.

Although prevention of posttraumatic epilepsy is universally desired, the use of prophylactic anticonvulsants to achieve this goal is controversial. Although some earlier nonrandomized studies had suggested that the risk of late seizures after trauma was reduced with prophylactic AEDs (class III data),[12,13] more recent and better-controlled studies do not support this conclusion.

Young et al[14] performed a randomized, double-blind, placebo-controlled study to determine whether phenytoin administered soon after injury decreases the incidence of early PTS (class I data). In this study 244 patients received phenytoin or placebo within 24 hours of hospital admission; 78% of the patients receiving phenytoin had plasma concentrations of at least 10 μg/mL at 1, 3, and 7 days after injury. The percentages of patients having early seizures were not significantly different between groups, and the intervals from injury to first seizure were likewise not significantly different. The authors suggested that anticonvulsant drugs be given only after an early seizure had occurred.

Temkin et al[15] performed a double-blind, randomized, placebo-controlled study of 404 patients with serious head injury (class I data). The patients were given an intravenous loading dose of phenytoin within 24 hours of trauma, and they then maintained a high therapeutic blood level for 1 year. Follow-up was continued for a total of 2 years from the time of injury. The results showed that the patients assigned to phenytoin had a seizure rate of 3.6% between drug loading and day 7 (early PTS), as compared with 14.2% in the patients receiving placebo. Between day 8 and the end of the first year, 21.5% of the phenytoin group and 15.7% of the placebo group had seizures. At the end of the second year, the rates were 27.5% and 21.1%, respectively. It was concluded that phenytoin exerted a beneficial effect by reducing seizures only during the first week after serious brain injury.

Temkin et al[4] reviewed studies of prophylaxis for early and late posttraumatic epilepsy (class III data). This meta-analysis found that the three placebo-controlled studies of phenytoin, including those of Young and Temkin, were compatible, and combined they showed a decrease in early seizures of 67%. A similar analysis also estimated that phenytoin was associated with no significant decrease in the development of late seizures.

In a systematic review of the use of drugs to prevent seizures after head injury, Schierhout and Roberts[16] identified 10 randomized controlled trials that reported data from a total of 1405 patients. Early treatment with AEDs (phenytoin, carbamazepine, or phenobarbital) was consistently associated with a significant decrease in the relative risk of early PTS. However, mortality was not decreased. The decrease in early seizures was not accompanied by a reduction in late posttraumatic epilepsy.

Haltiner and coworkers[17] concluded that although phenytoin was effective in preventing early PTS, and although patients with early seizures had a higher death rate, the reduction of early seizures in and of itself did not have a detectable impact on mortality (class II data). This result suggests that early seizures are markers of more severe head injuries, rather than being part of a pathogenetic process that leads from severe head injury to either late posttraumatic epilepsy or death (class III data).[17,18]

Pearl

Early treatment with phenytoin, carbamazepine, or phenobarbital seems to significantly decrease the relative risk of early PTS, but without a decrease in mortality or in late posttraumatic epilepsy.

Temkin and colleagues[19] conducted a double-blind study of valproate for the prevention of late posttraumatic epilepsy (class I data). In their study 132 patients were randomized to a 1-week course of phenytoin, 120 to a 1-month course of valproate, and 127 to a 6-month course of valproate. The entry criteria consisted of immediate posttraumatic seizure, depressed skull fracture, penetrating brain injury, or evidence of cortical contusion or subdural, epidural, or intracerebral hemorrhage on computed tomography scan. Patients received antiseizure medication (with monitoring of plasma levels of drug) for 1 year, after which they were followed until 24 months after injury. No differences were seen between the phenytoin group and the valproate groups in the frequency of early seizures. Similarly, late-seizure rates did not differ significantly between groups. A trend toward a higher mortality rate was present in valproate-treated patients.

Recommendations

1. Head-injured patients should receive a 1-week course of prophylactic AEDs to reduce the likelihood of early PTS (level I recommendation for prevention of early PTS).
2. A 1-week course of prophylactic AEDs has never been shown to reduce mortality or morbidity (level III recommendation for improving outcome).
3. Continuation of AED prophylaxis should not extend beyond the first postinjury week because such treatment does not prevent the development of late posttraumatic epilepsy (level I recommendation).

References

1. Kalsbeek WD, McLaurin RL, Harris BS III, Miller JD. The National Head and Spinal Cord Injury Survey: major findings. J Neurosurg 1980;S19–S31.
2. Young B. Post-traumatic epilepsy. In: Barrow DL, ed. Complications and Sequelae of Head Injury, 1st ed. Park Ridge, IL: AANS Publications, 1992:127–132.
3. Jennett B. Epilepsy After Non-Missile Head Injuries, 2nd ed. Chicago: Year Book Medical Publishers, 1975.
4. Temkin NR, Haglund M, Winn HR. Post-traumatic seizures. In: Youmans JR, ed. Neurological Surgery, 4th ed. Philadelphia: WB Saunders, 1996:1834–1839.
5. Annegers JF, Hauser WA, Coan SP, et al. A population-based study of seizures after traumatic brain injuries. N Engl J Med 1998;338:20–24.
6. Salazar AM, Jabbari B, Vance SC, et al. Epilepsy after penetrating head injury, I: Clinical correlates: a report of the Vietnam Head Injury Study. Neurology 1985;35:1406–1414.
7. Weiss GH, Salazar AM, Vance SC, et al. Predicting posttraumatic epilepsy in penetrating head injury. Arch Neurol 1986;43: 771–773.
8. Jennett B. Epilepsy and acute traumatic intracranial haematoma. J Neurol Neurosurg Psychiatry 1975;38:378–381.
9. Annegers JF, Grabow JD, Groover RV, et al. Seizures after head trauma: a population study. Neurology 1980;30:683–689.
10. Hahn YS, Fuchs S, Flannery AM, et al. Factors influencing posttraumatic seizures in children. Neurosurgery 1988;22: 864–867.
11. Rapport RL II, Penry JK. A survey of attitudes toward the pharmacological prophylaxis of posttraumatic epilepsy. J Neurosurg 1973;38:159–166.
12. Servit Z, Musil F. Prophylactic treatment of posttraumatic epilepsy: results of a long-term follow-up in Czechoslovakia. Epilepsia 1981;22:315–320.
13. Wohns RN, Wyler AR. Prophylactic phenytoin in severe head injuries. J Neurosurg 1979;51:507–509.
14. Young B, Rapp RP, Norton JA, et al. Failure of prophylactically administered phenytoin to prevent early posttraumatic seizures. J Neurosurg 1983;58:231–235.
15. Temkin NR, Dikmen SS, Wilensky AJ, et al. A randomized, double-blind study of phenytoin for the prevention of posttraumatic seizures. N Engl J Med 1990;323:497–501.
16. Schierhout G, Roberts I. Anti-epileptic drugs for preventing seizures following acute traumatic brain injury. Cochrane Database Syst Rev 2001;(4):CD000173.
17. Haltiner AM, Newell DW, Temkin NR, et al. Side effects and mortality associated with the use of phenytoin for early posttraumatic seizure prophylaxis. J Neurosurg 1999;91:588–592.
18. Chadwick D. Seizures and epilepsy after traumatic brain injury. Lancet 2000;355:334–336.
19. Temkin NR, Dikmen SS, Anderson GD, et al. Valproate therapy for prevention of posttraumatic seizures: a randomized trial. J Neurosurg 1999;91:593–600.

◆ 21 ◆

Are Steroids Indicated in the Treatment of Head Injury?

John L.D. Atkinson

Brief Answer

With a high degree of clinical certainty (level I), steroids are not indicated in the treatment of head injury. However, putative steroid-related neuronal salvage mechanisms make this an intriguing area of continuing interest. Further clinical and laboratory research will doubtless be forthcoming in the future.

Background

The chemical synthesis of cortisone by Nobel laureate Dr. Edward Kendall[1] at the Mayo Clinic led to its rapid dissemination into multiple and diverse medical fields. The results were often astounding. Initially used to treat rheumatoid arthritis, cortisone was subsequently adopted by neurologic surgery for perioperative management during pituitary surgery in the 1950s. It markedly altered the morbidity and mortality associated with hypopituitary states. Its use also made adenohypophysectomy a viable neurosurgical treatment option for endocrinologically driven malignancies that produced severe pain from widespread metastatic disease. In the early 1960s, cortisone proved remarkably successful as a treatment for peritumoral brain edema. For several decades, glucocorticoids remained the single most utilized pharmacologic agent in the medical management of neurosurgical patients. The often remarkable perceived or actual patient improvement that steroids effected in a variety of neurosurgical diseases resulted in a deep entrenchment of their universal use by a whole generation of neurosurgeons.

Chapter 12 of the original *Guidelines for the Management of Severe Head Injury* summarized the literature of steroid use in traumatic brain injury (TBI) up to 1995.[2] Based on the strength of the data, the authors concluded that a standard of care exists: the use of corticosteroids is not recommended for improving outcome or reducing intracranial pressure in patients with severe head injury.

However, entrenched medical practice is not so easily defeated, and underlying questions remain. Specifically, if steroids are reported to be efficacious for spinal cord injury, then shouldn't they also be efficacious for head injury?

Literature Review

The following is a laboratory and clinical review of the literature since the publication of the *Guidelines for the Management of Severe Head Injury*.

Administration of high-dose steroids after severe head injury in rats reduces lipid peroxidation, which is also reported to be a major mechanism underlying the efficacy of high-dose steroids in spinal cord injury.[3,4] However, glucocorticoids do not appear to be beneficial in the treatment of cerebral insults involving glutamate toxicity.[5]

Pearl

In the laboratory, high-dose steroids given after brain injury reduce lipid peroxidation but do not appear to affect glutamate-mediated toxicity.

Assumptions about clinical benefit of steroids in TBI are all based on laboratory and clinical studies [conducted after the first National Acute Spinal Cord Injury Study (NASCIS 1)] that suggested the existence of a therapeutic window for high-dose steroid therapy. To review, the NASCIS 1 trial suggested no clear benefit of higher-dose over lower-dose peri-injury glucocorticoids (level I), and early fatality and wound infection were more prevalent in the higher-dose arm of the trial.[6] However, subsequent laboratory evidence strongly suggested that a pharmacologic window exists for remarkably high doses of methylprednisolone.[4] The subsequent NASCIS 2 trial became a benchmark in the medical management of acute spinal cord injury, with purported neuroprotective effects occurring by a variety of possible mechanisms (class II data).[7] This led to the NASCIS 3 trial, which suggested mild additional benefit in select time frames (class II data).[8] It is of note, however, that a retrospective review of glucocorticoid use in the setting of gunshot wounds to the spine revealed no benefit and a higher complication rate, similar to the NASCIS 1 results (class III data).[9]

One might think that the encouraging results of the NASCIS 2 trial could logically be applied to the treatment of severe head injury. However, there are differences in pathophysiology between these two polar regions of the central nervous system. Severe closed head injury is frequently associated with a variable degree of brainstem-derived apnea and catecholamine surge, affecting oxygen and carbon dioxide levels and pH, with potentially significant change in the cellular milieu over and above the contusions, lacerations, and hematomas that both spinal cord and brain may acquire by primary injury mechanisms.[10,11] Despite these potential differences in secondary injury mechanisms, a prospective, controlled, multicenter trial suggested clinical benefit from peri-injury use of glucocorticoids after head injury based on a retrospective subgroup analysis (class III data).[12] However, a subsequent systematic review of randomized controlled trials reveals considerable uncertainty as to whether peri-injury steroid use has any benefit, not to mention harmful effects.[13] The most informative multicenter trial utilized tirilazad mesylate, a 21-aminosteroid derivative specifically designed to be a powerful antioxidant, which is reportedly the most significant mechanism by which glucocorticoids improve posttraumatic neuronal salvage. Overall efficacy in patients with moderate and severe head injury could not be demonstrated, but there were some problems inherent in the trial (class II data).[14]

In conjunction with this negative trial, serious questions regarding the validity of the NASCIS 2 results have been raised. An in-depth review of the trial suggests that methylprednisolone use in acute spinal cord injury is not a proven standard of care; in fact, it should not even be considered a recommended treatment.[15] The uncertainty of the literature as to any benefit, a recent designer drug trial proving no benefit, and questions regarding the validity of the NASCIS 2 spinal cord injury results support not using glucocorticosteroids in the management of severe head injury. Despite these reasons, another randomized trial of glucocorticoid use in head injury is currently under way.[16]

Pearl

Differences in posttraumatic pathophysiology between brain and spinal cord suggest that a treatment that is effective in one of these parts of the central nervous system may not necessarily be effective in the other.

Pearl

A large-scale study of the use of glucocorticoids in head injury is in progress.

Complications of high-dose steroids are in part an augmentation of stress injuries acquired soon after the injury itself, such as gastric mucosal ulcerations, resulting in increased risk of gastrointestinal hemorrhage or perforation.[10,17–21] Other known complications include avascular necrosis of the femoral head and infectious complications.[22,23] Concerns also exist about glucocorticoids directly increasing serum glucose levels, which may worsen any ischemic brain process in evolution.[24,25]

Recommendations

In summary, there exists no good evidence that steroids are beneficial in traumatic brain injury. Furthermore, steroids may cause a variety of complications that can worsen patient outcomes. Concerns over the validity of the NASCIS 2 conclusions and the failure of the 21-aminosteroid trial to demonstrate benefit lead to the conclusion that the 1995 published *Guidelines* recommendations remain unchanged: the use of corticosteroids is not recommended for improving outcome or reducing intracranial pressure in patients with severe head injury (level I).

References

1. Hench PS, Kendall EC, Slocumb CH, et al. The effect of cortisone and of ACTH on rheumatoid arthritis and acute rheumatic fever. Proceedings of Seventh International Congress on Rheumatic Diseases. Edited by Committee on Publications, American Rheumatism Association. Philadelphia: W.B. Saunders, 1952: 131–148.

2. Brain Trauma Foundation, American Association of Neurological Surgeons, Joint Section on Neurotrauma and Critical Care. Guidelines for the management of severe head injury. J Neurotrauma 1996;13:641–734.
3. Ildan F, Polat S, Öner A, et al. The effect of the treatment of high-dose methylprednisolone on NA^{+}-K^{+}/Mg^{+2} ATPase activity and lipid peroxidation and ultrastructural findings following cerebral contusion in rat. Surg Neurol 1995;44:573–580.
4. Hall ED. The neuroprotective pharmacology of methylprednisolone. J Neurosurg 1992;76:13–22.
5. Uhler TA, Frim DM, Pakzaban P, et al. The effects of megadose methylprednisolone and U-78517F on toxicity mediated by glutamate receptors in the rat neostriatum. Neurosurgery 1994;34:122–128.
6. Bracken MB, Collins WF, Freeman DF, et al. Efficacy of methylprednisolone in acute spinal cord injury. JAMA 1984;251: 45–52.
7. Bracken MB, Shepard MJ, Collins WF, et al. A randomized, controlled trial of methylprednisolone or naloxone in the treatment of acute spinal-cord injury. The results of the Second National Acute Spinal Cord Injury Study. N Engl J Med 1990; 322:1405–1411.
8. Bracken MB, Shepard MJ, Holford TR, et al. Administration of methylprednisolone for 24 or 48 hours or tirilazad mesylate for 48 hours in the treatment of acute spinal cord injury. Results of the Third National Acute Spinal Cord Injury Randomized Controlled Trial. National Acute Spinal Cord Injury Study. JAMA 1997;277:1597–1604.
9. Heary RF, Vaccaro AR, Mesa JJ, et al. Steroids and gunshot wounds to the spine. Neurosurgery 1997;41:576–584.
10. Atkinson JLD. The neglected prehospital phase of head injury: apnea and catecholamine surge. Mayo Clin Proc 2000;75: 37–47.
11. Atkinson JLD, Anderson RE, Murray MJ. The early critical phase of severe head injury: importance of apnea and dysfunctional respiration. J Trauma 1998;45:941–945.
12. Grumme T, Baethmann A, Kolodziejczyk D, et al. Treatment of patients with severe head injury by triamcinolone: a prospective, controlled multicenter clinical trial of 396 cases. Res Exp Med (Berl) 1995;195:217–229.
13. Alderson P, Roberts I. Corticosteroids in acute traumatic brain injury: systematic review of randomised controlled trials. BMJ 1997;314:1855–1859.
14. Marshall LF, Maas AIR, Marshall SB, et al. A multicenter trial on the efficacy of using tirilazad mesylate in cases of head injury. J Neurosurg 1998;89:519–525.
15. Hurlbert RJ. Methylprednisolone for acute spinal cord injury: an inappropriate standard of care. J Neurosurg 2000;93:1–7.
16. Kmietowicz Z. Trial of steroids for treating head injury begins. BMJ 1999;318:1441.
17. Weiner HL, Rezai AR, Cooper PR. Sigmoid diverticular perforation in neurosurgical patients receiving high-dose corticosteroids. Neurosurgery 1993;33:40–43.
18. Lu WY, Rhoney DH, Boling WB, et al. A review of stress ulcer prophylaxis in the neurosurgical intensive care unit. Neurosurgery 1997;41:416–426.
19. Brown TH, Davidson PF, Larson GM. Acute gastritis occurring within 24 hours of severe head injury. Gastrointest Endosc 1989;35:37–40.
20. Larson GM, Koch S, O'Dorisio TM, et al. Gastric response to severe head injury. Am J Surg 1984;147:97–105.
21. Fadul CE, Lemann W, Thaler HT, et al. Perforation of the gastrointestinal tract in patients receiving steroids for neurologic disease. Neurology 1988;38:348–352.
22. Keogh P, Masterson E, Quinlan W. Bacterial arthritis in the neurosurgical patient: report of four cases. Neurosurgery 1994; 34:364–368.
23. Nagashima G, Suzuki R, Asai J, et al. Avascular necrosis of the femoral head caused by steroid treatment in neurosurgery. No Shinkei Geka 2000;28:523–528.
24. Rovlias A, Kotsou S. The influence of hyperglycemia on neurological outcome in patients with severe head injury. Neurosurgery 2000;46:335–343.
25. Chiaretti A, De Benedictis R, Langer A, et al. Prognostic implications of hyperglycaemia in paediatric head injury. Childs Nerv Syst 1998;14:455–459.

◆ 22 ◆

Does Following the Recommendations in the Guidelines for the Management of Severe Traumatic Brain Injury *Make a Difference in Patient Outcome?*

Roger Hartl and Jamshid Ghajar

Whereof one cannot speak, thereof one must be silent.
—Ludwig Wittgenstein, *Tractatus Logico-Philosophicus*

Brief Answer

Because of the relatively meager scientific evidence supporting the individual recommendations in the *Guidelines*, one would not expect protocols based on the *Guidelines* to have a significant effect on patient outcome. However, several studies demonstrate that the possibility of significant improvement in outcome does exist. Reduction in mortality as seen in one of the three reported studies may be related to detailed and comprehensive management protocols for intracranial hypertension and cerebral perfusion. Data on hospital costs are difficult to interpret because authors use different methods to generate the published numbers. Clinical pathways that focus on the organizational management of patient care, as in the study by Vitaz et al (discussed below), see a significant reduction in costs, whereas Palmer et al (discussed below) advocate very intensive patient management with expensive monitoring technology that entailed higher costs. Higher costs in the acute care setting, however, can result in significant cost reductions later on if overall outcome is improved.

Pearl

Although *Guidelines*-based treatment protocols may raise acute care costs in institutions that previously had not practiced aggressive treatment or sophisticated monitoring of brain-injured patients, overall improvement in patient outcomes may offset the initially increased costs.

Background

Patient management guidelines document the current scientific basis of clinical practice. In keeping with Wittgenstein's above statement from 1918, the guidelines explicitly state and emphasize what can be discussed based on scientific evidence, and they avoid recommendations that are based only on expert opinion. Their ultimate purpose is to improve and standardize delivery of care and to stimulate research that will not only identify superior treatment modalities, but also improve the methods of clinical research.

The guideline movement in neurosurgery first attracted attention in 1995 when the *Guidelines for the Management of Severe Head Injury* were published as a joint effort of the Brain Trauma Foundation, the American Association of Neurological Surgeons, and the Joint Section on Neurotrauma and Critical Care. An update was published in 2000 as *Guidelines for the Management of Severe Traumatic Brain Injury* (*Guidelines*).[1] The *Guidelines* consisted of 14 topics ranging from trauma systems and prehospital resuscitation to monitoring and treatment of intracranial hypertension and other related topics. Since then, the *Guidelines* have been adopted by neurosurgeons around the world. A Medline search reveals a multitude of articles that deal with implementation of the *Guidelines* into clinical practice. The frequency with which the *Guidelines* are cited in the literature suggests that they have had a significant impact on how patients with severe traumatic brain injury (TBI) are treated.

It is important to understand that guidelines per se are not a practical clinical tool, but rather a summary and review of scientific evidence. They have to be part of a more comprehensive, multidisciplinary treatment protocol that embraces all aspects of patient care, including geographic and infrastructure-related characteristics of a particular trauma center. This chapter reviews the literature that explores whether or not treatment protocols for severe TBI based on the *Guidelines* make a difference in patient outcome.

Literature Review

Only three of the *Guidelines'* recommendations (about hyperventilation, steroids, and anticonvulsants) are based on prospective, randomized, controlled trials that demonstrated a significant effect (or lack thereof) on patient outcome; that is, they are based on class I evidence that can support a "standard."

Hyperventilation in Patients with Severe Traumatic Brain Injury

The recommendation that "in the absence of increased intracranial pressure (ICP), chronic prolonged hyperventilation therapy should be avoided after severe TBI" is based on a prospective study by Muizelaar et al.[2] In their study, 77 patients with severe TBI were randomized to a group treated with chronic prophylactic hyperventilation for 5 days or to a group that was kept normocapneic during that time. Six months after trauma, patients with an initial Glasgow Coma Scale (GCS) motor score of 4 to 5 who had been hyperventilated had a significantly worse outcome.

Steroids for the Treatment of Patients with Severe Traumatic Brain Injury

The use of steroids is not recommended for improving outcome or reducing ICP in patients with severe TBI. This standard was based on nine class I trials in which the preponderance of evidence demonstrated that steroids did not reduce ICP or improve outcome after TBI. The largest study was published in 1994 by Gaab et al.[3] The authors conducted a randomized, prospective, double-blind, multicenter trial investigating the efficacy and safety of very high dose dexamethasone on outcome in 300 patients with moderate and severe TBI. At 12 months, no differences were found between the treatment groups.

Antiseizure Medication in Patients with Severe Traumatic Brain Injury

Antiseizure prophylaxis is not recommended for the prevention of late posttraumatic seizures. This recommendation is supported by eight class I studies. The largest of these is a prospective, randomized, placebo-controlled trial with 404 patients published by Temkin et al.[4] Patients were randomized to a group treated with phenytoin or to a group that received placebo. The incidence of early posttraumatic seizures, that is, those occurring during the first week after injury, was significantly lower in the treated group. No effect was seen on the occurrence of late posttraumatic seizures, and survival was the same in both groups.

Clinical Protocols Based on the Guidelines

Three class III studies have addressed the impact of *Guidelines*-based protocols on patient management. Their main results are summarized in Table 22–1.

Palmer et al[5] compared outcomes from the 42-month period preceding implementation of a *Guidelines*-based TBI protocol (37 patients) to those from the 30-month period after implementation of the protocol (56 patients). Patients age 8 years or older with a closed head injury and GCS score of 3 to 8 or patients who deteriorated to that level within 48 hours of admission were included. Data from the 37 preimplementation patients were obtained retrospectively, whereas concurrent data collection was performed on the 56 postimplementation patients. The initial treatment protocol emphasized fluid restriction, hyperventilation to a $PaCO_2$ between 25 and 30 mmHg, liberal use of vasopressors to keep systolic blood pressure above 90 mmHg, and treatment of ICP >20 mmHg with cerebrospinal fluid (CSF) drainage and mannitol. No minimum target for cerebral perfusion pressure (CPP) was specified. In contrast, the *Guidelines*-based protocol emphasized fluid resuscitation, hemodynamic monitoring with continuous cardiac output pulmonary artery catheters, and jugular bulb oximetry in addition to ICP monitoring. Specific treatment goals included maintenance of the following physiologic parameters: CPP >70 mmHg, ICP <20 mmHg, central venous pressure 5

Table 22-1 Summary of the Effect of Implementation of *Guidelines*-Based Severe TBI Management Protocols on Mortality, ICU Length of Stay, and Hospital Charges at Three Centers

Series	Palmer et al[5]	Vitaz et al[7]	Trask et al[6,8]
Patients (before/after protocol)	*N*=37/56	*N*=43/119	*N*=219/93 (high compliance group)
Class of study	III	III	III
Mortality (%)	At 6 months	At discharge	At discharge
Before *Guidelines* protocol	43	39	18
With *Guidelines* protocol	16*	47	12
ICU days			
Before *Guidelines* protocol	21.0	21.2	9.7
With *Guidelines* protocol	22.0 (not significant)	16.8*	7.1*
Hospital Costs per patient ($)			
Before *Guidelines* protocol	196,128	Not recorded	Not recorded
With *Guidelines* protocol	293,065*	14,551 less than before protocol	9,498 less than before protocol*

*Significantly different than before protocol implementation.

to 10 mmHg, pulmonary capillary wedge pressure 10 to 15 mmHg, jugular venous oxygen saturation 55 to 75%, SaO_2 >95%, $PaCO_2$ 35 mmHg, and aggressive, early nutritional support.

The protocol covered patient care in the emergency room, in the operating room, and in the intensive care unit (ICU). Age, admission GCS score, length of stay in the ICU, and total number of ventilator days were not different between groups. Score on the dichotomized Glasgow Outcome Scale at 6 months was significantly better in patients treated with the protocol. The proportion of deaths decreased by more than 50%, and the proportion of patients with good outcomes more than doubled. Hospital costs, however, were more than $97,000 higher in patients treated according to the *Guidelines*. This result was attributed mainly to the use of more expensive drugs (e.g., propofol) and monitoring technology (jugular bulb oximetry, fiberoptic ICP monitors, etc.). The authors speculated that higher hospital costs may be more than compensated for by improved patient outcomes, with reduced need for rehabilitation and quicker reintegration into society.

Pearl

The *Guidelines for the Management of Severe TBI* should serve as the basis of a multidisciplinary treatment protocol.

Trask et al[6] studied the impact of the implementation of a *Guidelines*-based protocol on length of stay, mortality, and hospital charges in severe TBI patients. Inclusion criteria were blunt head injury, age >14 years, GCS score ≤8, and survival for at least 48 hours after admission. The protocol consisted of a set of standard orders and a pathway for patient management.

The study population was divided into two groups based on protocol compliance. Analysis of patients from 1995 and 1996 indicated only 50% compliance with the protocol (186 patients, "low-compliance group"), which increased to 85% in 1997 (93 patients, "high-compliance group"); 219 patients treated from 1991 to 1994 (before the protocol was implemented) served as a control group. The groups did not differ in terms of injury severity score, GCS score, or age. Total hospital days and ICU days were significantly reduced after implementation of the protocol, and hospital costs (as determined by data obtained from institutional financial records) were also cut. Overall mortality dropped from 18% in the control group to 12% in the high-compliance group. To control for general factors that may have affected results, the authors analyzed 686 patients who presented during the same time period without head injuries, but who otherwise met the inclusion criteria (Fakhry et al, unpublished data). In this subgroup of patients, hospital stay increased, mortality doubled, and total hospital charges increased. These findings indicate that improved outcomes among the severe TBI patients can be attributed to implementation of the protocol.

A slightly different approach was taken by Vitaz et al,[7] who developed a clinical pathway based on the *Guidelines*. The authors compared length of stay, number of ventilator days, incidence of pneumonia, mortality, and hospital charges in a prospectively collected data set of 119 severe TBI patients managed by the pathway to a retrospectively studied group of 43 patients. Their pathway was developed in collaboration with a multidisciplinary task force and consisted of four treatment phases. Phase 1 comprised admission of the patient to the ICU, phase 2 covered the acute critical care phase (~4 days), phase 3 was termed the "mobility and weaning" phase, and during phase 4 the patient was prepared for rehabilitation ("prerehab" phase). Treatment goals during the admission and critical care phases eventually included maintenance of $PaCO_2$ between 35 and 40 mmHg; ICP monitoring with ventricular catheters; treatment of ICP >20 mmHg (and, eventually, CPP <70 mmHg) with CSF drainage and mannitol; monitoring of wedge pressures; initiation of enteral feeding within the first 4 days after trauma; and antiseizure prophylaxis with phenytoin for 7 days.

No differences were found between the groups in age, GCS score at 24 hours, or injury severity score. No difference was seen in mortality rates between groups. Total hospital length of stay, ICU length of stay, and number of ventilator days was less in the clinical pathway group than in the historical control group. Based on the reductions in hospital and ICU lengths of stay and in number of ventilator days, the total reduction of hospital charges effected by implementation of the pathway was estimated to be $14,551 per patient.

The main purpose of the clinical pathway in this publication was to standardize patient care and use ancillary services to provide all patients with the highest level of care. Important components included involvement of different clinical services early in a patient's stay, mobilization of patients as soon as possible after trauma, and initiation of discharge planning at the time of admission to expedite placement in rehabilitation facilities. By focusing on the organizational aspects of patient management, the authors were able to cut hospital costs. This is in contrast to the pathway by Palmer et al and Trask et al, in which the main emphasis was on treatment algorithms for elevated ICP and compromised CPP.

Pearl

Clinical pathways based on the *Guidelines* should streamline and standardize patient management in order to make it more cost effective.

Conclusions and Recommendations

Integration of the *Guidelines* recommendations into a multidisciplinary, comprehensive clinical pathway that streamlines patient care and standardizes critical care management can significantly improve patient outcome and reduce hospital costs.

References

1. Brain Trauma Foundation, American Association of Neurological Surgeons, Joint Section on Neurotrauma and Critical Care. Management and prognosis of severe traumatic brain injury. J Neurotrauma 2000;17:449–554.
2. Muizelaar JP, Marmarou A, Ward JD, et al. Adverse effects of prolonged hyperventilation in patients with severe head injury: a randomized clinical trial. J Neurosurg 1991;75: 731–739.
3. Gaab MR, Trost HA, Alcantara A, et al. "Ultrahigh" dexamethasone in acute brain injury: results from a prospective randomized double-blind multicenter trial (GUDHIS). German Ultrahigh Dexamethasone Head Injury Study Group. Zentralbl Neurochir 1994;55:135–143.
4. Temkin NR, Dikmen SS, Wilensky AJ, et al. A randomized, double-blind study of phenytoin for the prevention of post-traumatic seizures. N Engl J Med 1990;323:497–502.
5. Palmer S, Bader MK, Qureshi A, et al. The impact on outcomes in a community hospital setting of using the AANS traumatic brain injury guidelines. J Trauma 2001;50:657–664.
6. Trask AL, French KB, Burgess JE, et al. Trauma service management of brain injured patients by protocol improves outcomes. Presented at the 12th Annual Scientific Assembly of the Eastern Association for the Surgery of Trauma, Orlando, Florida, January 1999.
7. Vitaz TW, McIlvoy L, Raque GH, et al. Development and implementation of a clinical pathway for severe traumatic brain injury. J Trauma 2001;51:369–375.
8. Fakhry SM, Trask AL, Waller MA, et al. Management of brain-injured patients by an evidence-based medicine protocol improves outcomes and decreases hospital charges. J Trauma 2004;56:492–499.

◆ 23 ◆

Why Have Therapeutic Trials in Head Injury Been Unable to Demonstrate Benefits?

Azadeh Farin and Lawrence F. Marshall

The topic of this chapter does not lend itself to the class I, II, or III format for the analysis of published studies.

Brief Answer

The Decade of the Brain saw several dramatic advances in our understanding of the pathophysiology of traumatic brain injury (TBI) and focal and global cerebral ischemia. Unfortunately, however, with the exception of tissue plasminogen activator (tPA) for ischemic stroke, these advances in our understanding of the biologic mechanisms that produce brain damage have not translated into success in the clinical arena. Reasons for our failure to improve the outcomes of our patients are multifactorial and include the following:

- Failure to adequately test therapeutic agents in animal models
- Presence of multiple mechanisms of brain damage at the cellular level
- Complexity of head injury, making it unlikely that any single treatment will be efficacious, and therefore requiring either drugs with multiple mechanisms of action or sequential therapy with different drugs
- Inappropriate mechanism of action of investigational drugs in terms of the types of injuries in patients selected for clinical trials
- Incomplete understanding of drug mechanism of action, with the result that reasons for failure of clinical trials were incorrectly assigned
- Inadequate understanding of required duration of treatment
- Lack of sufficiently sensitive measures to detect favorable changes in neurobehavioral outcome

The complexity of brain injury is a consequence of a myriad of neurochemical processes that begin after the damage of the initial injury. Unlike stroke, in which the damage is initiated some time after the initial ictus, much of the damage in head injury (perhaps more than we would like to admit) occurs at the time of impact, particularly in more severe injuries. A chain of neurochemical events is then superimposed upon an already damaged brain. Coupled with the brain's unique and still very poorly understood vulnerability to ischemia, the incredible complexity and dynamic nature of brain injury have thus far thwarted our overly simplistic therapeutic initiatives.

Background

Phase I trials attempt to establish the safety of the maximum tolerated dose of a drug. Because neuroprotective agents are often tested earlier in patients with stroke or subarachnoid hemorrhage (SAH), phase I trials are not always conducted in head-injured patients. A major weakness of this strategy is the fact that dose-limiting side effects in patients without head injury (such as depressed consciousness, depressed respiration, and development of hallucinations) may be irrelevant in head-injured patients, who may be comatose or mechanically ventilated. Phase II trials are blinded and enroll 25 to 50 randomized patients per group to demonstrate preliminary efficacy. Phase II findings enable power calculations for later phase III trials. Phase I and phase II studies have defined entry criteria, an outcome measure (typically clinical recovery for phase II studies), and multiple secondary end points. Phase III trials are also randomized but, in addition, are placebo-controlled and double-blind. They often include at least 400 patients per group to test whether a drug improves outcome over the current standard of care or over placebo.

The main objective of the treatment of patients with head injury is prevention of secondary damage. Causes of secondary damage include systemic insults such as hypotension and hypoxia, delayed or recurrent intracranial mass lesions, and biochemical processes leading to cell membrane dysfunction and disturbed circulation in the microvasculature. Appropriately, recent clinical trials have involved several agents believed to be neuroprotective against these putative mechanisms of secondary damage. For reasons outlined above, however, none of the 10 published reports of clinical trials performed during the past decade has proven any agent to be efficacious in the general head injury population. Of the 10 studies, four were terminated early, and only six were actually completed.

Pearl

A drug's dose-limiting side effects in patients without head injury may be irrelevant in comatose or mechanically ventilated head-injured patients.

Literature Review of Head Injury Trials

Corticosteroids

Although corticosteroids have a known role in controlling tumor-related edema, no clear indication for their use in head injury has been identified.[1] Several prospective randomized clinical trials have failed to show that corticosteroid use was associated with statistically significant improvement in outcome for the general study population.[2] In the triamcinolone study, however, a statistically significant effect was noted in a subgroup of patients with focal lesions and Glasgow Coma Scale scores (GCS) ≤ 8 on admission.[3] A meta-analysis of both published and unpublished trials of corticosteroids in head injury showed a possible 2% reduction in mortality and also determined that a prospective trial of 20,000 would be necessary to confirm or exclude this possibility.[2] The Corticosteroid Randomization After Significant Head Injury (CRASH) Trial is now attempting to test the efficacy of corticosteroids in an appropriately sized sample.[4,5]

Pearl

Treatment of head injury with corticosteroids may be associated with a 2% reduction in mortality.

Calcium Channel Antagonists

Nimodipine is known to reduce the risk of ischemia after spontaneous SAH[6] but has not yet been shown to be effective in traumatic SAH. The British/Finnish Cooperative Head Injury Trial Group study (HIT I) of 351 patients with severe head injury showed an 8% relative but statistically insignificant improvement in 6-month outcome.[7] The HIT II study was a prospective, multicenter, placebo-controlled trial of 852 patients with severe head injury. Again, nimodipine showed a relative but statistically insignificant increase in favorable outcome and decrease in unfavorable outcome for the overall population.[8] Nimodipine did, however, significantly reduce unfavorable outcome in a subgroup with traumatic SAH. The HIT III trial was a prospective, multicenter, randomized trial of 123 patients with traumatic SAH. Although a statistically significant effect was noted,[9] the finding was not accepted universally because the presence of SAH could not be reconfirmed later in one fifth of patients.

Analysis of pooled data from all three trials shows a significant benefit from nimodipine in traumatic SAH. However, given the different inclusion criteria for the three trials, the validity of such a result is questionable. Furthermore, a retrospective analysis of HIT I patients with traumatic SAH did not show nimodipine to be protective.[10] Results from the HIT IV trial, which was focused on the efficacy of nimodipine for traumatic SAH, showed no effect of the drug in this targeted population.[11]

Free Radical Scavengers

Tirilazad mesylate is an inhibitor of free radical–mediated lipid peroxidation.[12] In phase I and phase II trials, it was shown to have a good safety profile and to be effective in experimental models of head injury even when hypoxia was present. Two prospective multicenter trials were then launched to study its efficacy. The North American study was terminated before full enrollment was attained because of higher mortality in the treatment group, although this increase was found not to be significant when 6-month outcomes were analyzed.[13] The European/Australian trial included 957 patients with severe head injury and 163 with moderate head injury; a statistically significant effect in the full population was not demonstrated, though a significant effect in males with traumatic SAH was noted.[14]

Polyethylene glycol-conjugated superoxide dismutase (PEG-SOD) is another free radical scavenger that significantly improved outcome in phase II studies. Two consecutive phase III trials were initiated in patients with severe head injury. Although the treatment group had a more favorable outcome profile, outcomes in the two groups were not significantly different.[15] Improved trial design may have improved the chances of attaining significance in a subsequent trial, but the sponsoring American company was bought out by a French company that had little interest in pursuing studies of a drug extracted from cow liver because of fear of potential transmission of bovine spongiform encephalopathy ("mad cow disease").

N-*Methyl-D-Aspartate (NMDA)/Glutamate Receptor Antagonists*

The competitive NMDA receptor antagonist Selfotel (CGS 19755) was tested in two multicenter phase III trials of patients with severe head injury[16] after investigators reported that excessive concentrations of excitatory amino acids, especially glutamate, can lead to secondary damage[17] and, further, that NMDA antagonists can block ischemia-induced neuronal degeneration.[18,19] Before full enrollment was attained, however, the head injury trials were stopped because of concern over increased deaths and serious adverse events in the treatment groups of two concurrent stroke trials.[20] Though the head injury data did not show an increased frequency of serious adverse events, the data suggested that efficacy could not be demonstrated even if the trials were allowed to continue to completion. Subsequent studies revealed that up to 40% of patients enrolled in these trials had no intracranial mass lesions, such as focal contusions and acute subdural hematomas, and therefore constituted groups with a low likelihood of excess glutamate release as part of their pathophysiology.[21,22]

The noncompetitive NMDA receptor antagonist Cerestat (CNS 1102) was also tested in a phase III trial of patients with severe head injury after it was found to exhibit neuroprotection in laboratory models of ischemic brain injury and head trauma. In animals with cortical impact injury, Cerestat reduced contusion volume, decreased hemispheric swelling and water content, lowered intracranial pressure, and improved cerebral perfusion pressure. During the phase III trial in head-injured patients, concerns about the effects of Cerestat in stroke patients and about the futility of continuing the trial led to the termination of the study before full enrollment was attained.[22] However, subsequent analysis suggested that a subset of stroke patients may in fact have benefited from Cerestat.

Pearl

Although interim analyses in stroke trials have raised concerns about potential adverse effects of NMDA receptor antagonists, such concerns do not seem to have been justified in head injury trials.

The confidence intervals for the aforementioned trials are plotted in Fig. 23-1. Although it can be argued that the neuroprotective agents in general appear to be somewhat efficacious in the total population of head-injured patients, a beneficial effect is much more obvious in the subgroup of patients with traumatic SAH or focal contusions. A meta-analysis of the previous trials to estimate the pooled effect of the neuroprotective agents in the total population of head-injured patients yielded an odds ratio of 0.9 (95% confidence interval 0.70–1.06).[22]

Recommendations Based on Lessons Learned from Head Injury Trials

Perform Adequate Preclinical Studies

Before phase III trials are initiated, investigational agents must undergo adequate preclinical testing to answer key questions. Conclusions about dose–response curves, time window response curves, length of treatment, therapeutic range, target organ drug availability, and drug metabolism must be accurately extrapolated from experimental models. Specifically, the tirilazad and Selfotel examples demonstrate the importance of phase I and II studies for characterizing pharmacokinetics and hence target organ drug availability, for identifying the appropriate group of patients in whom pathophysiology matches the drug's mechanism of action, and for demonstrating safety. Only after termination of the tirilazad and PEG-SOD trials was it recognized that both agents fail to demonstrate significant crossing of the blood–brain barrier (BBB) after severe head injury.[14,15] It was also discovered that women had lower plasma levels of tirilazad than men, sometimes below the therapeutic range,[23] and that metabolism of tirilazad was increased by phenytoin.[24] This latter issue is of concern because seizure prophylaxis with phenytoin is common in head injury management in the United States. The fact that tirilazad was shown to have significant efficacy in men with traumatic SAH may indicate that therapeutic concentrations were achieved in appropriate compartments, including the microvascular bed and cerebrospinal fluid, as a consequence of the traumatic SAH. Selfotel was also found to have poor brain penetration. Furthermore, in TBI, the frequent occurrence of low

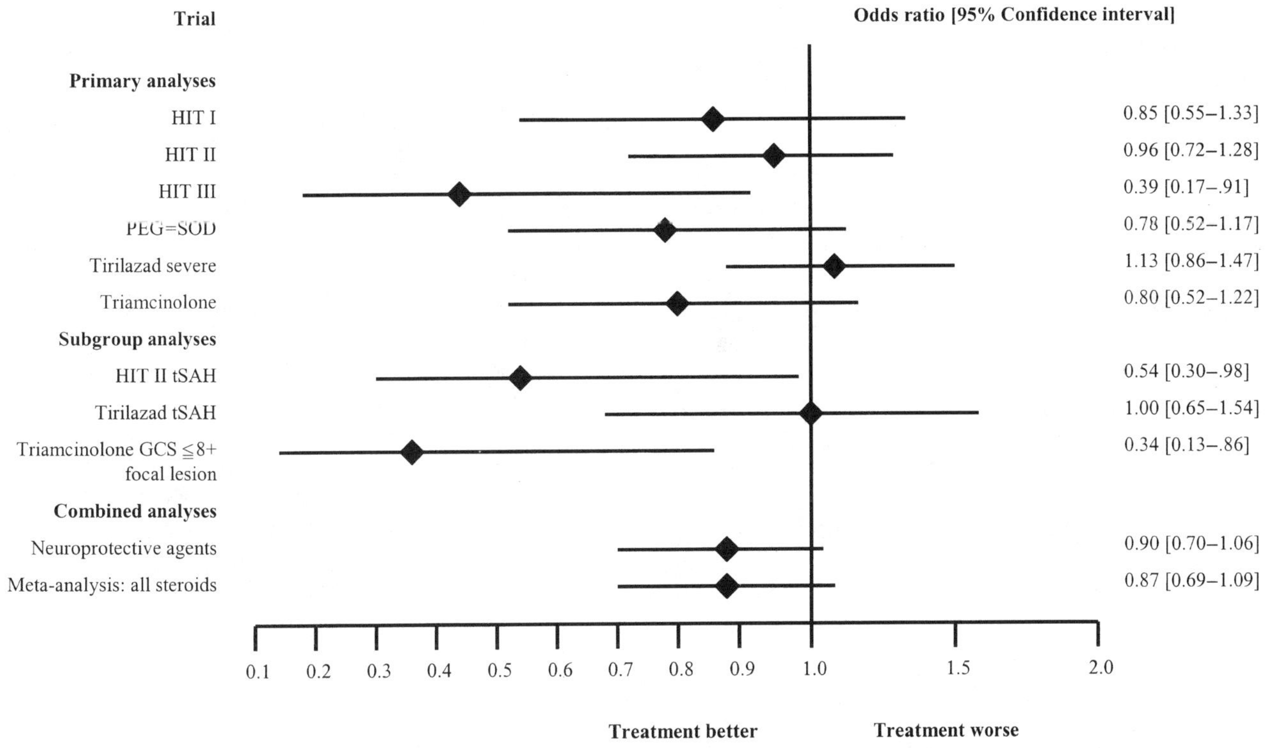

Figure 23-1 Summary of treatment results of several head injury trials. From Maas AI, Steyerberg EW, Murray GD, et al. Why have recent trials of neuroprotective agents in head injury failed to show convincing efficacy? A pragmatic analysis and theoretical considerations. Neurosurgery 1999;44:1286–1298.

cerebral blood flow early after injury would reduce drug delivery to the brain even more.[25] Without adequate crossing of the BBB, this competitive NMDA receptor antagonist would not be expected to interfere with the binding of endogenous glutamate to its receptor.

Pearl

Basic pharmacokinetic studies might have predicted that some large clinical trials would have failed.

Improve Targeting of Therapy

The multiplicity of mechanisms of brain damage at the cellular level is partly responsible for the complex nature of head injury. Single-agent treatment creates the potential problem that the therapeutic mechanism by which a drug works may not address the most critical aspect of the pathophysiology of a particular patient. Therefore, single-agent treatment is less likely to be efficacious for the total population than treatment directed at several potential mechanisms via sequential therapy or administration of several drugs. This problem may partly explain why the trials described above failed to show significantly improved outcomes in the overall treatment populations. Instead, single agents may be efficacious only in specific subgroups of head-injured patients, as with triamcinolone and nimodipine. Because of the complexity of head injury, a more time-sensitive and strategic approach to designing therapies applicable to the total population may be beneficial. Efforts should perhaps focus on characterizing the chronologic sequence of activation of certain pathophysiologic mechanisms. These may then serve as appropriate targets for drugs with matched mechanisms of action at various postinjury time points.

Draw Meaningful Conclusions from a Heterogeneous Population

Despite strict inclusion and exclusion criteria, the head-injured patients included in clinical trials remain heterogeneous, especially with respect to their mechanisms of damage, pathophysiology, and clinical condition. Even with randomization and enrollment of more than 800 patients, imbalances in the distribution of prognostic variables, including age, GCS scores, pupillary reactivity, computed tomography (CT) classification, and pretreatment hypotension or hypoxia, are still quite possible. The treatment and control groups in the North American tirilazad trial were retrospectively found to be unequal in several prognostic criteria, including motor scores, pretreatment CT classification, and prevalence of bilaterally unreactive pupils. Results were further confounded by the fact that patients with pretreatment hypotension who received placebo had an unexpectedly good outcome. Despite a large sample size ($n = 1120$) and block randomization in the European trial, the unequal distributions of patients with pretreatment hypotension, hypoxia, or epidural hematoma acted to improve outcome in the placebo group.

Pearl

Despite proper randomization, placebo and control groups may often differ in important baseline characteristics.

The tirilazad trial also underscored the importance of gender in affecting overall outcome from brain injury. The studies of tirilazad in aneurysmal SAH initially demonstrated a marked difference in outcome based on gender, with males faring substantially better than females. A similar and significant difference in outcome between men and women was also identified in the tirilazad head injury trial, particularly if the women had also suffered traumatic SAH. The subsequently recognized accelerated metabolism of the drug in females may explain these findings. In retrospect, unbalanced randomization of traumatic SAH may have acted as an additional confounding factor in the tirilazad trial.

Because of the heterogeneity of head-injured patients, clinical trials should classify baseline risk variables from the outset and should stratify patients accordingly so that frequencies of baseline risk variables are similar in treatment and placebo groups. Randomization should also be stratified by center to ensure balance in treatment assignment. The method of minimization and the use of a central telephone randomization system provide effective means of increasing comparability of groups when many variables are present.[26]

Some argue that randomizing patients according to specific prognostic variables is not sufficient and that patients should also be randomized by the probability that they will achieve a certain recovery.[22] Patients entering a trial with a low risk of unfavorable outcome are unlikely to enjoy a large benefit from the drug. Conversely, other patients may be in such poor condition that the drug has little possibility of improving outcome. Clearly, expectation for improvement is linked to initial clinical condition. The ability to predict outcome soon after injury would identify patients whose outcome is uncertain. Focusing on this "intermediate risk" group, that is, patients whose likelihood of either a good or bad outcome is not high, would enable investigators to obtain results more reflective of the therapeutic effect, rather than a dominant prognostic effect. Trials focusing on patients with such an "intermediate prognosis" can reduce sample size by up to 30% without reducing power.[27] Prognostic equations might improve comparability of groups by more accurately distributing the risk of adverse outcomes among treatment groups, as opposed to using analyses of distributions of prognostic variables across groups only to check for comparability after the fact. Also, prerandomization stratification by expected outcome will allow, for example, movement of patients from an expected outcome of death to an actual outcome of vegetative state to be considered as an improvement in outcome. In other types of illnesses, clinical trial results have been analyzed with prognostic equations that predict survival or death in ~30 to 40% of patients, although equations from different databases have not been cross-validated.[28] Also, these equations may not take into account the fact that death after head injury usually occurs within the first few days. However, use of an accelerated log-normal method to develop prognostic equations could account for this fact.[28]

Pearl

Future studies might consider randomization of patients by predicted outcome.

Multivariable data analysis, including regression analysis, can adjust for imbalanced baseline characteristics and can yield findings that apply to patients with a specific risk profile. Standard error may increase, but by less than the increase in treatment effect, therefore increasing power.[29]

Although every effort should be taken to minimize the number of confounding factors that exist, the importance of known confounders should not be overemphasized. Just as known confounders may explain some differences in outcome between treatment and placebo groups, other unknown or unreported imbalances may eliminate differences between treatment and placebo groups.

Develop Realistic Success Criteria

Some investigators argue that criteria for success in head injury trials are unreasonably strict and therefore almost impossible to meet, especially given the lack of an adequately sensitive measure to detect favorable changes in outcome. Head injury trials generally employ the 6-month Glasgow Outcome Scale (GOS) as the primary outcome measure. Often, outcomes are dichotomized as favorable (combining good recovery and moderate disability) and unfavorable (combining severe disability, vegetative state, and death.). Clinical trials involving head-injured patients commonly define success by a 10 to 12% improvement in favorable outcome at 6 months or more after injury. Approximately 800 patients (two groups of 400) are required to detect such an improvement in favorable outcome with a power of 80% and significance level of .05. The distribution of outcomes in unselected populations of severely head-injured patients tends to assume a U-shape, with a low incidence of patients with severe disability or vegetative state. Most patients either die or demonstrate substantial recovery. Favorable and unfavorable outcomes occur with approximately equal frequency. Among survivors, however, favorable outcome approaches 70 to 80%; many investigators blame this high frequency of favorable outcome a priori for part of the difficulty in demonstrating success. First, it is difficult to achieve a 10% increase in the rate of favorable outcome solely by improving the state of survivors; that is, without a decrease in mortality. As mentioned earlier, prerandomization stratification by expected outcome may make it possible to meet such a criterion of success by allowing, for example, those patients moving from an expected outcome of death to an actual outcome of vegetative state to be considered as having an improvement in outcome. Second, any improvement in the group with favorable outcome may not be captured on the dichotomized GOS unless an extended eight-point GOS is utilized.

Pearl

It may be unrealistic for a trial to expect a 10% improvement in favorable outcome.

Further problems associated with use of the dichotomized GOS were illustrated by a recent analysis calculating the hypothetical effect of increasing the number of improved patients over one, two, or three categories by 25 to 50% with respect to the placebo population, using data from the HIT II nimodipine trial as an example.[22] The authors found that improving outcomes enough to move 50% of patients into the next best outcome category would increase favorable outcome on the dichotomized GOS by only 5%. If 25% of all patients improved by two levels, favorable outcome increases only 3%. Upgrading outcome by three categories in 25% of patients increases favorable outcome by only 9%—less than the 10% improvement in favorable outcome required by most clinical trials. Admittedly, this analysis does not account for the possibility that a drug may worsen outcomes in some patients, or that outcome shifts are not uniform. If a similar type of analysis is performed using the data from the traumatic SAH subgroup of the HIT II study, a greater percentage increase in favorable GOS is seen because of the different distribution of outcome in this subgroup, which had a more unfavorable outcome initially. The authors also determined that the results obtained in the nimodipine trial with traumatic SAH were similar to the effect that would have been obtained by upgrading 25% of patients by three categories and that the results obtained in the triamcinolone trial, though not statistically significant, were analogous to what would have been obtained had 25% of patients in each category been upgraded by two levels. The authors recommended assessing the feasibility of attaining a certain improvement in outcome by performing a sample calculation to estimate the percentage of patients who would need to be upgraded by a certain number of outcome levels to meet their stated goal in a population with intermediate risk, or that a goal of 5 to 8% improvement be sought in the total population.

Further, the authors reported that a modest but statistically significant improvement in outcomes using the HIT II data would not be reflected in the dichotomized GOS; in this situation, an ordinal analysis according to the five categories of the Glasgow Outcome Scale (good recovery, moderate disability, severe disability, vegetative state, death) would be more useful. The authors then hypothesized that the possibility of statistical significance being reflected as an improvement in favorable GOS by 10% or more is greater when there is a larger change in outcome with respect to the placebo population, such as upgrading patients by three categories. However, by analyzing data from other completed trials, the authors found that the dichotomized GOS yielded significance, when ordinal analysis did not, in the previously analyzed subgroups of the HIT II and triamcinolone trials. Because the effect of treatment in the subgroups was to reduce mortality, favorable outcomes may have been increased because of survival of some patients who may have otherwise died without treatment. On the other hand, given that placebo outcomes in both trials were nearly identical, the authors raise the question of whether such an outcome distribution in the placebo group is an accommodating backdrop against which to demonstrate treatment efficacy. Still, subgroups were not specified in advance, and consequently no definite conclusion can be drawn.

Minimize Other Factors That May Complicate Clinical Trials

Some point out that the failure to demonstrate efficacy in specialized centers does not necessarily translate to ineffectiveness in less specialized centers, where facilities are often limited and secondary insults may occur with greater frequency. Patients in such centers may serve as better subjects for demonstrating efficacy of neuroprotective agents.

Data from preclinical and clinical trials of stroke or subarachnoid hemorrhage often influence whether head injury trials are initiated or continued with the same neuroprotective agent. It is questionable whether conclusions about the role of a neuroprotective agent in one arena are applicable to another arena. For example, enrollment in the Selfotel head injury trial was curtailed after increased deaths and severe adverse events were noted in patients treated with Selfotel in two stroke trials, even though the head injury data showed no excess of serious adverse events in the treatment group. Similar concern about the effect of Cerestat in stroke patients led to early termination of the phase III head injury trial of that agent.

In some trials, sample sizes may have been too small to permit either detection or exclusion of a subtle but clinically relevant finding.

Conclusions

Without exception, no head injury clinical trial conducted in the past decade has shown a statistically significant improvement in outcome in the total treatment population. It must be noted, however, that this failure is only valid in the context of defining success as a 10% improvement in favorable outcome on the dichotomized GOS. The neuroprotective agents studied may indeed be effective, but not to the extent necessary to achieve such a degree of outcome improvement in the total population. Some agents may be more effective in specific subgroups of patients. Halting trials prematurely prevents investigators from answering the question of efficacy (either positively or negatively) either in the full population or in a subgroup. This chapter outlined several challenges faced by head injury trials and described possible ways of improving the preclinical phases of information gathering and design and analysis of clinical trials to maximize the possibility of obtaining conclusive findings.

References

1. Brain Trauma Foundation. American Association of Neurological Surgeons, Joint Section on Neurotrauma and Critical Care. Guidelines for the management of severe traumatic brain injury. J Neurotrauma 2000;17:449–554.
2. Alderson P, Roberts I. Corticosteroids in acute traumatic brain injury: systematic review of randomised controlled trials. BMJ 1997;314:1855–1859.
3. Grumme T, Baethmann A, Kolodziejczyk D, et al. Treatment of patients with severe head injury by triamcinolone: a prospective, controlled multicenter clinical trial of 396 cases. Res Exp Med (Berl) 1995;195:217–229.
4. Yates D, Roberts I. Corticosteroids in head injury: it's time for a large simple randomised trial. CRASH trial management group. Corticosteroid randomisation after significant head injury. BMJ 2000;321:128–129.
5. Roberts I. Design of CRASH trial. Trial is best way to elucidate effectiveness of corticosteroids in acute severe head injury. BMJ 1999;319:1069.
6. Robinson MJ, Teasdale GM. Calcium antagonists in the management of subarachnoid haemorrhage. Cerebrovasc Brain Metab Rev 1990;2:205–226.
7. Bailey I, Bell A, Gray J, et al. A trial of the effect of nimodipine on outcome after head injury. Acta Neurochir (Wien) 1991;110: 97–105.
8. European Study Group on Nimodipine in Severe Head Injury. A multicenter trial of the efficacy of nimodipine on outcome after severe head injury. J Neurosurg 1994;80:797–804.
9. Harders A, Kakarieka A, Braakman R. Traumatic subarachnoid hemorrhage and its treatment with nimodipine. German tSAH Study Group. J Neurosurg 1996;85:82–89.
10. Kakarieka A. Traumatic Subarachnoid Haemorrhage. Berlin: Springer-Verlag, 1997.
11. Sprenger K, Farrell D, Servadei F. et al. Nimodipine in head injury: results of the HIT IV study. Presented at the 5th International Neurotrauma Symposium, Garmisch-Partenjirchen, Germany, October 5, 2000.
12. Hall ED, Yonkers PA, McCall JM, et al. Effects of the 21-aminosteroid U74006F on experimental head injury in mice. J Neurosurg 1988;68:456–461.
13. Straw RN, Means ED, Kitt TM, et al. Preliminary Efficacy and Safety Results from Protocol P/2700/0017: Tirilazad Mesylate in the Treatment of Acute Head Injury (North American study)—Technical Report. Kalamazoo, MI: Pharmacia & Upjohn Co.; 1995.
14. Marshall LF, Maas AI, Marshall SB, et al. A multicenter trial on the efficacy of using tirilazad mesylate in cases of head injury. J Neurosurg 1998;89:519–525.
15. Young B, Runge JW, Waxman KS, et al. Effects of pegorgotein on neurologic outcome of patients with severe head injury: a multicenter, randomized controlled trial. JAMA 1996;276: 538–543.
16. Morris GF, Bullock R, Marshall SB, et al. Failure of the competitive N-methyl-D-aspartate antagonist Selfotel (CGS 19755) in the treatment of severe head injury: results of two phase III clinical trials. The Selfotel Investigators. J Neurosurg 1999;91: 737–743.
17. Hayes RL, Jenkins LW, Lyeth BG. Neurotransmitter-mediated mechanisms of traumatic brain injury: acetylcholine and excitatory amino acids. J Neurotrauma 1992;9(suppl 1):S173–S187.
18. Chen MH, Bullock R, Graham DI, et al. Ischemic neuronal damage after acute subdural hematoma in the rat: effects of pretreatment with a glutamate antagonist. J Neurosurg 1991; 74:944–950.
19. Mcintosh TK, Vink R, Soarez H, et al. Effects of the N-methyl-D-aspartate receptor blocker MK-801 on neurologic function after experimental brain injury. J Neurotrauma 1989;6:247–259.
20. Davis SM, Albers GW, Diener HC, et al. Termination of Acute Stroke Studies Involving Selfotel Treatment. ASSIST Steering Committee. Lancet 1997;349:32.
21. Bullock R, Zauner A, Woodward JJ, et al. Factors affecting excitatory amino acid release following severe human head injury. J Neurosurg 1998;89:507–518.
22. Maas AI, Steyerberg EW, Murray GD, et al. Why have recent trials of neuroprotective agents in head injury failed to show convincing efficacy? A pragmatic analysis and theoretical considerations. Neurosurgery 1999;44:1286–1298.
23. Fleishaker JC, Hulst-Pearson LK, Peters GR. Effect of gender and menopausal status on the pharmacokinetics of tirilazad mesylate in healthy subjects. Am J Ther 1995;2:553–560.
24. Fleishaker JC, Straw RN, Cross CJ. Pharmacokinetics of tirilazad and U-89678, an active, reduced metabolite, following acute head trauma in adults. J Pharm Sci 1997;86:434–437.
25. Bouma GJ, Muizelaar JP, Stringer WA, et al. Ultra-early evaluation of regional cerebral blood flow in severely head-injured patients using xenon-enhanced computerized tomography. J Neurosurg 1992;77:360–368.

26. Treasure T, MacRae KD. Minimisation: the platinum standard for trials? Randomisation doesn't guarantee similarity of groups; minimisation does. BMJ 1998;317:362–363.

27. Machado SG, Murray GD, Teasdale GM. Evaluation of designs for clinical trials of neuroprotective agents in head injury. European Brain Injury Consortium. J Neurotrauma 1999;16:1131–1138.

28. Knaus WA, Harrell FE Jr, LaBrecque JF, et al. Use of predicted risk of mortality to evaluate the efficacy of anticytokine therapy in sepsis. The rhIL-1ra Phase III Sepsis Syndrome Study Group. Crit Care Med 1996;24:46–56.

29. Steyerberg EW, Bossuyt PM, Lee KL. Clinical trials in acute myocardial infarction: should we adjust for baseline characteristics? Am Heart J 2000;139:745–751.

Brain Injury

Treatment of Elevated Intracranial Pressure

◆ 24 ◆

At What Level Should I Start Treating Elevated Intracranial Pressure?

Juan Sahuquillo

Brief Answer

Intracranial pressure (ICP)-targeted therapy remains the gold standard in the management of severely head-injured patients. No robust evidence is available to support a level I recommendation about a specific ICP threshold. However, our recommendation is that the optimal ICP at which treatment should be started is 20 mmHg (level II). The threshold for treating ICP should be reduced from 20 to 15 mmHg in patients who have had a decompressive craniotomy and in those who have a mass lesion in the temporal lobe (level III recommendation). Further research is needed to determine whether the outcome of patients treated at the lower threshold of 15 mmHg is better than that of patients treated at a threshold of 20 mmHg (as suggested by class III evidence). To improve accuracy and to avoid suboptimal care in patients with mass lesions or midline shift, the ICP monitor should be placed in the hemisphere with the greatest lesional volume when a neurosurgeon uses a parenchymal device to monitor ICP (level II).

Background

ICP monitors, *per se*, do not save lives. The people who judiciously use the data obtained from ICP monitoring can save lives and alter outcomes in patients with severe head injuries.

—T.G. Saul and T.B. Ducker, 1982[1]

The goals of the clinical management of severe head injury consist of controlling ICP and maintaining sufficient cerebral perfusion pressure (CPP) and cerebral blood flow (CBF) to avoid brain ischemia. However, the best way to achieve these goals is still debated because most of the management of ICP and CPP takes place in those gray areas of practice that still lack class I evidence that would provide answers to many questions.

Ever since the beginning of neurointensive care, the main targets of the management of severe head injury have generally been the prevention of high ICP and the prompt and aggressive treatment of its elevations; that is, ICP-based management. ICP has traditionally been defined as elevated if it crosses a threshold that is variously described as 15 to 25 mmHg.[2,3]

Because of the emphasis on CPP as the main force driving blood flow to the brain, many clinicians focus on that parameter as the main target of the management of severe head injuries; that is, CPP-based management.[4–6] For many practitioners of this approach, achieving an adequate CPP is much more important than maintaining tight control of ICP. CPP has been empirically considered to be sufficient when the difference between mean arterial blood pressure (MABP) and ICP exceeds 70 mmHg. It is assumed that keeping CPP above this threshold indicates that brain perfusion, and consequently CBF, is adequate. This approach is based on the unproven notion that a higher CPP can maintain an adequate CBF even if ICP is high. Consequently, the MABP-ICP gradient is considered more important than the absolute values of both ICP and MABP.

Following this line of thought, the second edition of the *Guidelines for the Management of Severe Traumatic Brain Injury* recommends (as an option), that "cerebral perfusion pressure should be maintained at a minimum of 70 mmHg."[7] However, this recommendation is based on class III data and, thus, a CPP threshold of 70 mmHg cannot be considered a better therapeutic option than any other level. Despite the lack of strong evidence, word has been spread in the international neurocritical care community that maintaining CPP below 70 mmHg cannot be considered good clinical practice. Ninety-seven percent of a group of board-certified North American neurosurgeons who participated in a recent survey on the management of severe head injuries felt that CPP should be maintained above 70 mmHg (class III data).[8] Another survey of neuroanesthesiologists in Germany showed that 69% of patients with a severe head injury were managed with a CPP between 70 and 90 mmHg (class III data).[9]

Pearl

Recommendations to use 70 mmHg as a threshold for CPP are based on class III data, and therefore 70 mmHg cannot be considered a better therapeutic option than any other threshold.

To add more fuel to the fire, much has been written in the last decade on a completely different and almost opposite approach for managing CPP that is advocated by investigators working at the University of Lund.[10] The Lund concept is based on the strict prevention of increases in—or even the reduction of—MABP to maintain CPP at 50 to 60 mmHg. The aim is to reduce capillary hydrostatic pressure and thus avoid edema in a brain with impaired autoregulatory mechanisms and an altered blood–brain barrier.

As is clear from the above discussion, there exist no universally accepted guidelines for manipulating CPP. Consequently, the concept of so-called CPP-based management has different meanings for different authors. Several other important questions in the ICP-CPP debate also remain unanswered. This chapter investigates one such question by reviewing available data about the threshold at which an increase in ICP should trigger therapeutic interventions.

Literature Review

Is Increased Intracranial Pressure a Good Predictor of Outcome?

Several authors have reported a strong correlation between sustained high ICP and high morbidity and mortality. The relationship between high ICP and poor outcome has been very consistent in both single-center and multicenter studies, and the ability to bring elevated ICP under control has long been considered a requirement for improving outcome of severely head-injured patients. Since the earliest work of Miller et al in the late 1970s, the threshold most frequently used in outcome studies has been 20 mmHg.[2,11–13] In an analysis of data from the Traumatic Coma Data Bank (TCDB), Marmarou et al[14] found that poor outcome after severe head injury was strongly related to high ICP (>20 mmHg) (class II data). In that study, age, admission motor score, and the presence of pupillary abnormalities correctly explained 46% of the observed outcomes when modeled alone. Beyond these three factors, the proportion of ICP measurements greater than 20 mmHg was the factor that was most indicative of outcome. This threshold was identified by testing critical ICP levels from 0 to 80 mmHg in increments of 5 mmHg.

Pearl

Beyond age, admission motor score, and the presence of pupillary abnormalities, the factor most indicative of outcome is the proportion of ICP measurements greater than 20 mmHg.

Is There an Optimal Threshold for Treating Intracranial Pressure?

If we accept that the "gold standard" method for answering questions in medicine is the randomized, controlled trial, one of the most important problems in practicing evidence-based care in the management of severe head injuries is the lack of unambiguous evidence justifying many routinely used treatments or even basic neuromonitoring methods.[15] One of the most obvious examples is choosing the most appropriate threshold at which to start treating elevated ICP.

However, debate on thresholds seems paradoxical because of the lack of class I evidence that ICP monitoring improves the outcome of patients with severe head injuries. No trials have randomized patients with severe head injury to ICP monitoring versus no ICP monitoring. The negative side of using a dogmatic approach to evidence-based medicine is that strict adherence to evidence-based care management (i.e., only accepting unambiguous evidence) may result in the modern treatment of severe head injuries being subjected to a moratorium that will completely paralyze currently accepted protocols used in clinical practice, as is happening in other areas of critical care. Such a situation might provoke such undesirable effects as flipping the coin to the other side; that is, all therapeutic strategies are valid because nothing has been adequately proved. If scientific fundamentalism can be avoided, however, a positive aspect that may emerge from the current emphasis on evidence-based care is that every single treatment is placed under careful scrutiny. Such a process favors a more rigorous and scientific approach to the management of traumatic brain injuries. Refraining from "expert opinions" and unproven hypotheses promotes scientific progress and improves clinical practice.

Although for many the last word on the subject of ICP monitoring has not been said, there is a general consensus that the low risk:benefit ratio of this monitoring technique is obvious and that a randomized trial on this topic could be considered unethical, not to mention very difficult to implement methodologically.[3] One of the several problems the clinician would confront in conducting such a trial is similar to that faced by participants in a consensus conference on the use of pulmonary artery catheters (PAC) in critical care. To summarize the problem, these authors asked, "Can a clinician ethically enroll patients in such a trial, knowing that the patient may not receive a PAC, despite subsequent hemodynamic (or cardiopulmonary) deterioration?"[16]

The morbidity of ICP monitoring, which is quite low, is overshadowed by the fact that ICP monitoring provides essential and continuous cerebral hemodynamic information that cannot be supplied by comprehensive neurologic examination or even by serial computed tomography (CT) scans. Furthermore, ICP is used to calculate CPP and therefore to protect the brain from ischemia, evidence of which is observed very commonly in postmortem examination of patients who die after head injury.[17] For all these reasons, ICP monitoring was recommended by the Brain Trauma Foundation's (BTF's) *Guidelines* as a guideline (i.e., between a standard and an option) for the management of all patients with a severe head injury and an abnormal CT scan.[18] However, in practice, ICP monitoring is considered a "standard of care" in the majority of centers managing patients with severe head injuries.

Pearl

Based on a review of available evidence, the Brain Trauma Foundation recommended as a guideline (i.e., between a standard and an option) that ICP be monitored in patients with a severe head injury and an abnormal CT scan. However, in practice, ICP monitoring is considered a "standard of care" in the majority of centers managing patients with severe head injuries.

When Should Elevated Intracranial Pressure Be Treated?

The second edition of the BTF *Guidelines* recommends, "ICP treatment should be initiated at an upper threshold of 20–25 mmHg."[19] This recommendation is believed to reflect a moderate degree of clinical certainty and is consequently offered at the level of a therapeutic guideline, not a standard or option. However, a reappraisal of the reviewed articles included in the evidentiary table of this chapter of the *Guidelines*[19] raises certain points that warrant comment (Table 24-1). In brief, the primary hypothesis of the study by Eisenberg et al[2] was that the addition of high doses of pentobarbital would improve control of ICP; the study was not designed to define ICP treatment thresholds. Although this study should be regarded as class I evidence for making recommendations on the use of barbiturates in the treatment of refractory intracranial hypertension, it should be reclassified as class III evidence for answering questions about ICP treatment thresholds.

The other study listed as class II in this chapter of the *Guidelines*, by Marmarou et al,[14] was a post hoc logistic regression analysis in which elevated ICP (above the threshold of 20 mmHg) was found to be the strongest predictor of poor outcome after severe head injury. However, this study was not specifically designed to identify the most appropriate threshold at which to start treating elevated ICP. One of the problems in this study is that only 295 of the initial group of 654 patients met minimum monitoring criteria and also had sufficient data available for an analysis of outcome. Furthermore, as pointed out by the authors, the variability in thresholds used to treat ICP among the four participating centers may have introduced bias into the analysis.

The only study that has specifically addressed the issue of ICP treatment thresholds was published by Saul and Ducker[1] in 1982 and was already included in the BTF *Guidelines*' evidentiary table.[19] To summarize this class III study, 106 head-injured patients with a Glasgow Coma Scale (GCS) score of 7 or less were treated according to a very strict protocol in which ICP treatment was started at a threshold of 15 mmHg. The mortality in this group (28%) was compared with that of a historical control group treated at the same institution during the preceding 2 years. The treatment protocol was similar except for the fact that ICP in the earlier group was treated at the higher threshold of 20 to 25 mmHg. Mortality in the historical control group was 46% (p <.0005). Unfortunately, this study has many flaws. The most important are the use of historical controls, the lack of a clear description of the patients' primary lesions, and the inclusion of patients treated at the lower threshold in a randomized barbiturate study. For these reasons, this study should be

Table 24-1 Evidentiary Table for Optimal ICP Treatment Threshold*

Reference	Study Description	Class of Evidence	Study Conclusions
Chambers et al. 2001[30]	Observational study of 291 severely head-injured patients (207 adults). Receiver-operating characteristic (ROC) curves were used to analyze whether significant threshold levels for ICP and CPP exist for predicting outcome.	II	When outcome was categorized as either independent (good recovery or moderate disability) or poor (severe disability, vegetative state, or death), a 2-minute rolling average ICP of 35 mmHg appeared to be the best predictor of outcome in adults. Different thresholds may exist for different types of lesions.
Eisenberg et al. 1988[2]	Multicenter randomized trial in 73 patients to test the hypothesis that the addition of high doses of pentobarbital (37 cases) would improve the ability to control ICP compared with a rigorous protocol applying "conventional" therapies (36 patients). Control of ICP (<20 mmHg) was chosen as the primary outcome variable.	III (II in BTF *Guidelines*)	When intracranial hypertension is refractory to conventional treatments (sedation, analgesia, severe hyperventilation, mannitol, etc.), high-dose pentobarbital is an effective adjunctive therapy.
Marmarou et al. 1991[14]	Post hoc analysis of 1030 severely head-injured patients in the Traumatic Coma Data Bank study. Of the total series, 428 patients met minimum monitoring criteria for entry into the study. Logistic regression was used to determine the ICP cutoff point that was most indicative of outcome.	II	A 20 mmHg threshold was found to be the best independent predictor of outcome. A potential bias in this study is that the ICP level used to start treatment varied from 15 to 25 mmHg among the participating centers.
Saul and Ducker, 1982[1]	The only study designed to answer the specific issue of ICP thresholds. One hundred six severely head-injured patients were treated according to a strict protocol in which therapeutic measures were started at an ICP >15 mmHg. Mortality in this group (28%) was compared with that of a historical control group treated at the same institution during the two preceding years, when treatment for elevated ICP was initiated at 20–25 mmHg. Mortality in the latter group was 46%.	III	A significant reduction in mortality was found when patients treated at an ICP threshold of 15 mmHg were compared with historical controls in whom ICP was treated at 20–25 mmHg. Analysis of the data in this report demonstrates a sizable reduction in the odds of death at three months (OR 0.47, 95% confidence interval 0.26 to 0.84).

*During the creation of this table, only papers not included in the evidentiary table of the chapter "Intracranial Pressure Treatment Threshold" in the second edition of the BTF *Guidelines* were reviewed. In addition, studies are listed if they have been discussed in the text or if the class of evidence differs from that of the *Guidelines*. For a more complete list, the reader is referred to reference 19. CPP, cerebral perfusion pressure; ICP, intracranial pressure; OR, odds ratio.

considered class III evidence. Nevertheless, analysis of the data for an ICP treatment threshold of 15 mmHg demonstrates a significant reduction in the odds of death at three months [odds ratios (OR) 0.47, 95% confidence interval 0.26 to 0.84]. The magnitude of the effect is important enough to suggest the need for a multicenter, randomized trial in which the effect on outcome of these two different levels of treatment can be evaluated.

In an attempt to find additional evidence to support a clinical recommendation about the optimal ICP treatment threshold, the same electronic search strategy used to answer this question in the second version of the BTF *Guidelines* was used to search the Medline database for publications appearing between 1995 and 2001. No restrictions on language of publication were included in the query. This search produced 72 references that were inspected one by one, including nine papers not included in the evidentiary table of the BTF *Guidelines*. Of these nine papers, only one (in addition to the studies already identified by the BTF) was considered appropriate for inclusion in this updated review (Table 24-1).

Should Different Lesions Be Treated at Different Intracranial Pressure Thresholds?

In the TCDB report, elevated ICP (<20 mmHg) was observed in 72% of severely head-injured patients (class II data).[20] However, pupillary abnormalities suggestive of brainstem compression from transtentorial herniation have been described at a relatively low or even normal ICP.[21] Herniation can occur at the flat part of the pressure-volume curve during the phase of spatial compensation. This is particularly important in patients with temporal mass lesions and in those who have undergone decompressive craniotomy. Eisenberg et al[2] suggested that the threshold to treat elevated ICP should be reduced from 25 to 15 mmHg in patients with an "opened skull" (craniectomy >25 cm^2 and dura left open). Again, no class I or II evidence can be cited to support this particular approach. It therefore should be treated as a level III recommendation.

Where Should an Intracranial Pressure Monitor Be Inserted?

According to the BTF's recommendations, "the ventricular catheter connected to an external strain gauge is the most accurate, low-cost, and reliable method of monitoring intracranial pressure."[22] The *Guidelines* state that the accuracy of intraparenchymal fiberoptic or strain gauge devices is similar to that of ventriculostomy catheters, but at a higher cost and with the potential for baseline drift because these devices cannot be recalibrated once inserted.[22]

Although the ventriculostomy catheter is still considered the gold standard for ICP monitoring, over the last few years it has been replaced in many centers by brain tissue pressure monitoring. In the survey by Ghajar et al[23] on current practices in the monitoring and treatment of patients with severe head injury in the United States, 48% of the trauma centers used intraparenchymal devices to monitor ICP (class III data). A survey by Marion and Spiegel[8] on the impact of the BTF *Guidelines* in changing the management of severe head injuries showed that 48% of the respondents used a transducer-tip white matter probe for ICP monitoring and 50% used a ventriculostomy catheter, in some cases (21%) in combination with a transducer-tip probe (class III data). Several reasons may be offered to explain this shift from ventriculostomy catheters to transducer-tip white matter probes. Perhaps the most important reasons are that these transducers may be inserted quickly and easily at the bedside, the learning curve is faster, and they are easier to insert than ventriculostomy catheters when brain swelling or midline shift is present. Furthermore, the nurses' workload is reduced, and the rate of complications, especially infection, is less than that of ventriculostomy. The main disadvantages of these methods are that they do not permit recalibration and they do not allow cerebrospinal fluid drainage as a first-tier measure for the treatment of elevated ICP. In addition, the cost of disposable transducers and monitoring equipment is high.

The increased use of compartmental methods (intraparenchymal, subdural, and epidural) to measure ICP has reopened the debate on the uniformity of pressures across the intracranial space. Traditionally, the intracranial space has been viewed as a unicameral compartment, with pressure equally distributed throughout the chamber.[24] Under normal conditions there should be little difference in pressures between the cerebral hemispheres. However, brain shifts or blocks in the subarachnoid spaces may disrupt the equilibrium between these freely communicating compartments, causing interhemispheric ICP gradients. Clinical studies using different methods of measurement have reached contradictory conclusions on this important issue (class III data).[25–28] Using subarachnoid catheters, Weaver et al[27] observed unilateral ICP gradients in four of 20 patients with mass lesions (class III data). In contrast, Yano et al[28] reported that ICP was identical throughout the supratentorial space in patients with head injuries and mass lesions (class III data).

Sahuquillo et al[24] prospectively studied this issue in 50 moderately or severely head-injured patients in whom bilateral intraparenchymal ICP monitors were implanted (class II data). No patient with a diffuse brain lesion (midline shift <3 mm and total volume of lesions in a hemisphere <25 mL) demonstrated clinically significant supratentorial ICP gradients. Therefore, in patients with diffuse injury, the intracranial compartment behaves as a unicameral space, and ICP is nearly identical in both hemispheres. However, clinically significant interhemispheric pressure gradients were present for various time periods in 50% of patients with focal lesions (summed hemispheric lesional volumes >25 mL and/or midline shift >3 mm). In almost 25% of patients with focal lesions, CPP differed significantly when calculated separately for each hemisphere. Management of these patients might have been different if the available data had been obtained only from the hemisphere with a lower lesional volume.

The main pitfall of intraparenchymal pressure monitoring is that it may overestimate the actual CPP.[24] To optimize ICP monitoring when intraparenchymal catheter-tipped transducers are used in patients with intradural mass lesions larger than 25 mL and/or midline shift, the monitor by probe or sensor should be implanted on the side with the greatest lesional volume.

Pearl

To optimize ICP monitoring when intraparenchymal catheter-tipped transducers are used in patients with intradural mass lesions larger than 25 mL and/or midline shift, the monitor by probe or sensor should be implanted on the side with the greatest lesional volume.

Recommendations

Because of the lack of robust evidence, no strong general recommendations can be made about the optimal level at which ICP should be treated. No randomized trials have been performed to define the optimal ICP threshold. However, based on class II and III evidence, our recommendation is that ICP-lowering treatment should be started at an ICP of 20 mmHg (level II). Further research is needed to determine whether the outcome of patients treated at a lower threshold (15 mmHg) is better than that of patients treated at 20 mmHg. In addition, controlled studies are required to determine whether some patients with mass effect should also be treated at a lower threshold. We recommend that a threshold of 20 mmHg be used for diffuse lesions, whereas 15 mmHg be used as the threshold for patients with mass lesions in the temporal lobe or with a decompressive craniotomy (level III). To improve accuracy and to avoid suboptimal care in patients with mass lesions or midline shift, the transducer should always be placed in the hemisphere with the greatest lesional volume when intraparenchymal devices are used to monitor ICP (level III). Although protracted intracranial hypertension (ICP >20 mmHg) is a predictor of bad outcome, the reader should bear in mind that some studies have shown that a good outcome after head injury is still possible despite persistently high ICP (class III data).[29]

Acknowledgments

The author gratefully acknowledges the assistance of Gail Craigie in translating the manuscript. This work was supported by grant 00/0827 from the Fondo de Investigaciones Sanitarias de la Seguridad Social (FIS) to Dr. J. Sahuquillo.

References

1. Saul TG, Ducker TB. Effect of intracranial pressure monitoring and aggressive treatment on mortality in severe head injury. J Neurosurg 1982;56:498–503.
2. Eisenberg HM, Frankowski RF, Contant CF, et al. High-dose barbiturate control of elevated intracranial pressure in patients with severe head injury. J Neurosurg 1988;69:15–23.
3. Brain Trauma Foundation. American Association of Neurological Surgeons, Joint Section on Neurotrauma and Critical Care. Guidelines for the management of severe traumatic brain injury. J Neurotrauma 2000;17:449–554.
4. Rosner MJ, Rosner SD. Manipulation of cerebral perfusion pressure and management of the head-injured patient. J Neurosurg 1992;76:399A.
5. Rosner MJ. Therapeutic increase of cerebral perfusion pressure and the management of traumatic brain injury. Neurosurgery 1992;30:803.
6. Rosner MJ, Rosner SD, Johnson AH. Cerebral perfusion pressure: management protocol and clinical results. J Neurosurg 1995;83:949–962.
7. Brain Trauma Foundation, American Association of Neurological Surgeons, Joint Section on Neurotrauma and Critical Care. Guidelines for the management of severe traumatic brain injury. Guidelines for cerebral perfusion pressure. J Neurotrauma 2000;17:507–511.
8. Marion DW, Spiegel TP. Changes in the management of severe traumatic brain injury: 1991–1997. Crit Care Med 2000;28: 16–18.
9. Himmelseher S, Pfenninger E. Neuroprotection in neuroanesthesia: current practices in Germany. Anaesthesist 2000;49: 412–419.
10. Asgeirsson B, Grände PO, Nordström CH. The Lund concept of post-traumatic brain oedema therapy. Acta Anaesthesiol Scand 1995;39:103–106.
11. Miller JD, Becker DP, Ward JD, et al. Significance of intracranial hypertension in severe head injury. J Neurosurg 1977;47:503–516.
12. Narayan RK, Kishore PR, Becker DP, et al. Intracranial pressure: to monitor or not to monitor? A review of our experience with severe head injury. J Neurosurg 1982;56:650–659.
13. Marshall LF, Smith RW, Shapiro HM. The outcome with aggressive treatment in severe head injuries, II: Acute and chronic barbiturate administration in the management of head injury. J Neurosurg (Suppl.) 1979;50:26–30.
14. Marmarou A, Anderson RL, Ward JD, et al. Impact of instability and hypotension on outcome in patients with severe head trauma. J Neurosurg 1991;75:S59–S66.
15. Sahuquillo J. Evidence-based medicine and clinical practice guidelines for traumatic brain injury. In: Gonzalez-Feria L, von Wild KRH, Diemath HE (eds). Quality Management in Head Injuries Care: Critical Approaches to Health Economics, Patient Selection and Acute Treatment. La Laguna, Spain: El Productor, S.L.; 2000:109–117.
16. Pulmonary Artery Catheter Consensus Conference. Consensus Statement. Crit Care Med 1997;25:910–925.
17. Graham DI, Ford I, Adams JH, et al. Ischaemic brain damage is still common in fatal non-missile head injury. J Neurol Neurosurg Psychiatry 1989;52:346–350.
18. Brain Trauma Foundation, American Association of Neurological Surgeons, Joint Section on Neurotrauma and Critical Care. Guidelines for the management of severe traumatic brain injury. Indications for intracranial pressure monitoring. J Neurotrauma 2000;17:479–491.
19. Brain Trauma Foundation, American Association of Neurological Surgeons, Joint Section on Neurotrauma and Critical Care. Guidelines for the management of severe traumatic brain injury. Intracranial pressure treatment threshold. J Neurotrauma 2000;17:493–495.
20. Marmarou A, Anderson RL, Ward JD, et al. NINDS Traumatic Coma Data Bank: intracranial pressure monitoring methodology. J Neurosurg (Suppl.) 1991;75:S21–S27.
21. Marshall LF, Barba D, Toole BM, et al. The oval pupil: clinical significance and relationship to intracranial hypertension. J Neurosurg 1983;58:566–568.
22. Bullock RM, Chesnut RM, Clifton GL, et al. Management and prognosis of severe traumatic brain injury: recommendations for intracranial pressure monitoring technology. J Neurotrauma 2000;17:497–506.
23. Ghajar J, Hariri RJ, Narayan RK, et al. Survey of critical care management of comatose, head-injured patients in the United States. Crit Care Med 1995;23:560–567.
24. Sahuquillo J, Poca MA, Arribas M, et al. Interhemispheric supratentorial intracranial pressure gradients in head-injured patients: are they clinically important? J Neurosurg 1999;90:16–26.
25. Gambardella G, d'Avella D, Tomasello F. Monitoring of brain tissue pressure with a fiberoptic device. Neurosurgery 1992;31: 918–922.
26. Mindermann T, Reinhardt H, Gratzl O. Significant lateralisation of supratentorial ICP after blunt head trauma. Acta Neurochir (Wien) 1992;116:60–61.
27. Weaver DD, Winn HR, Jane JA. Differential intracranial pressure in patients with unilateral mass lesions. J Neurosurg 1982; 56:660–665.
28. Yano M, Ikeda Y, Kobayashi S, et al. Intracranial pressure in head-injured patients with various intracranial lesions is

identical throughout the supratentorial intracranial compartment. Neurosurgery 1987;21:688–692.

29. Resnick DK, Marion DW, Carlier P. Outcome analysis of patients with severe head injuries and prolonged intracranial hypertension. J Trauma 1997;42:1108–1111.

30. Chambers IR, Treadwell L, Mendelow AD. Determination of threshold levels of cerebral perfusion pressure and intracranial pressure in severe head injury by using receiver-operating characteristic curves: an observational study in 291 patients. J Neurosurg 2001;94:412–416.

◆ 25 ◆

Is There a "Best" Way to Give Mannitol?

Rudolph J. Schrot and J. Paul Muizelaar

Brief Answer

The only level I recommendation supported by the evidence is the use of high-dose mannitol (at least 1.2–1.4 g/kg) in comatose trauma patients with operative acute subdural hematoma or operative intraparenchymal temporal lobe hemorrhage. Use of mannitol (0.25–1.0 g/kg) to control elevated intracranial pressure (ICP) in severely head-injured patients is a level II recommendation. In this setting, mannitol may be especially effective when cerebral perfusion pressure (CPP) is below 70 mmHg (level III recommendation). Additional level III recommendations include administering bolus doses of mannitol at a rate not exceeding 0.1 g/kg/min, replacing urinary losses of fluid, and maintaining serum osmolarity below 320 mOsm/L and serum osmolar gap below 55 mOsm/L.

Background

Mannitol, an inert six-carbon alcohol of the corresponding sugar mannose, causes cellular dehydration by increasing serum osmolarity. Wise and Chater[1] pioneered the use of hypertonic mannitol to reduce cerebral swelling (class III data). Although the use of mannitol in head injury has been recommended as a guideline,[2] the optimal use of mannitol remains a complicated issue about which the data are incomplete. Questions persist about such issues as bolus versus continuous administration, ICP-directed dosing versus regularly scheduled boluses, optimal rate of infusion, optimal dosage, fluid replacement of urinary losses, clinical thresholds for treatment, role of serum osmolarity monitoring, and timing of treatment after entrance into the trauma care system. Because of this paucity of data, nearly all recommendations about the best method of mannitol administration in head injury (except for treatment of operative acute subdural hematoma or intraparenchymal temporal lobe hemorrhage in comatose head-injured patients) must be considered level III with respect to both ICP control and clinical outcome.

Literature Review

Mechanism of Action

The original model to explain mannitol's effects proposed that ICP reduction occurred through an osmotic gradient created between the blood and the brain. This gradient reduced brain water content. Therefore, mannitol therapy has classically been directed toward establishing and maintaining this gradient.[3] More recently, however, this paradigm has shifted. The time course of reduction in ICP after bolus mannitol infusion is not explained by its osmotic effects. Experiments in cats showed that the ICP decline from mannitol was greatest 30 minutes after a bolus, even though brain water content remained stable.[4] Subsequent laboratory studies showed that mannitol decreased blood viscosity and caused a decrease in the diameter of pial arterioles in a manner similar to the vasoconstricting effect of hyperventilation.[5]

Although mannitol-induced osmotic tissue dehydration may still play an important role in reducing ICP (class III data),[6] mannitol's primary mechanism of

Pearl

Mannitol's primary mechanism of action is its rheologic effect. For this reason, mannitol can have dramatic effects on cerebral blood flow (CBF) even in cases in which it has only minimal effects on ICP.

action is its rheologic effect. Mannitol dilutes the blood and increases the deformability of erythrocytes (class II data),[7] thereby decreasing blood viscosity. CBF is augmented both by the decreased viscosity and by the favorable effect of the mannitol bolus on mean arterial pressure (MAP). The sudden increase in CBF causes autoregulatory vasoconstriction of cerebral arterioles, decreasing the intracerebral blood volume and lowering the ICP (Fig. 25-1). This vasoconstriction in the presence of maintained CBF may explain the lasting effects of mannitol on ICP (class II data),[8] even after mannitol has been excreted.

It is important to realize that even in cases in which mannitol does not reduce ICP (much), it can markedly increase CBF through its rheologic effect (class II data).[9,10] This augmentation of CBF may have important clinical consequences (class III data).[11]

Bolus versus Continuous Infusion

No clinical studies have compared bolus to continuous mannitol infusion. Becker and Vries[12] presented a retrospective case series of 18 patients treated with either bolus or continuous infusion of mannitol, but no information was given as to which method was used in each case (class III data). James[13] reported that, in a series of 60 patients, mannitol boluses of at least 1.0 g/kg always reduced ICP by at least 10%, but smaller doses did not always reduce ICP. James also reported that continuous infusion was successful in keeping ICP below 25 mmHg in 16 of 18 patients (class III data). Marshall et al[3] reported that mannitol boluses alone were effective in reducing ICP (class II data).

Arguments in support of bolus dosing are based on the postulated mechanism of action of mannitol; that is, on a rheologically mediated autoregulatory response. Muizelaar et al[10] demonstrated that mannitol boluses (0.66 g/kg over 3 minutes) were effective in reducing

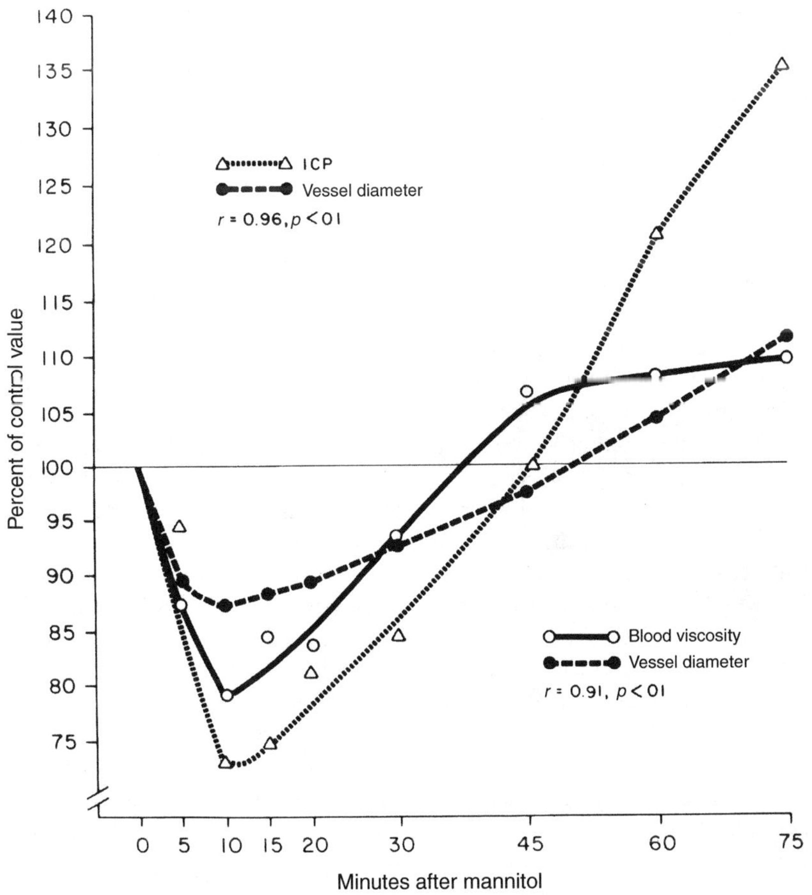

Figure 25-1 Graph showing the effects of mannitol in an experimental model. Changes in blood viscosity, pial vessel diameter, and intracranial pressure are plotted versus time.

ICP (class II data). Furthermore, in patients with intact autoregulation, ICP was reduced by 27%, but CBF remained unchanged. In patients with defective autoregulation, ICP dropped by only 4.7%, and CBF increased by 18%. This differential response is consistent with a rheologic mechanism of action for mannitol. The effect on clinical outcome of mannitol bolus treatment for elevated ICP is less clear. In patients in whom ICP was above 20 mmHg, Unterberg et al[14] reported significant improvement in ICP and CPP after infusion of mannitol (125 cc of 20% mannitol over 30 minutes), but not in brain tissue oxygenation ($PbtO_2$) or jugular venous oxygen saturation (class II data). No changes were seen in these parameters when ICP was below 20 mmHg. In a separate communication from this same group, Hartl et al[15] (class II data) found that mannitol had little effect on $PbtO_2$.

Arguments against continuous infusion are based on expert opinion[16] (class III data) that prolonged high levels of serum mannitol result in rebound brain edema as mannitol leaks into the interstitium. Experimental evidence in cats has shown that repeated dosing of mannitol leads to an increased accumulation of mannitol in the brain, especially in areas with injury-induced vasogenic edema.[17] Becker and Vries[12] reported a very high mortality rate in patients in whom mannitol therapy was associated with high serum osmolarity (class III data). This high mortality was probably attributable to high serum mannitol levels. Mannitol can produce acute renal failure (class III data),[18] and bolus dosing would presumably prevent chronic exposure of the renal tubule to mannitol.

Rate of Infusion

Very rapid infusion of mannitol has been reported to cause hypotension via decrease in peripheral vascular resistance from vasodilation in skeletal muscle (class III data).[19] In a study by Ravussin et al,[20] 1 g/kg of mannitol infused over 4 minutes (0.25 g/kg/min) to three human subjects caused a drop in MAP of 12 mmHg and a rise in heart rate of 30 beats per minute (both statistically significant) (class III data). The blood pressure returned to baseline within 2 minutes, whereas the heart rate required 15 to 30 minutes to normalize. In a series of six craniotomy patients, mannitol delivered at a very fast rate of infusion (20% mannitol at 60–80 mL over 15–20 seconds, or roughly 0.8 g/kg/min for a 70-kg adult) caused a mean drop in MAP of 30 mmHg. Blood pressure generally returned to normal within 2 minutes when the infusion rate was slowed (class III data).[21] The authors suggested that hypotension occurs when the infusion rate of mannitol is "much more rapid" than 1.0 g/kg administered over 10 minutes (0.1 g/kg/min). Because sudden hypotension associated with mannitol infusion times of less than 5 minutes (0.2 g/kg/min) has been observed in head-injured patients as well (class III data), Rosner and Coley[8] "prefer 15- to 30-minute rapid drips"; that is, infusion rates of 0.033 to 0.067 g/kg/min. To avoid the risk of sudden hypotension from rapid infusion of mannitol while still preserving its plasma-expanding effects, mannitol should probably be bolused at a rate not exceeding 0.1 g/kg/min, or 10 minutes for a dose of 1 g/kg.

Pearl

To avoid the risk of sudden hypotension from rapid infusion of mannitol, it should be bolused at a rate not exceeding 0.1 g/kg/min, and urinary losses of fluid should be replaced.

Dose

The optimal dose of mannitol has been addressed both with regard to emergency resuscitation and with regard to ICP control in the neuromonitoring unit. Class I evidence supports use of high-dose mannitol (1.2–1.4 g/kg) in the preoperative treatment of acute subdural hematoma. Thus, such treatment should be considered a level I recommendation in this circumstance. Cruz et al[22] (class I data) prospectively randomized patients with operative acute subdural hematoma into conventional-dose and high-dose mannitol treatment groups. All patients received an initial mannitol bolus of 0.6 to 0.7 g/kg in the emergency room. After computed tomography (CT) scanning revealed an acute subdural hematoma, patients were randomized to one of two groups. In the conventional-dose group, no additional mannitol was given, regardless of pupillary changes. In the high-dose group, treatment was based on the pupillary exam; patients in the high-dose group without anisocoria received an additional 0.6 to 0.7 g/kg of mannitol prior to operation, whereas patients in the high-dose group with anisocoria received an additional 1.2 to 1.4 g/kg of mannitol. To prevent hypotension from mannitol-induced osmotic diuresis, patients in all groups received normal saline boluses after each administration of mannitol. Preoperative improvement in pupillary widening was significantly better in the high-dose treatment group. The two groups did not differ significantly in the incidence of refractory intracranial hypertension requiring barbiturates or decompressive surgery. A significantly increased likelihood of low cerebral oxygen extraction and brain swelling was seen in the control group. At 6 months, Glasgow Outcome Scale scores were significantly better in the high-dose group.

These same authors have also reported a study of the effects of high-dose versus conventional-dose mannitol in patients with traumatic intraparenchymal temporal lobe hemorrhages.[23] In that study, comatose head-injured patients were eligible if they presented with abnormal pupillary widening and normal or elevated blood pressure. Half the patients were randomized to receive a conventional dose of mannitol, or ~0.7 g/kg. The other half were randomized to receive the high dose; that is, 1.4 g/kg. Mannitol infusion was followed by normal saline boluses. As in the above study, the high-dose mannitol patients demonstrated a significantly greater degree of early improvement in pupillary widening and also had higher cerebral oxygen extraction, less frequent brain swelling, and better 6-month outcomes than the conventional-dose patients.

Pearl

Prehospital administration of relatively large doses of mannitol may have significantly beneficial effects, at least in specific groups of severely head-injured patients.

This marked improvement in pupillary abnormality after aggressive early mannitol use is not surprising. Ritter et al[11] showed a positive correlation between pupillary reactivity in head-injured patients and brainstem blood flow as assessed by xenon CT (class II data). The failure of pupils to respond did not depend on the presence of uncal herniation or mass effect on the brainstem. Mannitol improves the blood flow to all parts of the brain, including the brainstem; thus, mannitol-induced reversal of abnormal pupillary widening may be at least partially attributed to the effect on CBF instead of to the reversal of uncal herniation.

With regard to management in the intensive care unit (ICU), there is no consensus regarding the optimal dose of mannitol. McGraw et al[24] (class III data) established a dose–response relationship between mannitol and ICP reduction when mannitol was given in doses ranging from 10 to 100 g. Less than 50% of patients responded to the 10-g dose, but over 80% of patients responded to a 50-g dose. Marshall et al[3] (class II data) found that in eight patients receiving at various times 0.25, 0.5, or 1.0 g/kg, the ICP reduction at smaller doses was equivalent to that at higher doses. Conversely, James[13] (class III data) reported that doses of 1.0 g/kg/dose or higher were always effective in reducing ICP, but doses below 1.0 g/kg were not always effective.

Pearl

In ICU patients, elevated ICP may decrease after as little as 0.25 g/kg of mannitol, but some patients may require as much as 1.0 g/kg or even more.

ICP-Directed versus Empiric Therapy

With respect to whether mannitol therapy should be ICP-directed or empiric, the available class I data are simply too limited to support any firm conclusions. Smith et al[25] (class I data) prospectively randomized 80 patients with a Glasgow Coma Scale (GCS) score of 8 or less into two groups. Group I was treated with a bolus of 0.75 g/kg followed by incremental boluses of 0.25 g/kg up to a maximum of 1.5 g/kg/h as needed for ICP >25 mmHg until serum osmolarity exceeded 310 mOsm/L. Pentobarbital coma was used for ICP elevations >35 mmHg. Group II received an initial mannitol bolus of 0.75 g/kg and then regular boluses of 0.25 g/kg every 2 hours, regardless of the ICP. An extra bolus of 0.75 g/kg was given in the event of neurologic deterioration. No pentobarbital was used in the second group. ICP tended to be higher in group I, but outcomes did not differ between the two groups. However, the number of patients enrolled in this trial may have been too small to demonstrate an effect of treatment regimen.

Clinical Thresholds for Treatment

Several class III studies suggest that mannitol is most effective when ICP is high or when CPP is low. These studies support a level III recommendation that mannitol therapy be guided by ICP and/or by CPP. Mendelow et al[26] (class III data) demonstrated that mannitol boluses (0.25–0.5 g/kg over 10–15 minutes) effectively reduced ICP and increased CPP and that a mannitol-related increase in CBF was more likely when ICP was below 40 mmHg or when CPP was at or below 50 mmHg. Similarly, Rosner and Coley[8] suggested that mannitol controls ICP best when CPP is below 70 mmHg (class III data). Presumably, when perfusion pressure is lower, cerebral arterioles are maximally dilated to the limit of autoregulatory reserve and are most responsive (i.e., by constriction) to the increase in CBF effected by the mannitol bolus.

Pearl

Mannitol may be most effective in controlling ICP when CPP is below 70 mmHg.

Prehospital and Pre–Intensive Care Unit Treatment

As clearly demonstrated by Cruz et al[22,23] (class I data), administration of large doses of mannitol (up to 1.8–2.1 g/kg) should be regarded as a level I recommendation during neuroresuscitation of comatose trauma patients with operative acute subdural hematoma or with dilated pupils subsequently found to be caused by an operative intraparenchymal temporal lobe hemorrhage.

Nonetheless, recommendations for a liberal policy of prehospital mannitol administration are tempered by the fear that mannitol might frustrate cardiovascular resuscitation efforts by causing or exacerbating hypotension.[27] To test this hypothesis, Sayre et al[28] (class II data) prospectively randomized 44 head-injured patients to receive either mannitol (1.0 g/kg) or normal saline before arrival at the hospital. The groups did not differ in systolic blood pressure or heart rate during a 2-hour observation period following administration of mannitol or saline ($p = .80$ and .41, respectively). In this study, "the flight crew was instructed [to give mannitol] over as little as five minutes," but it is not clear if this goal was accomplished. A small increase in mortality was seen in the mannitol patients, but the number of patients enrolled in this trial was too small to demonstrate an effect of treatment regimen on mortality. In a larger study, Abbott et al[29] evaluated the effect on mortality of a neuroresuscitation protocol that included mannitol (infusion over 10–15 minutes of 1.0 g/kg in adult and 0.5 g/kg in pediatric patients) (class III data); 196 study patients and 1090 control patients were enrolled. A statistically significant 11% decrease in mortality was seen in the study group. This result, however, is confounded by the study design, which included air transport and rapid sequence intubation with neuromuscular blockade exclusively in the treatment arm. Despite their weaknesses, the above studies nevertheless suggest that reluctance to give mannitol early during neuroresuscitation or in the face of hypotension may be unwarranted.

Contraindications and Complications

Hypotension

Hypotension is often considered an absolute contraindication to mannitol therapy. However, investigations on the effectiveness of mannitol as a small-volume resuscitation fluid seem to contradict this view. In a study employing a canine model of hypovolemic shock and elevated ICP, mannitol infusion consistently decreased ICP and improved cardiac index.[30] Hypotension associated with mannitol can have several causes. Mannitol causes an osmotic diuresis, which can lead to loss of free water from the intravascular space.[16,18] Meticulous replacement of urinary water and electrolyte losses is critical to modern mannitol therapy. Conversely, the intravascular volume expansion caused by bolus mannitol administration can precipitate congestive heart failure, with resultant hypotension and pulmonary edema.

Mannitol Intoxication and the "Rebound Effect"

When the infusion rate of mannitol exceeds the rate of hourly excretion in the urine, mannitol accumulates in the extracellular space. Sequelae may include cellular desiccation, hyponatremia, hyperkalemia, low serum bicarbonate, and serum hyperosmolarity with high osmolar gap.[18] Breakdown of the blood–brain barrier and extravasation of mannitol into the interstitium of the brain is thought to result in a reverse osmotic gradient that can cause cerebral edema, a phenomenon that is sometimes referred to as the "rebound effect." This risk may be greater with continuous as opposed to bolus infusions of mannitol.[17] Some studies have shown that frequent dosing of mannitol is associated with decreased effectiveness of subsequent doses (class III data).[24] It is possible that the classic "rebound" phenomenon could actually result from the traditional reluctance to replace fluid losses in the effort to "run patients dry" during classic osmotherapy, causing volume depletion, hypotension, hemoconcentration, and autoregulatory increases in cerebral blood volume. Again, the importance of fluid replacement must be emphasized.

Renal Failure

Renal failure is only rarely associated with mannitol use. In fact, mannitol is sometimes used to prevent and treat nephrotoxicity from radiocontrast or platinum.[18] In the classic series by Becker and Vries,[12] renal failure developed in three of nine patients in whom ICP was controlled after serum osmolarity exceeded 320 mOsm/L. The volume status of the patients is not given, but the peak osmolarity in most of these patients exceeded 400 mOsm/L. Dorman et al[18] reported a series of patients undergoing mannitol therapy for increased ICP (seven stroke patients and one head-injured patient) who developed acute oliguric renal failure after daily doses of mannitol of 189 ± 64 g over 3.5 ± 1.5 days, with a peak osmolal gap of 74 ± 39 mOsm/kg water (see below for calculation of osmotic gap). Experimental evidence suggests that small doses of mannitol that produce plasma mannitol concentrations below 1000 mg/dL decrease renal vascular resistance and increase renal blood flow,[18] but concentrations above 1000 mg/dL (corresponding to more than 55 mOsm/kg water) cause renal vasoconstriction[31] and consequently decrease renal blood flow. This decreased blood flow, in turn, may lead to acute tubular necrosis. Thus, renal failure from mannitol may be a function of the serum mannitol concentration instead of the serum osmolarity, as is usually assumed. Dorman et al suggest that monitoring the osmolal gap (to keep it below 55 mOsm/kg water) might be preferable to using the serum osmolarity to direct mannitol therapy.[18]

Pearl

Renal failure from mannitol may be due to high serum mannitol concentrations, not to high serum osmolarity.

Pearl

$$\begin{aligned}\text{Osmolar gap} &= \text{OSM}_{\text{measured}} - \text{OSM}_{\text{calculated}}\\ &= \text{OSM}_{\text{measured}} - [2\times(\text{Na}+\text{K})\\ &\quad + (\text{BUN}/2.8) + (\text{glucose}/18)]\\ &\quad [\text{Na and K in mEq/L;}\\ &\quad \text{BUN and glucose in mg/dL}]\end{aligned}$$

Recommendations

Empiric mannitol in relatively large doses (up to 1.8–2.1 g/kg) as guided by the neurologic exam and/or CT scan is of benefit early in the neuroresuscitative effort (level I recommendation). Once invasive ICP monitoring has begun, rational mannitol therapy should consist of bolus administration of 20% mannitol in doses ranging from 0.25 to 1.0 g/kg (level II recommendation) infused over at least 15 minutes (level III recommendation). Mannitol is most effective when CPP is below 70 mmHg (level III recommendation). Meticulous fluid replacement of urinary losses to avoid dehydration is important (level III recommendation). A serum osmolar gap below 55 mOsm/L or a serum osmolarity below 320 mOsm/L should be targeted (level III recommendation).

References

1. Wise BL, Chater N. The value of hypertonic mannitol solution in decreasing brain mass and lowering cerebrospinal-fluid pressure. J Neurosurg 1962;19:1038–1043.
2. Brain Trauma Foundation, American Association of Neurological Surgeons, Joint Section on Neurotrauma and Critical Care. Guidelines for the management of severe head injury. Indications for intracranial pressure monitoring. J Neurotrauma 2000;17:479–492.
3. Marshall LF, Smith RW, Rauscher LA, et al. Mannitol dose requirements in brain-injured patients. J Neurosurg 1978;48:169–172.
4. Takagi H, Saitoh T, Kitahara T, et al. The mechanism of the ICP reducing effect of mannitol. In: Ishii S, Nagai H, Brock M, eds. Intracranial Pressure V. Berlin: Springer-Verlag, 1982:729–733.
5. Muizelaar JP, Wei EP, Kontos HA, et al. Mannitol causes compensatory cerebral vasoconstriction and vasodilation in response to blood viscosity changes. J Neurosurg 1983;59:822–828.
6. Nath F, Galbraith S. The effect of mannitol on cerebral white matter water content. J Neurosurg 1986;65:41–43.
7. Burke AM, Quest DO, Chien S, et al. The effects of mannitol on blood viscosity. J Neurosurg 1981;55:550–553.
8. Rosner MJ, Coley I. Cerebral perfusion pressure: a hemodynamic mechanism of mannitol and the postmannitol hemogram. Neurosurgery 1987;21:147–156.
9. Bruce DA, Langfitt TW, Miller JD, et al. Regional cerebral blood flow, intracranial pressure, and brain metabolism in comatose patients. J Neurosurg 1973;38:131–144.
10. Muizelaar JP, Lutz HA III, Becker DP. Effect of mannitol on ICP and CBF and correlation with pressure autoregulation in severely head-injured patients. J Neurosurg 1984;61:700–706.
11. Ritter AM, Muizelaar JP, Barnes T, et al. Brain stem blood flow, pupillary response, and outcome in patients with severe head injuries. Neurosurgery 1999;44:941–948.
12. Becker D, Vries J. The alleviation of increased intracranial pressure by the chronic administration of osmotic agents. In: Brock M, Dietz H, eds. Intracranial Pressure. Berlin: Springer-Verlag, 1972:309–315.
13. James HE. Methodology for the control of intracranial pressure with hypertonic mannitol. Acta Neurochir (Wien) 1980;51:161–172.
14. Unterberg AW, Kiening KL, Hartl R, et al. Multimodal monitoring in patients with head injury: evaluation of the effects of treatment on cerebral oxygenation. J Trauma 1997;42:S32–S37.
15. Hartl R, Bardt TF, Kiening KL, et al. Mannitol decreases ICP but does not improve brain-tissue pO2 in severely head-injured patients with intracranial hypertension. Acta Neurochir Suppl (Wien) 1997;70:40–42.
16. Damas F, Hans P. Management of severely head-injured patients during the first 24 hours: which specific therapeutics? Ann Fr Anesth Reanim 2000;19:326–332.
17. Kaufmann AM, Cardoso ER. Aggravation of vasogenic cerebral edema by multiple-dose mannitol. J Neurosurg 1992;77:584–589.
18. Dorman HR, Sondheimer JH, Cadnapaphornchai P. Mannitol-induced acute renal failure. Medicine (Baltimore) 1990;69:153–159.
19. Coté CJ, Greenhow DE, Marshall BE. The hypotensive response to rapid intravenous administration of hypertonic solutions in man and in the rabbit. Anesthesiology 1979;50:30–35.
20. Ravussin P, Archer DP, Tyler JL, et al. Effects of rapid mannitol infusion on cerebral blood volume: a positron emission tomographic study in dogs and man. J Neurosurg 1986;64:104–113.
21. Domaingue CM, Nye DH. Hypotensive effect of mannitol administered rapidly. Anaesth Intensive Care 1985;13:134–136.
22. Cruz J, Minoja G, Okuchi K. Improving clinical outcomes from acute subdural hematomas with the emergency preoperative administration of high doses of mannitol: a randomized trial. Neurosurgery 2001;49:864–871.
23. Cruz J, Minoja G, Okuchi K. Major clinical and physiological benefits of early high doses of mannitol for intraparenchymal temporal lobe hemorrhages with abnormal pupillary widening: a randomized trial. Neurosurgery 2002;51:628–638.
24. McGraw CP, Alexander E Jr, Howard G. Effect of dose and dose schedule on the response of intracranial pressure to mannitol. Surg Neurol 1978;10:127–130.
25. Smith HP, Kelly DL Jr, McWhorter JM, et al. Comparison of mannitol regimens in patients with severe head injury undergoing intracranial pressure monitoring. J Neurosurg 1986;65:820–824.
26. Mendelow AD, Teasdale GM, Russell T, et al. Effect of mannitol on cerebral blood flow and cerebral perfusion pressure in human head injury. J Neurosurg 1985;63:43–48.
27. Feldman JA, Fish S. Resuscitation fluid for a patient with head injury and hypovolemic shock. Review. J Emerg Med 1991;9:465–468.
28. Sayre MR, Daily SW, Stern SA, et al. Out-of-hospital administration of mannitol to head-injured patients does not change systolic blood pressure. Acad Emerg Med 1996;3:840–848.
29. Abbott D, Brauer K, Hutton K, et al. Aggressive out-of-hospital treatment regimen for severe closed head injury in patients undergoing air medical transport. Air Med J 1998;17:94–100.
30. Israel RS, Marx JA, Moore EE, et al. Hemodynamic effect of mannitol in a canine model of concomitant increased intracranial pressure and hemorrhagic shock. Ann Emerg Med 1988;17:560–566.
31. Temes SP, Lilien OM, Chamberlain W. A direct vasoconstrictor effect of mannitol on the renal artery. Surg Gynecol Obstet 1975;141:223–226.

◆ 26 ◆

Should I Use Hypertonic Saline to Treat High Intracranial Pressure?

Donald S. Prough

Brief Answer

The evidence supports a level III recommendation for the use of hypertonic saline to treat intracranial hypertension that is refractory to conventional interventions. The evidence also supports a level III recommendation for the use of hypertonic saline as an alternative to mannitol in the treatment of intracranial hypertension. There exists no evidence that the use of hypertonic saline improves outcome.

Background

The use of hypertonic saline solutions to reduce brain bulk and intracranial pressure (ICP) has been studied for almost a century, especially in experimental models. In the mid-1980s, experimental studies of hypertonic solutions for resuscitation of hemorrhagic shock accompanying traumatic brain injury (TBI) generated considerable interest in the clinical use of hypertonic solutions for prehospital resuscitation of hypotensive head-injured patients.[1,2] Enthusiasm for hypertonic resuscitation waned, however, at least in part because of emphasis in the United States on limiting any type of prehospital fluid resuscitation. Nevertheless, clinical investigators reported several series in which hypertonic saline solutions were used as primary fluid therapy in trauma patients (including those with TBI) or in which hypertonic solutions were used as rescue therapy for refractory intracranial hypertension. In general, these studies demonstrated that hypertonic saline solutions are effective in reducing ICP and usually improve cerebral perfusion pressure (CPP). Although authors of each of the studies noted that hypertonic saline has some theoretical advantages in comparison to mannitol, no convincing evidence demonstrated that hypertonic saline solutions are superior to mannitol. Moreover, because the designs of the studies varied so greatly and because the doses and compositions of the infused fluids were substantially different, no firm conclusions could be drawn.

Literature Review

Physiologic Effects

Hypertonic saline clearly reduces brain bulk and ICP. In a study in which patients undergoing elective craniotomy were randomly assigned to receive either 7.5% saline (1283 mEq/L) or 20% mannitol for reduction of brain bulk and lumbar cerebrospinal fluid pressure, Gemma et al[3] found that the two regimens had equal efficacy (class II data). Munar et al[4] (class II data) infused 1.5 mL/kg of 7.2% saline (1232 mEq/L) over 15 minutes in 14 patients aged >18 years with moderate or severe TBI. They demonstrated a significant reduction of ICP to 30% of baseline values without significant changes in mean arterial blood pressure or cerebral arteriovenous oxygen content difference. De Vivo et al[5] (class II data) also reported equivalent reductions of ICP in neurosurgical patients receiving mannitol, 3% hypertonic saline, or a combination of the two.

Fisher et al[6] randomized 18 head-injured children to receive 10 mL/kg of either 3% or 0.9% saline in a randomized crossover trial in which reduction of ICP was the primary end point (class II data). The hypertonic saline significantly reduced ICP in the majority of children, whereas 0.9% saline had no apparent effect. Suarez et al[7] (class III data) used 30 mL of 23.4% saline as rescue therapy in eight patients with 20 episodes of intracranial hypertension refractory to hyperventilation, mannitol, and furosemide; several patients had also received cerebrospinal fluid drainage or barbiturate infusion. ICP decreased from a median of 41.5 mmHg to a median of 17 mmHg at 1 hour and 14 mmHg at 3 hours after administration of hypertonic saline; significant decreases persisted for more than 6 hours. Hartl et al[8] (class II data) used a combination of 7.5% saline and 6% hydroxyethyl starch to treat six patients with refractory intracranial hypertension and reported that the average ICP decreased from 45 ± 15 mmHg to 25 ± 14 mmHg, although one of the six patients died of uncontrollable intracranial hypertension. Schatzmann et al[9] (class III data) used 10% saline to treat increased ICP in 42 episodes of intracranial hypertension in six patients and achieved a median ICP reduction of 43%; the reduction persisted for a median duration of 93 minutes. Horn et al[10] (class II data) demonstrated that 2.0 mL/kg of 7.5% saline effectively reduced ICP in 48 episodes of intracranial hypertension in 10 patients in whom ICP was increased secondary to TBI or subarachnoid hemorrhage. In eight stroke patients with 22 episodes of intracranial hypertension that did not respond to infusion of mannitol, Schwarz et al[11] (class II data) infused 75 mL of 10% saline and demonstrated prompt reduction of ICP that persisted throughout the 4-hour observation period. In a randomized, crossover study of nine stroke patients with 30 episodes of increased ICP, Schwarz et al[12] (class II data) infused either 100 mL of a combination of 7.5% saline and 6% hydroxyethyl starch or 200 mL of 20% mannitol and reported that the hypertonic saline/hydroxyethyl starch therapy seemed to reduce ICP at least as effectively as mannitol but was less effective at increasing CPP.

Pearl

Numerous studies have demonstrated the efficacy of hypertonic saline in reducing elevated ICP, but these studies are not directly comparable because the designs of the studies vary so greatly and because the doses, compositions, and infusion regimens of the saline solutions differ substantially.

Influence on Outcome

Qureshi et al[13] (class III data) infused 3% sodium chloride/acetate to treat 30 episodes of cerebral edema (with or without intracranial hypertension) in 27 consecutive patients, including eight patients with TBI. Retrospective analysis of the series demonstrated that the beneficial effect on ICP was short-lived (lasting less than 24 hours in TBI patients) but that lateral displacement of the brain was reduced in patients with TBI. In another retrospective analysis of 28 consecutive patients with a variety of intracranial pathologies (including four patients with TBI), Qureshi et al[14] (class III data) reported that reversal of herniation with a combination of hyperventilation, mannitol, thiopental for mean blood pressure increases beyond 150 mmHg, and (if needed) hypertonic saline was associated with survival to hospital discharge in 13 patients, two of whom died 6 and 7 months after discharge, respectively, from progression of brain tumor and from sepsis. Seven patients were able to function independently; however, all four TBI patients died.

Several investigators have used hypertonic saline solutions for maintenance fluid therapy in head-injured patients or have accepted much higher serum sodium concentrations when treating head-injured patients. Simma et al[15] (class II data) randomized severely head-injured children to maintenance fluids consisting of either lactated Ringer's solution (sodium concentration 131 mEq/L) or hypertonic saline (sodium concentration 268 mEq/L). They reported that the lactated Ringer's group exhibited trends toward a higher incidence of the acute respiratory distress syndrome and a higher number of complications and had a significantly longer mean stay in the intensive care unit (11.6 ± 6.1 days versus 8.0 ± 2.4 days). Peterson et al[16] (class III data) retrospectively reported on the use of 3% hypertonic saline to control ICP in 68 children with closed head injury and cerebral edema. Hypertonic saline effectively lowered ICP in all patients, perhaps in part because the authors used a sliding scale of targeted serum sodium levels, increasing the target level and titrating additional therapies as necessary to maintain control of ICP. Against a predicted survival of 41 patients, the authors reported an actual survival of 58 patients. In 10 children with increased ICP, Khanna et al[17] (class II data) used a continuous infusion of 3% saline to maintain ICP below a goal of 20 mmHg and concluded that sustained hypernatremia was an effective way to reduce ICP in head-injured children.

Pearl

No carefully designed prospective studies have investigated the effect of hypertonic saline on outcome from TBI, but retrospective and smaller prospective studies have suggested that there may be some benefit.

Complications

Although small studies have reported some encouraging results, it must be pointed out that use of hypertonic saline solutions to control intracranial hypertension has been associated with important complications. Qureshi et al[18] (class III data) reported two patients who had received hypertonic saline during treatment of cerebral edema caused by hypertensive intracerebral hemorrhage. Despite clinical improvement 24 hours after administration of hypertonic saline, both patients deteriorated, 48 and 96 hours, respectively, after the beginning of therapy, because of an increase in cerebral edema despite continued treatment with hypertonic saline, possibly because of a rebound effect. Although concerns about central pontine myelinolysis and acute renal failure have been repeatedly raised, these do not appear to be major risks. They have not been reported as complications in patients receiving hypertonic saline as part of resuscitation from hemorrhagic shock accompanying TBI or in normonatremic or hypernatremic patients receiving hypertonic saline to control ICP.[19]

Pearl

Central pontine myelinolysis and acute renal failure do not appear to be major risks of treatment with hypertonic saline, but some authors have reported subsequent increases in cerebral edema and possibly even an increase in mortality.

Recommendations

The above literature suggests that hypertonic saline may be of benefit in some patients with TBI. However, the evidence is insufficient to recommend specific protocols for using hypertonic saline. Thus, all recommendations are level III.

Indications

After severe TBI, intracranial hypertension refractory to moderate cerebrospinal fluid drainage, hyperventilation, mannitol, furosemide, and head elevation may respond to administration of hypertonic saline. The clinician must choose between hypertonic saline and other rescue therapies such as decompressive craniectomy and barbiturate coma.

Technique

Various concentrations have been used. Perhaps the most practical for use in the United States is 3% saline, which is stocked in most hospital pharmacies because it is occasionally used in the management of severe hyponatremia. An initial dose of 1.5 to 3.0 mL/kg is reasonable. A target serum sodium concentration less than 155 to 160 mEq/L appears prudent, although some investigators have accepted sodium concentrations as high as 180 mEq/L after previously effective levels of less pronounced hypernatremia lost effectiveness. Subsequent doses can be given if intracranial hypertension recurs.

References

1. Vassar MJ, Perry CA, Gannaway WL, et al. 7.5% sodium chloride/dextran for resuscitation of trauma patients undergoing helicopter transport. Arch Surg 1991;126:1065–1072.
2. Vassar MJ, Perry CA, Holcroft JW. Prehospital resuscitation of hypotensive trauma patients with 7.5% NaCl versus 7.5% NaCl with added dextran: a controlled trial. J Trauma 1993;34: 622–633.
3. Gemma M, Cozzi S, Tommasino C, et al. 7.5% hypertonic saline versus 20% mannitol during elective neurosurgical supratentorial procedures. J Neurosurg Anesthesiol 1997;9: 329–334.
4. Munar F, Ferrer AM, de Nadal M, et al. Cerebral hemodynamic effects of 7.2% hypertonic saline in patients with head injury and raised intracranial pressure. J Neurotrauma 2000; 17:41–51.
5. De Vivo P, Del Gaudio A, Ciritella P, et al. Hypertonic saline solution: a safe alternative to mannitol 18% in neurosurgery. Minerva Anestesiol 2001;67:603–611.
6. Fisher B, Thomas D, Peterson B. Hypertonic saline lowers raised intracranial pressure in children after head trauma. J Neurosurg Anesthesiol 1992;4:4–10.
7. Suarez JI, Qureshi AI, Bhardwaj A, et al. Treatment of refractory intracranial hypertension with 23.4% saline. Crit Care Med 1998;26:1118–1122.
8. Hartl R, Ghajar J, Hochleuthner H, et al. Hypertonic/hyperoncotic saline reliably reduces ICP in severely head-injured patients with intracranial hypertension. Acta Neurochir Suppl (Wien) 1997;70:126–129.
9. Schatzmann C, Heissler HE, Konig K, et al. Treatment of elevated intracranial pressure by infusions of 10% saline in severely head injured patients. Acta Neurochir Suppl (Wien) 1998;71: 31–33.
10. Horn P, Munch E, Vajkoczy P, et al. Hypertonic saline solution for control of elevated intracranial pressure in patients with exhausted response to mannitol and barbiturates. Neurol Res 1999;21:758–764.
11. Schwarz S, Georgiadis D, Aschoff A, et al. Effects of hypertonic (10%) saline in patients with raised intracranial pressure after stroke. Stroke 2002;33:136–140.
12. Schwarz S, Schwab S, Bertram M, et al. Effects of hypertonic saline hydroxyethyl starch solution and mannitol in patients with increased intracranial pressure after stroke. Stroke 1998; 29:1550–1555.
13. Qureshi AI, Suarez JI, Bhardwaj A, et al. Use of hypertonic (3%) saline/acetate infusion in the treatment of cerebral edema: effect on intracranial pressure and lateral displacement of the brain. Crit Care Med 1998;26:440–446.
14. Qureshi AI, Geocadin RG, Suarez JI, et al. Long-term outcome after medical reversal of transtentorial herniation in patients with supratentorial mass lesions. Crit Care Med 2000;28: 1556–1564.
15. Simma B, Burger R, Falk M, et al. A prospective, randomized, and controlled study of fluid management in children with severe head injury: lactated Ringer's solution versus hypertonic saline. Crit Care Med 1998;26:1265–1270.

16. Peterson B, Khanna S, Fisher B, et al. Prolonged hypernatremia controls elevated intracranial pressure in head-injured pediatric patients. Crit Care Med 2000;28:1136–1143.

17. Khanna S, Davis D, Peterson B, et al. Use of hypertonic saline in the treatment of severe refractory posttraumatic intracranial hypertension in pediatric traumatic brain injury. Crit Care Med 2000;28:1144–1151.

18. Qureshi AI, Suarez JI, Bhardwaj A. Malignant cerebral edema in patients with hypertensive intracerebral hemorrhage associated with hypertonic saline infusion: a rebound phenomenon? J Neurosurg Anesthesiol 1998;10:188–192.

19. Vassar MJ, Perry CA, Holcroft JW. Analysis of potential risks associated with 7.5% sodium chloride resuscitation of traumatic shock. Arch Surg 1990;125:1309–1315.

◆ 27 ◆

Does Barbiturate Coma Help to Improve Outcome from Head Injury?

Manuela Cormio and Claudia S. Robertson

Brief Answer

There is no evidence that barbiturate therapy for patients with severe head injury reduces mortality or disability. In the setting of uncontrollable intracranial hypertension refractory to all other conventional treatments, high-dose barbiturate therapy can be considered as a method to decrease intracranial pressure (ICP) in selected patients. It is a second-tier approach due to its attendant risks and to the intensity of care necessary to employ it successfully.

Background

Despite aggressive management to control elevated ICP, 10 to 25% of patients with severe traumatic brain injury develop intractable intracranial hypertension. The mortality rate is very high (84 to 100%) in this group of patients (class III data).[1–4] Barbiturate coma has been recommended as a last-ditch treatment after routine therapy fails to control elevated ICP.

The use of barbiturates for controlling refractory intracranial hypertension is based on the following two assumptions:

1. Barbiturates improve long-term ICP control when other treatments have failed.
2. ICP control improves ultimate outcome.

Cerebral Effects of Barbiturates

The mechanism of ICP reduction by barbiturates is not entirely clear but is almost certainly multifactorial. Because of the immediacy of the ICP-lowering effect, the mechanism is commonly thought to be hemodynamic. This immediacy of effect may be due to direct cerebral vasoconstriction (increased cerebral vascular resistance) since the reduction in ICP has been associated with reductions in cerebral blood flow (CBF) and cerebral blood volume (CBV) in laboratory studies.[5]

The immediacy of effect of barbiturates could also be explained by a metabolically coupled reduction in CBF. Barbiturates cause a reversible depression of neurologic function and reduce cerebral metabolic rate of oxygen ($CMRO_2$) by 50% in normal adults and by 58% in experimental studies.[6] This reduction in $CMRO_2$ is caused by inhibition of energy-dependent synaptic transmission. Therefore, reduction in $CMRO_2$ by pentobarbital is closely related to the pretreatment $CMRO_2$. Only those patients with a $CMRO_2 \geq 1.6\,mL/100\,g/min$ demonstrate a consistent reduction in $CMRO_2$ with barbiturates and a resulting reduction in ICP (class III data).[7] Patients with an extremely low $CMRO_2$ from overwhelming cerebral injury are not likely to benefit from barbiturate coma.

Other mechanisms by which barbiturates may exert cerebral protective effects in the injured brain have also been described: stabilization of lysosomal membranes, reduction of intracellular calcium concentrations, modification of release of amino acids and neurotransmitters, scavenging of free radicals, alteration of fatty acid metabolism, inhibition of phospholipase activation, reduction in cerebrospinal fluid (CSF) secretion, lowering of temperature, and suppression of seizures.[8–10] Using cerebral microdialysis, Goodman et al[11] described a 37% reduction of lactate, 59% reduction of glutamate, and 66% reduction in aspartate in the extracellular space of the brain when severely elevated ICP was managed with barbiturate coma (class III data). Stover et al[12] indicated that despite successful suppression of neuronal activity in patients with refractory intracranial hypertension, the use of barbiturate coma does not unequivocally preserve energetic stability (class III data). They reported that elevated levels of glutamate, presumably associated with ongoing anaerobic metabolism, may still be detected in some cases.

Indications

Indications for initiating barbiturate coma have not been consistently defined. It is used most commonly in selected patients in the setting of uncontrollable intracranial hypertension refractory to all other conventional treatments.[2,7,13] It should be instituted before irreversible brain injury has occurred. If barbiturates are started too late in the course of treatment, ICP may be controlled, but the patient is more likely to remain neurologically devastated.

Reasonable indications to begin high-dose barbiturates include 30 minutes of ICP over 30 mmHg with cerebral perfusion pressure (CPP) less than 60 mmHg, or ICP over 40 mmHg despite a CPP of 60 mmHg. Patients with overwhelmingly severe injuries are not likely to benefit from barbiturate coma, partly because their $CMRO_2$ is already markedly reduced by the injury and partly because their outcome is already predetermined by the injury. Patients with systemic hypotension are not likely to have a good response because hypotension limits the amount of barbiturates that can be given.

Pearl

Patients with systemic hypotension are not likely to have a good response to barbiturates because hypotension limits the amount that can be given.

Ethical issues may arise over how aggressively therapy for intracranial hypertension should be pursued and for how long. An ever-present concern is that prolonged barbiturate coma may prevent death, but with unacceptably severe disability.

Dose

A commonly used dosing regimen for pentobarbital is 10 mg/kg loading dose over 30 minutes, followed by 5 mg/kg/h over the next 3 hours. If systolic blood pressure decreases, the rate of loading dose infusion should be slowed. Maintenance infusion is usually begun at 1 to 3 mg/kg/h.[7,14]

Pearl

A common dosing regimen for pentobarbital is 10 mg/kg loading dose over 30 minutes, followed by 5 mg/kg/h over the next 3 hours. If systolic blood pressure drops, the rate of infusion should be slowed.

The lowest dose that effectively controls ICP should be utilized. When ICP control has been achieved for 24 hours, tapering of the barbiturate dose may be started. Such weaning should be performed slowly; decreasing the hourly infusion rate by 50% each day is a useful approach. Long-term administration may result in significant accumulation of barbiturates and may cause barbiturate levels in CSF and serum to remain elevated for days after administration is stopped. Clinical evaluation is impossible until these stores are eliminated. Thus, quantitative analysis of barbiturates in serum may be valuable in predicting the length of drug-induced neurologic impairment and in avoiding misinterpretation of the patient's neurologic status.

Complications and Adverse Effects

High-dose barbiturate therapy has a significant potential for serious complications that limit its utility. Continuous infusions are difficult to control because of accumulation of the drug over time. Systemic arterial hypotension is commonly observed in patients receiving barbiturates,[7,13,14] and this complication has the potential to offset beneficial effects of the drug on ICP. In fact, the one absolute contraindication to the initiation of barbiturate coma is the presence of cardiovascular compromise, including episodes of hypotension, before the administration of barbiturates.[14] Potential mechanisms of hemodynamic instability include a myocardial depressant effect, reduced ventricular filling pressure, reduced peripheral vascular resistance, reduced tone in venous capacitance vessels, redistribution of blood volume, impaired venous return, and inhibition of sympathetic activity.

Pearl

The one absolute contraindication to the initiation of barbiturate coma is the presence of cardiovascular compromise (including episodes of hypotension) prior to administration of barbiturates.

Another complication of barbiturate coma that may offset the beneficial effects on ICP is immunosuppression, leading to an increased risk of infection. A high incidence of infections (55%) and respiratory complications (76%) has been described in patients treated with barbiturate coma. Inhibition of lymphocytes, depression of lung mucociliary clearance, prolonged intubation, mechanical ventilation, immobilization, and/or loss of cough reflexes may be involved.[13] Hepatic (87%) and renal dysfunction (47%) are also very common.[13] Physiologic changes associated with the primary cerebral injury, combined with the pharmacodynamic influences of barbiturate therapy, contribute to the difficulties of initiating aggressive nutritional support.[15]

Management of Patients in Barbiturate Coma

The successful use of high-dose barbiturate therapy mandates vigilant and aggressive monitoring and management on the part of the physician and nurse. Hypotension and other potential complications associated with this form of therapy mandate that its use be limited to the intensive care unit (ICU) and that aggressive systemic hemodynamic support and monitoring be undertaken to avoid or treat any hemodynamic instability. A Swan-Ganz catheter is highly recommended, and cardiac filling pressure, systemic vascular resistance, and cardiac output should be optimized before initiation of barbiturate therapy. Throughout the time of barbiturate administration, blood pressure must be aggressively maintained with fluid and pressors.

The increased incidence of severe infection is a serious consequence of barbiturate coma. Patients are anergic, and, in conjunction with the poikilothermic effect of barbiturates, early signs of infection such as leukocytosis, fever, and tachycardia may be suppressed. A high degree of vigilance must be maintained, including clinical, laboratory, and radiologic monitoring to detect both common and uncommon sources of infection.

Pearl

Because patients in barbiturate coma may be anergic and poikilothermic, early signs of infection such as leukocytosis, fever, and tachycardia may be suppressed.

Electroencephalogram (EEG) monitoring may be used to titrate the dosage to burst suppression. In patients who have been titrated to burst suppression without adequate ICP control, further barbiturate administration may not be helpful.

Barbiturates alter cortical activity, resulting in difficulties in clinical evaluation. Loss of pupillary reactivity is common with high-dose pentobarbital therapy and should not be interpreted as irreversible loss of brainstem function from treatment failure.

Patients on barbiturate coma become poikilothermic, and although moderate hypothermia may provide some neuronal protection, a significant decrease in body temperature depresses the immune response, interferes with the coagulation system, alters systemic metabolism, and prolongs the half-life of drugs. Therefore, efforts should be made to keep the patient's body temperature above 35°C.

Skin care issues are also critical because patients are immobile and may also receive pressor agents that can decrease skin perfusion and increase the likelihood of pressure ulceration. Prolonged immobilization also increases the risk of deep venous thrombosis and pulmonary embolism.

Literature Review

Effect of Barbiturate Therapy on Intracranial Pressure

The majority of available literature on barbiturates and ICP control is in the form of case series (class III data). Most nonrandomized clinical studies have indicated a potential benefit of high-dose barbiturates for the control of otherwise unresponsive ICP.[3,4,7,14,16–20] Results from the most significant papers that describe use of barbiturates in brain-injured patients when elevated ICP remains unresponsive to other interventions are summarized in Table 27-1. The response rate (i.e., control of ICP) has ranged from 30 to 80% of treated patients.

Only three class I studies [well-conducted prospective, randomized clinical trials (PRCTs)] have evaluated effects of barbiturate coma after traumatic brain injury. These class I studies were very different in their objectives. Schwartz et al[21] compared the effectiveness of mannitol and barbiturates in controlling ICP. Ward et al[22] studied the routine addition of prophylactic barbiturate coma to a standard management protocol. This study included patients who never had elevated ICP. Eisenberg et al[14] studied the effects of barbiturate coma on ICP control in the 10 to 15% of severely head-injured patients with otherwise uncontrollable ICP.

The first of the PRCTs was published in 1984.[21] This study randomized patients to treatment with either barbiturates or mannitol. However, a double-crossover design was used so that if ICP control could not be achieved with the assigned drug, the patient went on to treatment with the second drug. This study found pentobarbital to be less effective than mannitol in controlling ICP. Absolute values for ICP were not provided; however, patients initially treated with pentobarbital were twice as likely to require crossover to mannitol.

Table 27-1 Results of the Most Important Studies Regarding High-Dose Barbiturates and Refractory Intracranial Hypertension

		Barbiturates, ICP control, and Outcome			
First Author (Year)	Class of Evidence	No. of Patients	ICP Responders (%)	Mortality Rate of Responders (%)	Mortality Rate of Nonresponders (%)
Rockoff (1979)	Class III	45	80	22	90
Marshall (1979)	Class III	25	76	21	83
Rea (1983)	Class III	27	56	33	75
Lobato (1988)	Class III	47	31	69	100
Nordstrom (1988)	Class III	19	42	25	64
Eisenberg (1988)	Class I	37	32	8	83
Lee (1994)	Class III	21	67	29	86
Cormio (1999)	Class III	67	84	52	9

"No. of patients" refers to number of patients included in the study. "Responders" refers to whether ICP decreased to the targeted level

Pearl

A prospective, randomized study found pentobarbital to be less effective than mannitol in controlling ICP.

In 1985, Ward[22] published a PRCT on prophylactic barbiturate coma for severe head injury. Fifty-three patients who were prospectively identified as being at risk for subsequent elevated ICP were randomized to receive either pentobarbital or no barbiturates; otherwise, all patients were managed by the same protocols. There were no significant differences between the treatment groups with respect to the occurrence of ICP >20 mmHg, the degree or extent of ICP elevation, or the response of ICP to therapy. Arterial hypotension occurred in more than half of the pentobarbital patients and in only two (7%) of the control patients.

Pearl

Prophylactic administration of pentobarbital to all head-injured patients lowers blood pressure without improving outcome.

The only PRCT to address the specific use of barbiturates to treat refractory ICP elevations was that of Eisenberg et al[14] in 1988. In this multicenter trial, 36 patients were randomly assigned to receive pentobarbital and 37 were assigned to a conventional treatment arm. However, of these 37, 32 eventually "crossed over" to barbiturate treatment because of refractory intracranial hypertension. In terms of the primary outcome measure of ICP control, patients receiving pentobarbital were twice as likely to have their ICP controlled.

Pearl

The only prospective, randomized trial that specifically addressed the use of barbiturates to treat refractory intracranial hypertension found that patients receiving pentobarbital were twice as likely to have their ICP controlled.

Two important literature reviews were performed in 2000: an update of the *Guidelines for the Management of Severe Traumatic Brain Injury* from the Brain Trauma Foundation[23] and a review from the Cochrane Collaboration.[24] Roberts[24] conducted the systematic Cochrane review of all unconfounded, randomized, or quasirandomized controlled trials of barbiturate therapy in the management of acute severe brain injury. The two studies that examined the effect of barbiturates on ICP and that met his review criteria were those of Eisenberg et al[14] and Ward et al.[22] From these studies, the relative risk for uncontrolled ICP associated with barbiturate treatment was 0.81 [95% confidence interval (CI) 0.62 to 1.06].[24]

Effect of Barbiturate Therapy on Outcome

Although it is clear that barbiturate coma can often reduce elevated ICP in head-injured patients, the influence of this effect on neurologic outcome remains controversial. It is intuitive to equate ICP control with survival. Several class III studies have been published regarding the ICP response to barbiturates and subsequent improved survival. Of those patients who respond to barbiturates, mortality was 21 to 69%, whereas in nonresponders, mortality ranged from 64 to 100%, as summarized in Table 27-1.[7,14,16–20,25]

However, because the patients with refractory intracranial hypertension have the most severe injuries, survival does not necessarily mean improved neurologic outcome. Schalen et al[26] studied cognitive impairment in patients with severe head injuries treated with barbiturate coma. Forty-two percent of the studied patients reached outcome levels of good recovery/moderate disability. However, almost all patients exhibited varying degrees of cognitive dysfunction, and many had signs of personality change.

Only three PRCTs have investigated effects of barbiturates in traumatic brain injury.[7,21,22] However, the intrinsic study designs and primary outcome measures were very different in the three PRCTs, making direct comparisons impossible. In addition, the crossover design of the studies makes any conclusions about the effect of barbiturates on outcome tenuous.

Pearl

Differences in intrinsic study designs and primary outcome measures, as well as effects of patient crossover into different treatment groups, make any conclusions about the effect of barbiturates on outcome tenuous.

Schwartz et al[21] reported that in patients requiring evacuation of intracranial hematomas, mortality with barbiturate treatment was 40%, compared with 43% with mannitol treatment. In patients not requiring neurosurgery, mortality in the pentobarbital group was 77%, compared with 41% in the mannitol group. In the report from Ward et al,[22] there was a similar incidence of deaths in each group from uncontrollable, elevated ICP. Thus, in these two PRCTs, no significant benefit was found from prophylactic administration of barbiturates.

Although the third randomized trial from Eisenberg et al demonstrated improved ICP control with barbiturate administration, the ultimate effects of this intervention on outcome are difficult to quantify because of the crossover study design.[14,24] Patients randomized to the control arm who then failed conventional treatment could be crossed over to receive barbiturates. Mortality in those patients whose ICP responded to barbiturate therapy was 8.3% in the primary treatment arm and 14.3% in the crossover group, compared with mortality of 88% and 84%, respectively, in those who did not respond.

The Roberts systematic review[24] of all class I studies regarding barbiturate coma in the management of acute severe brain injury investigated the associated mortality and morbidity of this therapy. In the three trials described that compared barbiturate therapy to treatment without barbiturates, the pooled relative risk of death was 1.09 (95% CI 0.81 to 1.47). The effect of barbiturates on adverse neurologic outcome, measured using the Glasgow Outcome Scale, was available in two of the three trials. The pooled relative risk for an adverse neurologic outcome (death, persistent vegetative state, or severe disability) was 1.15 (95% CI 0.81 to 1.64).

Effect of Barbiturate Therapy on Arterial Pressure

Cerebral perfusion pressure depends on both ICP and mean arterial blood pressure (CPP = mean arterial blood pressure − mean ICP). The hypotensive effect of barbiturates has the potential to offset the beneficial effect of reduction in ICP while leaving CPP unchanged.

In the three PRCTs available[14,21,22] there is a clear indication that arterial pressure is significantly affected by treatment. There are strong indicators that the beneficial effects of barbiturates on ICP control and mortality may be negated when their use is associated with hypotension. In the paper by Ward et al[22] there was a significantly higher incidence of hypotension in the barbiturate-treated group (54% vs 7%). Eisenberg et al[14] reported an association between a negative effect of pentobarbital and prerandomisation cardiovascular complications. In the absence of pretreatment hypotension, pentobarbital had a fourfold greater chance than conventional therapy of establishing ICP control, whereas when hypotension had occurred, both treatments had an equal chance of success.

In his review, Roberts[24] reported a substantial increase in the occurrence of hypotension in the barbiturate-treated group (relative risk = 1.80, 95% CI 1.19 to 2.70). For every four patients treated with barbiturate therapy, one will develop hypotension.

Effect of Barbiturate Therapy on Temperature

The study by Ward et al[22] examined the effect of barbiturate administration on mean body temperature. Mean body temperature was significantly lower in the barbiturate-treated group (class I study).

Recommendations

1. High-dose barbiturates should be considered for the treatment of elevated ICP that remains high despite maximal use of other medical measures to lower ICP. Patients should not be hypotensive and should be salvageable (level II).
2. Administration of barbiturates for the prophylactic treatment or prevention of intracranial hypertension is not indicated (level I).

References

1. Langfitt TW, Gennarelli TA. Can the outcome from head injury be improved? J Neurosurg 1982;56:19–25.

2. Miller JD, Butterworth JF, Gudeman SK, et al. Further experience in the management of severe head injury. J Neurosurg 1981;54:289–299.
3. Nordby HK, Nesbakken R. The effect of high dose barbiturate decompression after severe head injury: a controlled clinical trial. Acta Neurochir (Wien) 1984;72:157–166.
4. Saul TG, Ducker TB. Effect of intracranial pressure monitoring and aggressive treatment on mortality in severe head injury. J Neurosurg 1982;56:498–503.
5. Ogura K, Takayasu M, Dacey RG Jr. Differential effects of pentobarbital on intracerebral arterioles and venules of rats in vitro. Neurosurgery 1991;28:537–541.
6. Feustel PJ, Ingvar MC, Severinghaus JW. Cerebral oxygen availability and blood flow during middle cerebral artery occlusion: effects of pentobarbital. Stroke 1981;12:858–863.
7. Cormio M, Gopinath SP, Valadka AB, et al. Cerebral hemodynamic effects of pentobarbital coma in head-injured patients. J Neurotrauma 1999;16:927–936.
8. Cai Z, McCaslin PP. Acute, chronic and differential effects of several anesthetic barbiturates on glutamate receptor activation in neuronal culture. Brain Res 1993;611:181–186.
9. Smith DS, Rehncrona S, Siesjo BK. Barbiturates as protective agents in brain ischemia and as free radical scavengers in vitro. Acta Physiol Scand Suppl 1980;492:129–134.
10. Steen PA, Michenfelder JD. Mechanisms of barbiturate protection. Anesthesiology 1980;53:183–185.
11. Goodman JC, Valadka AB, Gopinath SP, et al. Lactate and excitatory amino acids measured by microdialysis are decreased by pentobarbital coma in head-injured patients. J Neurotrauma 1996;13:549–556.
12. Stover JF, Pleines UE, Morganti-Kossmann MC, et al. Thiopental attenuates energetic impairment but fails to normalize cerebrospinal fluid glutamate in brain-injured patients. Crit Care Med 1999;27:1351–1357.
13. Schalen W, Messeter K, Nordstrom CH. Complications and side effects during thiopentone therapy in patients with severe head injuries. Acta Anaesthesiol Scand 1992;36:369–377.
14. Eisenberg HM, Frankowski RF, Contant CF, et al. High-dose barbiturate control of elevated intracranial pressure in patients with severe head injury. J Neurosurg 1988;69:15–23.
15. Magnuson B, Hatton J, Zweng TN, et al. Pentobarbital coma in neurosurgical patients: nutrition considerations. Nutr Clin Pract 1994;9:146–150.
16. Lee MW, Deppe SA, Sipperly ME, et al. The efficacy of barbiturate coma in the management of uncontrolled intracranial hypertension following neurosurgical trauma. J Neurotrauma 1994;11:325–331.
17. Lobato RD, Sarabia R, Cordobes C, et al. Posttraumatic cerebral hemispheric swelling: analysis of 55 cases studied with computerized tomography. J Neurosurg 1988;68:417–423.
18. Marshall LF, Smith RW, Shapiro HM. The outcome with aggressive treatment in severe head injuries, II: acute and chronic barbiturate administration in the management of head injury. J Neurosurg 1979;50:26–30.
19. Nordstrom CH, Messeter K, Sundbarg G, et al. Cerebral blood flow, vasoreactivity, and oxygen consumption during barbiturate therapy in severe traumatic brain lesions. J Neurosurg 1988;68:424–431.
20. Rea GL, Rockswold GL. Barbiturate therapy in uncontrolled intracranial hypertension. Neurosurgery 1983;12:401–404.
21. Schwartz ML, Tator CH, Rowed D, et al. The University of Toronto head injury treatment study: a prospective, randomized comparison of pentobarbital and mannitol. Can J Neurol Sci 1984;11:434–440.
22. Ward JD, Becker DP, Miller JD, et al. Failure of prophylactic barbiturate coma in the treatment of severe head injury. J Neurosurg 1985;62:383–388.
23. Brain Trauma Foundation, American Association of Neurological Surgeons, Joint Section on Neurotrauma and Critical Care. Management and prognosis of severe traumatic brain injury. Use of barbiturates in the control of intracranial hypertension. J Neurotrauma 2000;17:527–530.
24. Roberts I. Barbiturates for acute traumatic brain injury. Cochrane Database Syst Rev 2000;(2):CD000033.
25. Rockoff MA, Marshall LF, Shapiro HM. High-dose barbiturate therapy in humans: a clinical review of 60 patients. Ann Neurol 1979;6:194–199.
26. Schalen W, Sonesson B, Messeter K, et al. Clinical outcome and cognitive impairment in patients with severe head injuries treated with barbiturate coma. Acta Neurochir (Wien) 1992;117:153–159.

◆ 28 ◆

Does Hypothermia Improve Outcome?

Guy L. Clifton

Brief Answer

Maintenance of hypothermia in the 23% of severely head-injured patients who are hypothermic on admission and who are less than 45 years of age may improve outcome. It is possible that very early induction of hypothermia (<3 hours after injury) may improve outcome.

Background

In 1993, phase II studies testing surface cooling in patients with severe brain injuries were completed in Houston[1] and Pittsburgh[2] (class I data). These trials were based on laboratory data in brain injury and were supported by an extensive experimental literature in stroke, as well as by a phase I safety trial (class II data).[3,4] The Houston cooling protocol achieved 33°C within 8 hours of injury and maintained hypothermia for 48 hours, resulting in a 15% absolute improvement in the percentage of patients with good outcome [good recovery/moderate disability on the Glasgow Outcome Scale (GOS)]. The Pittsburgh hypothermia protocol achieved 33°C within 10 hours after injury and used a 24-hour period of hypothermia. A 24% absolute improvement in the percentage of patients with good outcome was found in this study. No significant hypothermia-related toxicity occurred in either study. Based on the strength of the Houston and Pittsburgh studies, the National Acute Brain Injury Study: Hypothermia (NABIS:H) was funded by the National Institute of Neurological Disorders and Stroke (NINDS) in 1994.

Clinical Trial and Literature Review

The specific aim of NABIS:H, a randomized, prospective, multicenter trail, was to determine if surface-induced moderate hypothermia (33°C) begun within 6 hours of severe brain injury [Glasgow Coma Scale (GCS) score ≤ 8) and maintained for 48 hours would improve outcome, with low toxicity. The design of NABIS:H projected that an enrollment of 500 patients would be needed to detect a 10% absolute shift in the percentage of patients making a good outcome on the GOS score (good outcome = good recovery or moderate disability; poor outcome = severe disability, vegetative, or dead) at 6 months after injury. NABIS:H met its performance standards, but after enrolling 392 patients, the trial was stopped in May 1998 by the Patient Safety and Monitoring Board when a regularly scheduled futility analysis showed low probability of detecting a treatment effect (class I data).[5]

There was no difference in outcome measured at 6 months postinjury, with 57% of both groups showing a poor outcome.[5] The mortality rate was 28% in the hypothermia group and 27% in the normothermia group. Data analysis showed that treatment with hypothermia blunted major elevations of intracranial pressure (ICP), with a significantly lower percentage of hypothermia patients having ICP >30 mmHg (hypothermia group 41%, normothermia group 59%; $p < .02$). Older patients (age > 45 years, $n = 52$) had a higher percentage of poor outcomes than younger patients (hypothermia 88%, normothermia 69%; $p = .08$).

Patients were randomized at 4.2 ± 1.1 hours after injury; those assigned to hypothermia reached 33°C at

Pearl

Outcome did not differ between normothermia and hypothermia groups, but hypothermia blunted major elevations of intracranial pressure.

8.4 ± 3.1 hours after injury. There were no significant differences between the groups in age, admission GCS score, incidence of operated hematomas, subarachnoid hemorrhage, prehospital hypoxia, computed tomography (CT) classification or Injury Severity Score. The hypothermia treatment group had a higher cumulative fluid balance (intake − output) for the first 96 hours (hypothermia 3061 ± 5946 mL, normothermia 1947 ± 4586 mL, $p < .05$). Patients treated with hypothermia also received vasopressors for a higher percentage of the first 96 hours (hypothermia 48.5 ± 33.9%, normothermia 41.0 ± 37.8%, $p < .05$). This was anticipated in the trial design because volume expansion and vasopressors are often required during rewarming. All other aspects of management were similar in the two treatment groups.

Pearl

Volume expansion and vasopressors are often required during rewarming.

The hypothermia group had a higher percentage of hospitalization days with complications (hypothermia 78% ± 22% days, normothermia 70% ± 29% days, $p < .005$). Hypotension for two or more consecutive hours with organ failure recorded as a complication occurred in 10% of hypothermia patients and 3% of normothermia patients ($p = .01$). Ventricular arrhythmias occurred in 22 hypothermia patients and 19 normothermia patients. Mean ICP did not differ in the two treatment groups. The percentage of patients with ICP >30 mmHg in the hypothermia group was 41%, as compared with 59% in the normothermia group ($p = .02$). Mean arterial pressure (MAP) and cerebral perfusion pressure (CPP) levels were similar in both groups. The percentage of patients with occurrence of MAP <70 mmHg and CPP <50, <60, or <70 mmHg was the same in both treatment groups. There were no clinically significant differences in electrolyte balance between hypothermia and normothermia groups. Potassium levels in the groups differed by 0.1 mEq. Mean serum sodium values differed by 1 mEq. Mean serum glucose was 155 mg/dL in hypothermia patients and 151 mg/dL in normothermia patients.

Subgroup Analyses

We conducted subgroup analyses on variables known to influence outcome from severe brain injury, including age, initial GCS score, pupillary reactivity, presence of surgical mass lesions, hypoxia, hypotension, and initial CT classification. We also examined the effect of hypothermia treatment on those who were hypothermic on admission. In addition, the effects of the amount of time between injury and attainment of the target temperature of 33°C were examined.

Age and admission temperature were the only two variables that exerted a significant effect.[5] Patients age ≥ 45 years had a higher percentage of poor outcomes (hypothermia 88% poor outcome, normothermia 69% poor outcome, $p = .08$). This was most likely due to a higher percentage of hospital days with medical complications in the hypothermia group (hypothermia 82% ± 21%, normothermia 55% ± 29%, $p = .002$) (Table 28-1).

Table 28-1 Body Temperature on Admission and Poor Outcome* 6 Months After Severe Brain Injury

Treatment Group	No. of Patients with Admission Temp ≤ 35°C	% Poor Outcome	*p* Value	No. of Patients with Admission Temp > 35°C	% Poor Outcome	*p* Value
All patients	102		.09	264		.7
Hypothermia	62	61		127	54	
Normothermia	40	78		137	52	
Patients ≤ 45 years	81		.02	233		.84
Hypothermia	48	52		115	51	
Normothermia	33	76		118	50	
Patients ≥ 45 years	21		.60	31		.23
Hypothermia	14	93		12	83	
Normothermia	7	86		19	63	

*Poor outcome is severe disability, vegetative state, or death.

Twenty-eight percent of the NABIS:H patients had body temperatures ≤ 35°C as their first recorded temperature after arrival in the emergency department. In this subgroup, the percentage of patients with poor outcome was 78% for those patients assigned to normothermia. The percentage of patients with poor outcome was 61% in the group treated with hypothermia ($p = .09$), an absolute improvement of 17%. Patients older than 45 years were adversely affected by induction or maintenance of hypothermia regardless of admission temperature. Among patients aged 16 to 45 years, the hypothermia treatment effect was, therefore, even more pronounced, with a percentage of poor outcomes of 52% for patients assigned to hypothermia compared with 76% for patients assigned to normothermia ($p = .02$), an absolute improvement of 24%. In this subgroup there was no difference in percentage of hospital days with complications (hypothermia 78.9% ± 20%, normothermia 78.6% ± 25%; not significant). This treatment effect of maintaining hypothermia was found in patients at all temperatures below 35°C. The apparent benefit of maintaining hypothermia in those who were hypothermic on admission raises the question of what the treatment window for neuroprotective hypothermia might be. However, there are not sufficient data at this time to make a recommendation on the hypothermic treatment window for patients who are hypothermic on admission.

Pearl

The apparent benefit of maintaining hypothermia in patients who are hypothermic on admission raises the question of what the treatment window for neuroprotective hypothermia might be.

The Treatment Window for Hypothermia

A guiding principle of NABIS:H was that rapid cooling was essential to achieve a neuroprotective effect with hypothermia. The study was designed to reach target temperature (33°C) by 8 hours after injury. Target was reached by 8.4 ± 3.1 hours after injury. We found no effect of time required to reach target temperature on outcome. There was no relationship between admission temperature and time needed to reach 33°C.

The time between injury and attainment of 33°C was 8.1 ± 3.0 hours in 38 patients with hypothermia on admission (<35°C) who were randomized to hypothermia and 8.6 ± 3.1 hours in 69 patients with normothermia on admission who were randomized to hypothermia (not significant). The reason for the small difference in cooling times was spontaneous rewarming of hypothermia-on-admission patients prior to randomization. Those patients admitted to hypothermia and randomized to hypothermia were, however, significantly cooler in the first 8 hours after injury than those who were admitted normothermic and randomized to hypothermia. The mean temperature in the first 8 hours in hypothermia-on-admission patients randomized to hypothermia was 33.6° ± 1.3°C, compared with 36.5° ± 0.9°C ($p < .001$) in normothermia-on-admission patients randomized to hypothermia.

Cause of Hypothermia on Admission

Patients who were hypothermic on admission (<35°C) and normothermic on admission (≥ 35°C) did not have major differences in baseline variables or injury severity. Factors associated with low admission temperature were randomization in winter months (October to March), receipt of larger volumes of room-temperature intravenous fluids, a positive blood alcohol level, smaller body size, increased age, prehospital hypotension, and slightly increased injury severity. A similar pattern of risk factors is seen with multiple trauma patients (class II and III data).[6–11] These data suggest that most of the risk factors for admission hypothermia are environmental.

In NABIS:H, the percentage of patients that was hypothermic on admission varied from 17 to 36%. Paramedics and emergency medical technicians at all the centers reported that body temperature is rarely measured in the ambulance or at the scene because there are too many other lifesaving priorities. They indicate that there is little that they do to influence temperature other than placing a blanket over the patients. Also, ambulances have little equipment to control temperature. It can be concluded that cool ambient temperatures and exposure to room-temperature air in the ambulance reduce temperatures to varying degrees in all patients. Even normothermia-on-admission patients had a mean temperature of 36.5° ± 0.9°C. Anesthetics reduce the threshold for activation of the body's heat-generating mechanisms (e.g., shivering, vasoconstriction) to 35°C from the normal value of 37°C. It can be speculated that similar mechanisms occur immediately after severe brain injury.

Effect of Rewarming

Another explanation for the treatment effect of maintaining hypothermia in patients who are hypothermic on admission is that, since hypothermia occurs accidentally, it may be detrimental to rewarm hypothermic patients. In our experience with hypothermia in animal models of brain injury, rapid rewarming is associated with a marked increase in mortality, and recently published experimental data report a similar deleterious effect of rapid rewarming.[12] In NABIS:H, patients who were hypothermic on admission and assigned to normothermia were covered with blankets and allowed to rewarm passively. These patients required 16 to 20 hours to return to normothermia.

Pearl

It may be detrimental to rewarm patients who are hypothermic on admission.

There is another reason to believe that rapid rewarming is detrimental. A study from the University of Pittsburgh in 1997 reported a treatment effect of 24% with induction of hypothermia in patients with GCS of 5 to 7.[2] The discrepancy between those results and NABIS:H has puzzled many people. In this Pittsburgh trial, the percentage of poor outcome in the normothermia group was unexpectedly high, with 67% of patients having a poor outcome (severe disability, vegetative, or dead), as compared with 57% poor outcome in NABIS:H. In the Pittsburgh study, patients who arrived with low admission temperatures and who were then randomized to normothermia were actively rewarmed over a few hours (D. W. Marion, personal communication). This same Pittsburgh center participated in the NABIS:H study and had the highest percentage of patients with hypothermia on admission (36%). This indicates that the treatment effect in the 1997 study was most likely due to enrollment of a high percentage of patients with hypothermia on admission. Such patients may have been potentially responsive to hypothermia treatment, and they may have been vulnerable to worsened outcomes if they underwent rapid rewarming after assignment to the normothermic group.

Effect on Intracranial Pressure

Several studies have shown an effect of hypothermia on elevated ICP (class I and II data).[2,13–15] In NABIS:H, hypothermia reduced the incidence of ICP >30 mmHg in all patient groups: those over 45 years of age, those who were normothermic on admission who showed no treatment effect, and those who were hypothermic on admission who did show a treatment effect. Use of hypothermia to reduce elevated ICP may be a story reminiscent of that of barbiturate coma, in which ICP was reduced in extreme circumstances without a clear effect on outcome. There is evidence that use of hypothermia to control elevated ICP may improve outcome, as well as more evidence to support its ineffectiveness if used late after injury in the absence of elevated ICP (class I and II data).[15,16] In any event, the selective use of hypothermia to treat established elevations of ICP is a separate question from its use in all patients to treat the early biochemical cascade occurring immediately after injury.

Pearl

The selective use of hypothermia to treat established elevations of ICP is a separate question from its use in all patients to treat the early biochemical cascade occurring immediately after injury.

Effect on Outcome

Patients with hypothermia on admission showed a large treatment effect when hypothermia was maintained. The reason for this has not been determined. The treatment effect found in NABIS:H was a shift in patients from the severe disability category (poor outcome) to the moderate disability category (good outcome), with no change in the percentage of patients who were vegetative or dead.

Pearl

The treatment effect found in NABIS:H was a shift in patients from severe disability (poor outcome) to moderate disability (good outcome), with no change in the percentage of patients who were vegetative or dead.

Patients who were hypothermic on admission and treated with hypothermia showed improvement at 6 months after injury on the Disability Rating Scale, Neurobehavioral Rating Scale–Revised, Grooved Pegboard, Rey Complex Figure (copy, immediate recall, delayed recall), Verbal Selective Reminding (consistent long-term, delayed recall), and Symbol-Digit Modalities Test. Scores on the Galveston Orientation and Amnesia Test, the Controlled Oral Word Association Test, and the Trails B Test did not improve.

Recommendations (Level I)

Based on the evidence, it is not possible to make a recommendation regarding the use of hypothermia as a treatment for severe brain injury. Prospective study of the effect of maintaining hypothermia in patients who are hypothermic on admission is required. Hypothermia reduces markedly elevated ICP. Exactly how it could best be used for this purpose and whether or not its use for this purpose improves outcome have not been clinically documented.

References

1. Clifton GL, Allen S, Barrodale P, et al. A Phase II study of moderate hypothermia in severe brain injury. J Neurotrauma 1993;10:263–271.
2. Marion DW, Penrod LE, Kelsey SF, et al. Treatment of traumatic brain injury with moderate hypothermia. N Engl J Med 1997;336:540–546.
3. Clifton GL, Allen S, Berry J, Koch SM. Systemic hypothermia in treatment of brain injury. J Neurotrauma 1992;9 (suppl 2): S487–S495.
4. Clifton GL, Jiang JY, Lyeth BG, et al. Marked protection by moderate hypothermia after experimental traumatic brain injury. J Cereb Blood Flow Metab 1991;11:114–121.
5. Clifton GL, Miller ER, Choi SC, et al. Lack of effect of induction of hypothermia in acute brain injury. N Engl J Med 2001;344: 556–563.
6. Jurkovich GJ, Greiser WB, Luterman A, et al. Hypothermia in trauma victims: an ominous predictor of survival. J Trauma 1987;27:1019–1024.
7. Little RA, Stoner HB. Body temperature after accidental injury. Br J Surg 1981;68:221–224.
8. Luna GK, Maier RV, Pavlin EG, et al. Incidence and effect of hypothermia in seriously injured patients. J Trauma 1987;27: 1014–1018.
9. Gregory JS, Flancbaum L, Townsend MC, et al. Incidence and timing of hypothermia in trauma patients undergoing operations. J Trauma 1991;31:795–798.
10. Kurz A, Plattner O, Sessler DI, et al. The threshold for thermoregulatory vasoconstriction during nitrous oxide/isoflurane anesthesia is lower in elderly than in young patients. Anesthesiology 1993;79:465–469.
11. White MD, Ross WE, Mekjavid IB. Relationship between physique and rectal temperature cooling rate. Undersea Biomed Res 1992;19:121–130.
12. Suehiro A, Povlishock JT. Exacerbation of traumatically induced axonal injury by rapid posthypothermic rewarming and attenuation of axonal change by cyclosporin A. J Neurosurg 2001; 94:493–498.
13. Shiozaki T, Sugimoto H, Taneda M, et al. Effect of mild hypothermia on uncontrollable intracranial hypertension after severe head injury. J Neurosurg 1993;79:363–368.
14. Shiozaki T, Sugimoto H, Taneda M, et al. Selection of severely head injured patients for mild hypothermia therapy. J Neurosurg 1998;89:206–211.
15. Shiozaki T, Hayakata T, Taneda M, et al. A multicenter prospective randomized controlled trial of the efficacy of mild hypothermia for severely head injured patients with low intracranial pressure. Mild Hypothermia Study Group in Japan. J Neurosurg 2001;94:50–54.
16. Jiang J, Yu M, Zhu C. Effect of long-term mild hypothermia therapy in patients with severe traumatic brain injury: 1-year follow-up review of 87 cases. J Neurosurg 2000;93:546–549.

Does Decompressive Craniectomy Really Improve Outcome After Head Injury?

Brian T. Andrews

Brief Answer

The evidence supports classifying the performance of a decompressive craniectomy as a level II recommendation for lowering intracranial pressure (ICP) in cases of refractory intracranial hypertension. In terms of improving outcome, this practice should be considered a level III recommendation.

Background

From an evidence-based perspective, decompressive craniectomy has adequate class II support in recent literature to support its use as a level II recommendation for the treatment of refractory elevations in ICP after head injury. In terms of improving clinical outcome, it should be considered a level III recommendation because the only sound data that are available are limited to prospective or retrospective case series that often differ in the exact clinical time point at which decompression was performed. This limitation of the data makes it difficult to determine accurately the effect of decompression on clinical outcome. There exist no reliable prospective randomized controlled trials of this technique. Historical perspective gives us little useful information because decompressive craniectomy was generally applied in the past only as a last resort when all other options had been exhausted, and thus for patients beyond any reasonable hope for a functional recovery.

Literature Review

Physiologic Effects

In terms of ICP, persistent elevations of ICP after severe head injury are associated with poor outcome (class II data).[1] Miller et al[2] found that head-injured patients with uncontrollable elevations of ICP beyond 20 mmHg had a mortality rate of 100%, whereas those with ICP increases above 20 mmHg who responded to therapy had a mortality rate of 29%. Normal ICP throughout a patient's course was associated with a mortality rate of only 14% (class II data).

Decompression is an effective means of lowering elevated ICP. Yoo et al[3] measured ICP before and after bilateral craniectomy, as well as before and after the dura was opened, in 20 patients with massive brain swelling (class II data). The mean ICP decreased to 50.2% of the initial ICP after craniectomy alone and decreased an additional 34.5% after durotomy; the final pressure was reduced by an average of nearly 85%. Kunze et al[4] showed that, in 28 patients with an initial mean ICP of 41.7 ± 10.1 mmHg, postoperative ICP was reduced to 20.6 ± 15.3 mmHg (class III data). Polin et al[5] also noted a highly significant ($p = .0003$) reduction in ICP in 35 patients who underwent bifrontal decompression for diffuse traumatic cerebral swelling; postoperative reduction was also significant when compared with ICP values at 48 to 72 hours postinjury of weighted control patients from the Traumatic Coma Data Bank (class II data).

In a computed tomographic (CT) analysis, Münch et al[6] have shown that unilateral decompressive craniectomy for patients with acute subdural hematomas with severe mass effect significantly decreases midline shift and improves visibility of the mesencephalic cisterns (class III data).

Clinical Results

Available studies have used a variety of surgical techniques in small, heterogeneous groups of patients at differing time points after severe head injury.

In the study described above, Yoo et al[3] reported that in 20 patients with massive diffuse brain swelling and elevated ICP treated with bilateral decompression, the overall mortality rate was 20% (class II data). Fully 69% of survivors (11 of 16 patients) had a good outcome, defined as a Glasgow Outcome Scale (GOS)[7] score of 4 or 5. Importantly, persistent elevation of ICP above 35 mmHg during the first 24 hours after decompression correlated with 100% mortality.

Pearl

Persistent elevation of ICP above 35 mmHg during the first 24 hours after decompression has been associated with 100% mortality.

In the report by Polin et al,[5] bifrontal craniectomy was performed in 35 patients with "malignant posttraumatic cerebral edema" (class II data). The overall mortality rate was 23%, with 37% of patients achieving a good outcome or moderate disability (GOS 4 or 5); children had a higher rate of favorable outcome (44%). Patients who underwent surgery more than 48 hours after injury had worse outcomes than those who were decompressed within 48 hours.

Unilateral decompressive craniectomy has also been reported to be beneficial. In Kunze et al's[4] retrospective review of 28 patients with uncontrollable elevation of ICP, 17 of the 28 were treated with unilateral craniectomy for swelling that was primarily located in one hemisphere (class III data). Overall mortality was 11%, and 54% of patients had a good outcome (GOS 4 or 5) after 1 year. These authors found that patients under 30 years of age had particularly good outcomes and low mortality.

Guerra et al[8] prospectively treated 57 patients with unilateral (31 patients) or bilateral (26 patients) decompression (class II data). Overall mortality was 19%, and GOS scores of 4 or 5 were achieved by 58% of patients. These authors found that the Glasgow Coma Scale (GCS) score on the first day after trauma and the mean ICP were most predictive of outcome. Of interest, however, Münch et al[6] found that when unilateral decompression was performed for patients with a unilateral intracranial lesion and midline shift greater than 1 cm, the clinical results were no better than those reported in the Traumatic Coma Data Bank for similar patients treated without decompression (class III data).[9]

A recent study in pediatric patients concluded that early decompressive craniectomy was associated with better control of ICP and with better functional outcome in children with traumatic brain injury.[10] However, management protocols continually evolved and changed during the course of the study, including goals for cerebral perfusion pressure, use of hyperventilation and hypothermia, and administration of intravenous fluids. The decompressive craniectomies consisted only of limited bitemporal decompression, without opening of the dura in most cases. Other problems included the small number of patients ($n = 27$), the protracted time course of the study (7 years), and the method of obtaining outcome assessments. For these reasons, despite its laudable efforts to prospectively randomize patients, this trial may be regarded at best as a class II study.

Some authors have limited the use of decompression to patients younger than 50 years of age because of the generally poor prognosis of older trauma patients.[8,11] The author's experience, however, is that older patients may respond reasonably well to decompression, and therefore no specific age of exclusion for this technique is imposed.

Complications

Decompressive craniectomy has been associated with various complications (class II and class III data).[3–5,8] Leakage of cerebrospinal fluid (CSF) may occur after the craniectomy, and a small percentage of patients have difficulty with scalp breakdown at the bone edge after ICP normalizes and the scalp recedes. Wound infections may occur after reimplantation of the bone flap.[3] Delayed subdural hygromas at the site of decompression may require drainage and/or ventricular or lumbar shunting.

Surgical Technique

Decompression

Decompressive craniectomy can range from a simple subtemporal decompression (unilateral or bilateral) to subtotal calvariectomy.[3–5,8,12] Several authors describe large bifrontal craniectomies, particularly for patients with refractory elevations of ICP due to diffuse cerebral swelling.[3,5] The author prefers a large, unilateral craniectomy to include the frontal, parietal, and temporal bones, centered over the area of maximal brain injury as identified on the most recent preoperative CT scan. The bone flap should extend at least to or beyond the margins of injury or swelling and down to the floor of the middle fossa. This extension of the inferior margin of the craniectomy to the temporal skull base has been shown by Münch et al[6] to result in optimal decompression of the perimesencephalic cisterns (class III data).

Pearl

Decompression should extend down to the floor of the middle fossa to provide maximum decompression of the perimesencephalic cisterns.

The removed calvarium may be wrapped in antibiotic-soaked gauze, sealed in a sterile fashion in plastic, and carefully labeled and stored in a freezer until subsequent cranioplasty. Some neurosurgeons have described placement of the bone in a subcutaneous pocket in the abdominal wall for later use.[8]

At the time of decompression, the dura should be opened widely, with relaxing incisions placed at right angles along the dural edge.[12] Resection of hematomas or of infarcted, contused, or markedly edematous cerebral parenchyma may be performed, particularly in areas of noneloquent brain. Attempts should be made to preserve regions of eloquence, even if their viability is questionable. After the dura is laid back over the brain, the exposed cortex is covered with dural allograft or other type of dural substitute. A subgaleal drain may be placed if desired. The galea should be closed in a meticulous fashion with frequent interrupted sutures, and the skin closed with a running nylon suture to prevent leakage of CSF. If necessary, ICP monitoring may be performed with an ipsilateral intraventricular or parenchymal catheter. Measures to control ICP should be continued, including ventricular drainage, use of mannitol, hypothermia, and other measures as needed.[13]

Cranioplasty

After a successful decompressive craniectomy, the bone flap should be replaced reasonably promptly, for example, within 1 to 3 months after the initial procedure. Before reimplantation, the scalp edges should be fully healed and viable. If the edges remain marginal, one must consider wound revision at the time of bone replacement, with excision of the weakened scalp and approximation of healthy galeal edges. Great care must be taken while elevating the skin and galea away from the dura and away from any exposed brain. Rigid fixation is helpful for securing the bone flap in position.

It is likely that atmospheric pressure exerts a negative effect on the cortex underlying the scalp at the site of a craniectomy defect, with potentially adverse effects on neurologic function (class III data).[14] In addition, the literature contains numerous descriptions of the "syndrome of the trephined": complaints of severe headache, dizziness, fatigue, poor memory, depression, and intolerance of vibration in patients with a craniectomy defect (class III data).[14–16] These symptoms often improve after replacement of the bone flap. Winkler et al[16] have shown that cranioplasty improves postural blood flow regulation, cerebrovascular reserve, and cerebral glucose metabolism as measured by positron emission tomography (class II data). These results may be due to the restoration of a negative ICP above the foramen magnum when a patient assumes the upright position.

Pearl

The bone flap should be replaced after 1 to 3 months to restore normal cerebral blood flow and metabolism and to prevent the development of the "syndrome of the trephined."

Recommendations

Leaving the bone flap off and/or widening the craniectomy have long been recommended as potential options in cases of so-called malignant cerebral edema; that is, rapid and massive swelling of the brain into the craniotomy site immediately after removal of an acute subdural hematoma or other mass lesion.

For patients without operable mass lesions in whom ICP monitoring has been established, progressive elevation of ICP that is refractory to standard treatment measures should prompt consideration of decompressive craniectomy before cerebral perfusion becomes compromised (level II recommendation). Excessive delay in performing the procedure, with progressive regional and global secondary ischemic injury to the brain, may be the most important reason that decompressive craniectomy has often seemed to be fruitless in the past. Depending on the distribution of the cerebral edema, the craniectomy may be unilateral, bilateral, or bifrontal (level III recommendation).

Currently available modern evidence supports early decompressive craniectomy as a level II treatment recommendation for lowering ICP. In terms of improving outcome, this practice should be considered a level III recommendation. Failure of decompression to lower ICP to acceptable levels is associated with a high mortality rate.

References

1. Marmarou A, Eisenberg HM, Foulkes MA, et al. Impact of ICP instability and hypotension on outcome in patients with severe head trauma. J Neurosurg 1991;75:S59–S66.

2. Miller JD, Becker DP, Ward JD, et al. Significance of intracranial hypertension in severe head injury. J Neurosurg 1977;47: 503–516.
3. Yoo DS, Kim DS, Cho KS, et al. Ventricular pressure monitoring during bilateral decompression with dural expansion. J Neurosurg 1999;91:953–995.
4. Kunze E, Meixensberger J, Janka M, et al. Decompressive craniectomy in patients with uncontrollable intracranial hypertension. Acta Neurochir Suppl (Wien) 1998;71:16–18.
5. Polin RS, Shaffrey ME, Bogaev CA, et al. Decompressive bifrontal craniotomy in the treatment of severe refractory posttraumatic cerebral edema. Neurosurgery 1997;41:84–92.
6. Münch E, Horn P, Schürer L, et al. Management of severe traumatic brain injury by decompressive craniectomy. Neurosurgery 2000;47:315–322.
7. Jennett B, Bond M. Assessment of outcome after severe brain damage: a practical scale. Lancet 1975;1:480–484.
8. Guerra WKW, Gaab MR, Dietz H, et al. Surgical decompression for traumatic brain swelling: indications and results. J Neurosurg 1999;90:187–196.
9. Marshall LF, Gautille T, Klauber MR, et al. The outcome of severe closed head injury. J Neurosurg 1991;75:S28–S36.
10. Taylor A, Butt W, Rosenfeld J, et al. A randomized trial of very early decompressive craniectomy in children with traumatic brain injury and sustained intracranial hypertension. Childs Nerv Syst 2001;17:154–162.
11. Vollmer DG, Torner JC, Jane JA, et al. Age and outcome following traumatic coma: why do older patients fare worse? J Neurosurg 1991;75:S37–S49.
12. Valadka AB, Narayan RK. Surgical aspects of the head-injured. In: Narayan RK, Wilberger JE, Povlishock JT, eds. Neurotrauma. New York: McGraw-Hill; 1995:203–224.
13. Andrews BT. Head injury management. In: Andrews BT, ed. Intensive Care in Neurosurgery. New York: Thieme; 2003: 125–136.
14. Yamaura A, Makino H. Neurological deficits in the presence of the sinking flap following decompressive craniectomy. Neurol Med Chir (Tokyo) 1977;17:43–53.
15. Grantham EG, Landis HP. Cranioplasty and the post-traumatic syndrome. J Neurosurg 1948;5:19–22.
16. Winkler PA, Stummer W, Linke R, et al. Influence of cranioplasty on postural blood flow regulation, cerebrovascular reserve capacity, and cerebral glucose metabolism. J Neurosurg 2000; 93:53–61.

◆ 30 ◆

What Is the Best Algorithm for Treating Intracranial Hypertension?

Jürgen Meixensberger and Matthias Jaeger

Brief Answer

The evidence supports level II and level III recommendations for basic and extended treatment of intracranial hypertension. In terms of improving outcome, recommendations should be considered to be level III.

Background

Although various options are available for the treatment of elevated intracranial pressure (ICP), no consensus exists regarding the optimal therapeutic regime for patients with intracranial hypertension. The available options are usually applied as required in an escalating step-by-step fashion. The sequence of their application, however, may vary considerably at different neurotrauma centers.

The "optimal" treatment algorithm (according to the principles of evidence-based medicine) still needs to be defined. Ideally, prospective randomized trials generating class I evidence and level I recommendations should validate and compare the available treatment options in terms of their effectiveness for controlling ICP and improving patient outcome. A large amount of existing data does provide some guidance in choosing among different therapies. Unfortunately, little solid evidence is available to guide neurotraumatologists in the many ICP treatment decisions that they must make on a daily basis.

From a Medline search using "intracranial pressure AND treatment," we extracted those results that provided the best data for developing an evidence-based algorithm for the treatment of elevated ICP.

Literature Review

Basic Measures

Sedation and Artificial Ventilation

No studies have evaluated the effects on outcome of sedation and artificial ventilation by randomizing some patients with severe traumatic brain injury (TBI) and intracranial hypertension to control groups in which these interventions were not used. Nevertheless, expert opinion and widespread recognition of the ICP-lowering effects of these measures prompted the European Brain Injury Consortium to advocate their use as a level III recommendation.[1] Regarding the choice of sedative drugs, propofol and midazolam were both declared to be safe and effective for use in severely injured patients (some of whom had TBI) in class III studies,[2,3] but direct effects on ICP were not seen, possibly because all patients in these studies received some form of sedation. For analgesia, the opioids alfentanil, fentanyl, and sufentanil were all found to produce transient increases in ICP (8 mmHg for ~15 minutes) when administered by bolus injection, presumably reflecting an autoregulatory response to an associated decrease in mean arterial pressure; however, no cerebral ischemia was detected in measurements of jugular venous lactate-oxygen index (class II data).[4]

The ultrashort-acting opioid remifentanil was determined to be safe for analgesia in the neurosurgical intensive care unit (ICU), partly because it did not produce alterations in ICP or in blood pressure (class III data).[5] Despite the fact that ketamine has been largely abandoned for a long time in terms of analgesia in TBI patients, Kolenda et al[6] conducted a class II study in which the combination of midazolam plus ketamine had more beneficial effects than the combination of midazolam plus fentanyl in terms of vasopressor requirements and enteral food intake, but no major differences were seen in ICP or outcome.

Pearl

Various sedatives and analgesics have been shown to have comparable efficacy in lowering ICP, but no study has compared these medications to placebo.

In patients requiring artificial ventilation, use of positive end-expiratory pressure (PEEP) up to 10 cm H_2O was considered safe by Cooper et al[7] based on their study of 33 TBI patients (class II data). Schneider et al[8] observed that hyperventilation ($PaCO_2 < 30$ mmHg) produced decreases of brain tissue oxygen tension; in one of their 15 severe TBI patients, hyperventilation had to be stopped because the decrease in brain tissue oxygen tension was potentially of sufficient magnitude to cause cerebral tissue hypoxia (class II data). In a randomized trial reported by Muizelaar et al[9] (class II data), prolonged hyperventilation was associated with a trend toward worse outcomes in severe TBI patients with an initial Glasgow Coma Scale motor score of 4 to 5.

Patient Position

Correct patient positioning was the focus of a class II study of 25 patients by Schneider et al.[10] They investigated ICP and $SjvO_2$ at different head elevations ranging from 0 to 45 degrees. With 45 degrees of head elevation, an ICP reduction of almost 50% could be obtained without significant compromise of cerebral oxygenation or cerebral perfusion pressure (CPP), despite the potential for reduction in CPP upon head elevation. Although Schneider et al found that average CPP and $SjvO_2$ did not change significantly as head position varied, CPP responses of individual patients were unpredictable. Other investigators have reported that flexing the neck or turning the head to either side produces modest but statistically significant increases in ICP (class II data).[11]

Pearl

Keeping the head in a neutral position at 30 to 45 degrees of elevation is optimal for most head-injured patients.

Extended Measures

Hyperosmotic Solutions

Hyperosmotic solutions, such as mannitol, are still the most common "extended" treatment for posttraumatic ICP control. A randomized study reported by Schwartz et al[12] provided class I evidence supporting the use of mannitol prior to the use of barbiturates for the treatment of elevated ICP in head-injured patients. Additional class II studies have demonstrated that bolus doses of mannitol are effective for ICP treatment.[13,14] Infusable agents other than mannitol have also been found to reduce ICP effectively. Bolus infusions of hypertonic saline in concentrations ranging from 7 to 23% decreased mean ICP by at least 40% in several studies, without significant side effects (class II and class III data).[15–17] Furthermore, tromethamine (THAM) administered as a continuous infusion for 5 days after TBI was found to successfully reduce ICP in a multicenter class I trial reported by Wolf et al.[18] Beneficial effects on outcome, however, were not observed. THAM is also effective in lowering ICP when given as bolus infusion, with a reported reduction in ICP of 33% (class II data).[19]

Barbiturates

The use of barbiturates for ICP control has been studied extensively. Ward et al[20] investigated prophylactic barbiturate coma in 53 severely head-injured patients (class I data). They found no difference between groups in outcome or in ICP control, but the barbiturate-treated group was much more likely to experience arterial hypotension (54% versus 7%). Thus, the authors did not recommend prophylactic barbiturate coma for patients with severe TBI. On the other hand, Cormio et al[21] described a class II study that identified subgroups of patients who experienced considerable benefit from barbiturates. In particular, those patients in whom ICP decreased after the initial loading dose of barbiturates might benefit from the barbiturate-induced reduction of cerebral metabolism. As discussed above, however, Schwartz et al's[12] class I study comparing barbiturates and mannitol for ICP control found barbiturates to be less successful than mannitol for ICP reduction, at least at the earlier stage of intervention at which barbiturates were used in the Schwartz study.

Pearl

In a patient with refractory intracranial hypertension, the ICP response to an initial loading dose of barbiturates may indicate whether barbiturate therapy should be continued in that patient.

Invasive Measures

Invasive measures to counteract intracranial hypertension include drainage of cerebrospinal fluid (CSF) via ventriculostomy and decompressive craniectomy. CSF drainage is considered class II data, as assessed by Kerr et al,[22] who reported that this therapy significantly reduced ICP (mean decrease 4 mmHg) in a study of 31 severe TBI patients.

Early decompressive craniectomy for treatment of severely brain-injured children was investigated by Taylor et al[23] in a class II pilot study of 27 pediatric patients. Management protocols evolved during the course of the study, including changes in targeted CPP, use of hyperventilation and hypothermia, and management of fluids. The decompressive craniectomy consisted of limited bitemporal decompression without opening of the dura in most cases. Despite a strong tendency toward reduced ICP and improved outcome in the surgically treated group, results were not significant, most likely due to small cohorts. However, class II data from Yoo et al[24] found bilateral decompressive craniectomy with dural expansion to be highly successful for ICP reduction, producing immediate decreases in ICP to less than 20% of the initial values. However, because no patients were entered into a control group, the effects of these ICP decreases on outcome were unclear.

Lund Therapy

Contrary to commonly used strategies for treatment of TBI patients, which focus on avoiding cerebral ischemia by keeping CPP above 60 mmHg and ICP below 20 mmHg, the group from Lund University in Sweden advocates a different approach for treatment of posttraumatic brain edema.[25] Based on their understanding of principles of cerebral tissue and blood volume regulation, the Lund therapy protocol aims for normovolemia and reduction of intracapillary pressure. To achieve these goals, dihydroergotamine, clonidine, and metoprolol are administered. In addition, normal colloid osmotic pressure is maintained by albumin infusions and by administration of furosemide. The Lund investigators reported a series of 53 patients (class III data), of whom 79% achieved a favorable outcome (defined as good recovery or moderate disability). These results were better than those in a historical control group and in previously reported outcome studies.

Recommendations

Many of the options available for ICP control have been evaluated in different studies that have generated different classes of evidence justifying their use. However, in a treatment algorithm, it may not necessarily be reasonable to begin with those therapeutic options that have been validated in class I studies and therefore can be considered to be level I recommendations. Such practical considerations as invasiveness, expenditure of labor, and costs must also be weighed. For example, it may be preferable to follow a level III recommendation to administer a specific medication before following a level I recommendation to perform a major operation or other procedure that is more invasive, expensive, and time-consuming. Importantly, every algorithm for ICP control itself is class III, and, as a consequence, represents only level III recommendations.

Initiating ICP reduction with sedation and artificial ventilation of the severely brain-injured patient is a level III recommendation. Use of propofol, midazolam, and remifentanil is a level III recommendation, and administration of other opioids can be viewed as level III recommendations as long as they are not administered by bolus injection. The use of ketamine in neurotrauma should be reassessed. Based on the existing literature, a level III recommendation may be made to use it as an alternative to conventional opioid-based analgesia.

Regarding optimal ventilator settings, the avoidance of prophylactic and acute hyperventilation is a level II recommendation. In the situation of transtentorial herniation with impending irreversible brainstem damage, hyperventilation for ICP reduction through a decrease of intracranial volume is a level III recommendation. PEEP can be carefully elevated up to 10 cmH_2O (level II recommendation) to optimize pulmonary function and avoid systemic hypoxia.

In addition to sedation and artificial ventilation, TBI patients should be nursed with head and upper trunk elevation of 30 to 45 degrees, and the neck should be kept in a neutral position (level II recommendation).

If these basic measures fail to control ICP, extended measures should be undertaken. Use of mannitol can be advocated as a level II recommendation. THAM can effectively lower ICP when given either as a continuous infusion (level I recommendation) or as a bolus (level II recommendation), but beneficial effects on outcome have not been demonstrated. In addition, hypertonic saline has been reported to be highly effective for ICP control (level II recommendation).

In terms of invasive measures to lower ICP, CSF drainage and decompressive craniectomy are both considered to be level II recommendations. Decompression appears to be more successful for ICP reduction; however, CSF drainage is far less invasive and presumably less likely to cause complications and therefore may be preferable to decompression. The available literature suggests that surgical decompression is more effective than barbiturates for ICP control, but inconsistencies in patient selection criteria make comparison of different series difficult. However, if surgery is not possible, an

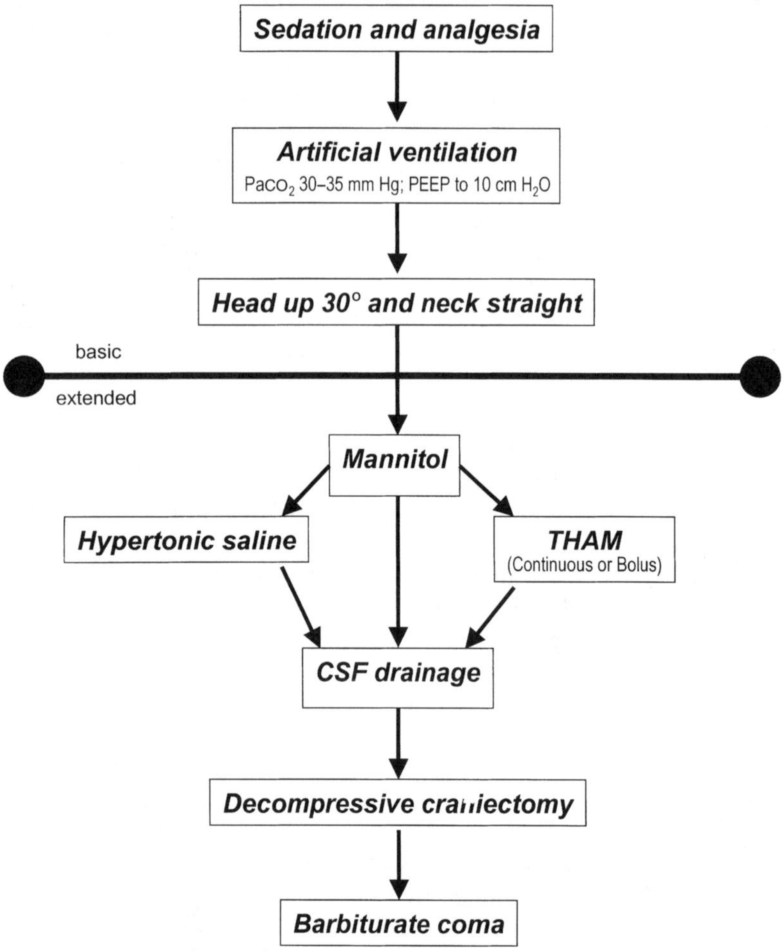

Figure 30-1 The algorithm for treating intracranial hypertension. CSF, cerebrospinal fluid; PEEP, positive end-expiratory pressure; THAM, tromethamine.

initial test bolus of pentobarbital may be considered to evaluate the potential for ICP reduction (level II recommendation). If ICP falls as desired, continuous barbiturate treatment may be considered.

The reports describing the Lund therapy support the use of this protocol as a level III recommendation.

Conclusions

From the conclusions drawn from this literature review, we developed the algorithm presented in Fig. 30-1.

References

1. Maas AI, Dearden M, Teasdale GM, et al. EBIC-guidelines for management of severe head injury in adults. European Brain Injury Consortium. Acta Neurochir (Wien) 1997;139:286–294.
2. Sanchez-Izquierdo-Riera JA, Caballero-Cubedo RE, Perez-Vela JL, et al. Propofol versus midazolam: safety and efficacy for sedating the severe trauma patient. Anesth Analg 1998;86: 1219–1224.
3. Kelly DF, Goodale DB, Williams J, et al. Propofol in the treatment of moderate and severe head injury: a randomized, prospective double-blinded pilot trial. J Neurosurg 1999; 90:1042–1052.
4. Albanese J, Viviand X, Potie F, et al. Sufentanil, fentanyl, and alfentanil in head trauma patients: a study on cerebral hemodynamics. Crit Care Med 1999;27:407–411.
5. Tipps LB, Coplin WM, Murry KR, et al. Safety and feasibility of continuous infusion of remifentanil in the neurosurgical intensive care unit. Neurosurgery 2000;46:596–601.
6. Kolenda H, Gremmelt A, Rading S, et al. Ketamine for analgosedative therapy in intensive care treatment of head-injured patients. Acta Neurochir (Wien) 1996;138:1193–1199.
7. Cooper KR, Boswell PA, Choi SC. Safe use of PEEP in patients with severe head injury. J Neurosurg 1985;63:552–555.
8. Schneider GH, Sarrafzadeh AS, Kiening KL, et al. Influence of hyperventilation on brain tissue-PO2, PCO2, and pH in patients with intracranial hypertension. Acta Neurochir Suppl (Wien) 1998;71:62–65.
9. Muizelaar JP, Marmarou A, Ward JD, et al. Adverse effects of prolonged hyperventilation in patients with severe head injury: a randomized clinical trial. J Neurosurg 1991;75: 731–739.
10. Schneider GH, von Helden GH, Franke R, et al. Influence of body position on jugular venous oxygen saturation, intracranial pressure and cerebral perfusion pressure. Acta Neurochir Suppl (Wien) 1993;59:107–112.
11. Williams A, Coyne SM. Effects of neck position on intracranial pressure. Am J Crit Care 1993;2:68–71.
12. Schwartz ML, Tator CH, Rowed DW, et al. The University of Toronto head injury treatment study: a prospective, randomized comparison of pentobarbital and mannitol. Can J Neurol Sci 1984;11:434–440.
13. Hartl R, Bardt TF, Kiening KL, et al. Mannitol decreases ICP but does not improve brain-tissue pO2 in severely head-injured

patients with intracranial hypertension. Acta Neurochir Suppl (Wien) 1997;70:40–42.

14. McGraw CP, Howard G. Effect of mannitol on increased intracranial pressure. Neurosurgery 1983;13:269–271.
15. Munar F, Ferrer AM, de Nadal M, et al. Cerebral hemodynamic effects of 7.2% hypertonic saline in patients with head injury and raised intracranial pressure. J Neurotrauma 2000;17:41–51.
16. Schatzmann C, Heissler HE, König K, et al. Treatment of elevated intracranial pressure by infusions of 10% saline in severely head injured patients. Acta Neurochir Suppl (Wien) 1998;71:31–33.
17. Suarez JI, Qureshi AI, Bhardwaj A, et al. Treatment of refractory intracranial hypertension with 23.4% saline. Crit Care Med 1998;26:1118–1122.
18. Wolf AL, Levi L, Marmarou A, et al. Effect of THAM upon outcome in severe head injury: a randomized prospective clinical trial. J Neurosurg 1993;78:54–59.
19. Gaab MR, Seegers K, Smedema RJ, et al. A comparative analysis of THAM (Tris-buffer) in traumatic brain oedema. Acta Neurochir Suppl (Wien) 1990;51:320–323.
20. Ward JD, Becker DP, Miller JD, et al. Failure of prophylactic barbiturate coma in the treatment of severe head injury. J Neurosurg 1985;62:383–388.
21. Cormio M, Gopinath SP, Valadka A, et al. Cerebral hemodynamic effects of pentobarbital coma in head-injured patients. J Neurotrauma 1999;16:927–936.
22. Kerr EM, Marion D, Sereika MS, et al. The effect of cerebrospinal fluid drainage on cerebral perfusion in traumatic brain injured adults. J Neurosurg Anesthesiol 2000;12:324–333.
23. Taylor A, Butt W, Rosenfeld J, et al. A randomized trial of very early decompressive craniectomy in children with traumatic brain injury and sustained intracranial hypertension. Childs Nerv Syst 2001;17:154–162.
24. Yoo DS, Kim DS, Cho KS, et al. Ventricular pressure monitoring during bilateral decompression with dural expansion. J Neurosurg 1999;91:953–959.
25. Eker C, Asgeirsson B, Grande PO, et al. Improved outcome after severe head injury with a new therapy based on principles for brain volume regulation and preserved microcirculation. Crit Care Med 1998;26:1881–1886.

Brain Injury

Special Circumstances

◆ 31 ◆

Simultaneous Intracranial and Abdominal Injury: Which Gets Operated on First, and Which Has the Higher Treatment Priority?

Colonel John B. Holcomb

Brief Answer

Prioritizing surgeries in trauma patients requiring surgery for both abdominal injuries and intracranial mass lesions is based on the initial hemodynamic status of the patient and on the response to fluid resuscitation. Stable patients with intraabdominal hemorrhage and severe head injury should undergo expeditious evaluation and treatment of their head injury, followed by more deliberate evaluation of their abdominal or thoracic injury. Those who are initially hypotensive but who stabilize after resuscitation should undergo a similar treatment plan. Patients who transiently respond but who again experience a drop in blood pressure should be moved rapidly to the operating room (OR) for treatment of their cavitary bleeding; evaluation of the head injury may proceed during treatment of the abdominal injury. Likewise, patients with persistent hypotension require immediate laparotomy, with intraoperative evaluation and possible treatment of the head injury. Avoiding secondary brain injury by preventing persistent hypotension and/or hypoxia is of primary concern. In many cases, these goals are best accomplished by surgical correction of ongoing abdominal bleeding. Effective communication between the trauma surgeon and neurosurgeon is critical to optimal outcome in these patients.

Pearl

In many cases, laparotomy to control ongoing abdominal bleeding is the best way to treat the secondary cerebral insult of hypotension.

Background

Patients who present to the emergency department (ED) with significant intraabdominal hemorrhage and concomitant large intracranial mass lesions are, fortunately, uncommon. These patients typically suffer from blunt vehicular trauma. Often, some element of illicit drug use confounds the hemodynamic and neurologic examinations. These severely ill patients require coordination of efforts by trauma surgeons and neurosurgeons. The main objective is to prevent or promptly treat hypotension, hypoxia, and other secondary brain insults. This goal is best achieved by balancing the devastating consequences of hypotension[1] from continued intraabdominal hemorrhage against those of untreated traumatic mass lesions.

The presence or absence of cavitary hemorrhage must be determined as expeditiously as possible. Although the method utilized will vary at different hospitals and even among different providers within the same hospital, the emphasis must remain on a safe yet rapid evaluation. Ultrasound or diagnostic peritoneal lavage (DPL) is used most commonly, largely because these tests may be performed without patients having to leave the ED. In many centers, obtaining computed tomography (CT) scans of the abdomen and head requires taking patients out of the ED. Such transport may be detrimental in hemodynamically unstable patients. However, the increasing presence of high-speed helical scanners in EDs may reduce the problem of hemodynamic deterioration in the radiology department or CT scanner by allowing extremely rapid evaluation of hemodynamically marginal patients. The ultimate solution to this problem may consist of portable CT scanners that can be wheeled into the ED.

The discussion of shock in the Advanced Trauma Life Support (ATLS) manual divides resuscitation of trauma patients into four categories based on their hemodynamic status and physiologic response to resuscitation.[2] The first group is hemodynamically stable, with minimal cavitary hemorrhage and severe head injury. The second group responds to fluid resuscitation and stabilizes at a normal blood pressure. The third group is initially hypotensive and transiently responds to fluid resuscitation, yet soon exhibits a return of hypotension. The fourth group is persistently hypotensive and does not respond to resuscitation. The last two physiologic patterns are consistent with ongoing bleeding and/or exsanguination. Patients' initial evaluation in the ED and their hemodynamic response to fluid resuscitation will determine whether they receive an emergency operation or a continuing radiologic evaluation followed by a more orderly progression to the OR. In the next section, the relative operative priorities of the intracranial lesion and the abdominal injury are evaluated in each group.

When combined with an operative head injury, a pelvic fracture causing hemodynamic compromise is an ominous finding. These patients require both rapid intervention for their intracranial lesion and external fixation and/or angiographic embolization for the pelvic fracture. Discussion of the timing and staging of these interventions would exceed the space allotted for this review. Also beyond the scope of this brief outline is the optimal combination of abdominal ultrasound, DPL, and CT in the evaluation of blunt abdominal trauma. The author routinely utilizes all three modalities because their distinct advantages suggest that they should be used in a complementary fashion.

Pearl

Ultrasound, DPL, and CT scanning should be used in a complementary fashion for the evaluation of blunt abdominal trauma.

Of utmost importance is early and ongoing communication between the neurosurgeon and the trauma surgeon concerning "who goes first." Optimally, these concepts have been coordinated ahead of time during the light of day so that minimal confusion will occur at 2 AM. Individual institutions and their medical staffs should have realistic expectations and goals concerning the availability of both trauma surgeons and neurosurgeons. The following discussion may provide a framework for such planning.

Early and ongoing communication between the neurosurgeon and the trauma surgeon is of utmost importance.

Literature Review and Recommendations

Group 1 patients are always hemodynamically stable despite the presence of intracavitary hemorrhage superimposed upon severe head injury. Because of the high probability that they will remain hemodynamically stable (class II data),[3,4] the head injury takes precedence in these patients. They should undergo CT scans of the abdomen and head before heading to the OR. Any solid organ injuries that are discovered can likely be managed nonoperatively (class III data).[5] Suspicion for a bowel injury should be high in those patients whose abdominal CT scans reveal intraabdominal fluid but no solid organ injury (class III data).[6] If the abdominal CT scan will unduly prolong operative treatment of the head injury, the abdominal evaluation may proceed either in the OR or postoperatively.

Group 2 patients demonstrate transient hypotension, which responds to minimal fluid resuscitation. These patients rapidly become hemodynamically stable. Although some studies have found that patients with reported prehospital hypotension (systolic blood pressure <90 mmHg) have an overall mortality rate >50% (emphasizing the grave prognostic implications of this isolated physiologic discriminator) (class III data),[7] those patients who exhibit only transient hypotension with subsequent stabilization after resuscitation constitute a subgroup with improved survival compared with those who are persistently hypotensive (class III data).[8] Patients who respond to fluid resuscitation with normalization and stabilization of vital signs have usually stopped bleeding. These patients should undergo rapid evaluation in the ED, followed by a head CT scan (class III data).[9] In the OR the head injury takes precedence, followed if necessary by the intraabdominal procedure. If the patient remains stable during the cranial procedure, immediate abdominal CT scanning is indicated after the craniotomy has been completed. During this sequence of evaluation and therapy, frequent communication between the neurosurgeon, trauma surgeon, and anesthesia personnel is critical. Any deterioration in hemodynamic stability must be ascribed to intracavitary hemorrhage, and immediate operative intervention must commence. This may require simultaneous laparotomy (and/or thoracotomy) and craniotomy.

Pearl

Patients who respond to fluid resuscitation with normalization and stabilization of vital signs have usually stopped bleeding.

Group 3 patients are initially hypotensive and respond only transiently to fluid resuscitation. They comprise a small group that presents a real dilemma for the evaluating physician in the EC. One of the hard-learned lessons in the initial evaluation of trauma patients is to avoid hemodynamic deterioration in the CT scanner. Unfortunately, these are the patients most likely to do just that as they initially respond to fluids, but soon afterward their blood pressure drops again. These patients should be moved rapidly to the OR after very minimal and rapid evaluation. Diagnostic and operative priority; that is, craniotomy versus laparotomy (or thoracotomy), should be established based on the amount of resuscitative fluid required, depth of hypotension, and size of intracranial hemorrhage. Good judgment, close communication, and recognition that the initial plan will change are all required for optimal care of these patients. Indicators of the likely need for a craniotomy include lateralizing neurologic signs (class III data),[10] prehospital intubation, and initial Glasgow Coma Scale score ≤ 8. Consideration should be given to performing simultaneous damage control laparotomy and craniotomy. These patients are at risk for developing life-threatening coagulopathy and hypothermia. Despite reports of its possible benefit in brain-injured patients, hypothermia is a dreaded complication of systemic trauma because it can result in uncontrolled microvascular hemorrhage.

Group 4 patients are critically ill, with persistent hypotension that does not respond to resuscitation. Because these patients are close to death from exsanguination, they should be moved from the ED to the OR within minutes of arrival. During the laparotomy or thoracotomy, the neurosurgeon will determine the need for intracranial pressure monitoring and/or exploratory burr holes. Simultaneous craniotomy and damage control laparotomy may be indicated. This group of patients has a mortality rate of ~50% (Class III data).[11] These patients will almost assuredly develop life-threatening coagulopathy and hypothermia. Small areas of previously nonbleeding cerebral contusion often expand rapidly after coagulopathy develops, resulting in significant morbidity. All efforts should be directed toward keeping the patients as warm as possible and to minimizing the time spent in the OR. These patients may require ICU rewarming and reversal of coagulopathy prior to postoperative CT scanning.

Summary of Recommendations

1. Hemodynamically stable patients with intracranial mass lesions should have their head injury addressed first (class II and level II).
2. Patients who are initially hypotensive but respond to fluid resuscitation and stabilize at a normal blood pressure should undergo CT scanning of the abdomen and head, with the head injury receiving operative priority (class III and level III).
3. Patients with an intracranial mass lesion who are initially hypotensive and respond only transiently to fluid resuscitation should progress directly to the OR (class III and level III). Decision making about laparotomy (or thoracotomy) versus craniotomy requires close communication between the trauma surgeon and neurosurgeon and the flexibility to respond appropriately to changes in the patient's condition. Most of these patients require either immediate laparotomy followed by craniotomy or simultaneous procedures.
4. Patients with a severe head injury whose persistent hypotension does not respond to resuscitation must be moved directly to the OR for a hemorrhage control procedure. These patients require immediate laparotomy or thoracotomy for hemorrhage control, with simultaneous craniotomy (class III and level III).

Conclusions

Fortunately, relatively few patients who need an emergency craniotomy also suffer from intraabdominal bleeding. Only class II or III data are available as a basis for making recommendations. Optimal management of such patients depends on many factors, the two most important being the severity of the initial injuries and the time to CT scanning and operative intervention. The specialties that will be making decisions about surgery should discuss these issues both prior to a patient's arrival and as an ongoing dialogue during a patient's evaluation and treatment.

Author's Note

The opinions expressed herein are the private views of the author and are not to be construed as official or as reflecting the views of the United States Army or the

References

1. Brain Trauma Foundation, American Association of Neurological Surgeons, Joint Section on Neurotrauma and Critical Care. Management and prognosis of severe traumatic brain injury. Hypotension. J Neurotrauma 2000;17: 591–595.
2. Shock. In: American College of Surgeons Committee on Trauma. Advanced Trauma Life Support Course Instructor Manual, 6th ed. Chicago: American College of Surgeons; 1997:109–110.
3. Huang MS, Shih HC, Wu JK, et al. Urgent laparotomy versus emergency craniotomy for multiple trauma with head injury patients. J Trauma 1995;38:154–157.
4. McKenney KL, McKenney MG, Cohn SM, et al. Hemoperitoneum score helps determine need for therapeutic laparotomy. J Trauma 2001;50:650–656.
5. Pachter HL, Knudson MM, Esrig B, et al. Status of nonoperative management of blunt hepatic injuries in 1995: a multicenter experience with 404 patients. J Trauma 1996;40:31–38.
6. Fakhry SM, Brownstein M, Watts DD, et al. Relatively short diagnostic delays (<8 hours) produce morbidity and mortality in blunt small bowel injury: an analysis of time to operative intervention in 198 patients from a multicenter experience. J Trauma 2000;48:408–415.
7. Heckbert SR, Vedder NB, Hoffman W, et al. Outcome after hemorrhagic shock in trauma patients. J Trauma 1998;45:545–549.
8. Franklin GA, Boaz PW, Spain DA, et al. Prehospital hypotension as a valid indicator of trauma team activation. J Trauma 2000;48:1034–1039.
9. Winchell RJ, Hoyt DB, Simons RK. Use of computed tomography of the head in the hypotensive blunt-trauma patient. Ann Emerg Med 1995;25:737–742.
10. Wisner DH, Victor NS, Holcroft JW. Priorities in the management of multiple trauma: intracranial versus intra-abdominal injury. J Trauma 1993;35:271–278.
11. Thomason M, Messick J, Rutledge R, et al. Head CT scanning versus urgent exploration in the hypotensive blunt trauma patient. J Trauma 1993;34:40–45.

◆ 32 ◆

When Should Head-Injured Patients with Long-Bone Fractures Undergo Surgical Treatment of Their Fractures?

Alex B. Valadka

Brief Answer

Surgical fixation of femur and other long bone fractures represents a major advance over earlier management strategies that used traction or plaster casts. Advantages of surgical fixation include improved ambulation and bony healing and fewer systemic complications, especially those affecting pulmonary function. Enthusiasm for prompt surgical treatment of these injuries has led some authors to call for very rapid surgery, sometimes within even a few hours of injury. Although in most cases fixation should probably not be put off for many days, the benefits of surgery performed within a few hours of injury instead of within a few days of injury remain unclear. Evidence both for and against very early surgery consists primarily of class III data. Because of the profound and permanent effects that secondary cerebral insults may have on recovery from brain injury, it seems reasonable to consider delaying fixation of long bone fractures until a brain-injured patient is stable in terms of both systemic and cerebral parameters.

Background

As recently as the middle of the 20th century, patients who sustained femur fractures had a good chance of never returning to gainful employment.[1] These injuries were generally managed by skeletal traction or plaster immobilization, with frequently poor results. Prolonged, forced immobilization in the supine position predisposes patients to the complications of immobility: deep vein thrombosis, pulmonary embolism, decubitus ulcers, generalized deconditioning, atelectasis, pneumonia, etc.[2] Moreover, continued motion of the ends of a fracture causes pain that may contribute to enforced immobility.[1] Persistent soft tissue injury from ongoing motion at the fracture site can also lead to the liberation of multiple inflammatory mediators.[1,2] Fat emboli syndrome was also said to be a frequent occurrence, partly because of entry of fat droplets and tissue thromboplastins into the bloodstream through torn marrow veins that remain open after injury because their walls remain adherent to bone.[3]

The development of effective methods of fracture fixation in the 1940s allowed for immediate anatomic reduction, with reduced pain and increased patient mobility.[1,2] By the late 1970s, the superiority of prompt operative fixation over traditional nonoperative management of femur fractures had become accepted.[1,2,4]

Pearl

As recently as the middle of the 20th century, patients who sustained femur fractures had a good chance of never returning to gainful employment because these injuries were generally managed by skeletal traction or plaster immobilization, with frequently poor results.

In some older studies, "early" surgery was defined as fixation within several weeks of injury. The time period that is considered "early" has become progressively shorter, with some studies extolling the virtues of fixation within 48 or even 24 hours of injury or of hospital admission.[5–7] Reported benefits include improved pulmonary function and shorter hospital and intensive care unit (ICU) stays. The acceptance of the concept of a trauma-activated systemic inflammatory response that may peak several days after injury has likely contributed to the shortening of the interval between injury and fixation because it has been suggested that fixation of fractures is of most benefit if performed early in the inflammatory cascade, perhaps because early fixation may help prevent or minimize the inflammatory response.

At about the same time that prompt fixation of these fractures became established as the preferred method of treatment, the concept of potential secondary brain injury from such insults as hypotension and hypoxia became firmly established. Impairment of cerebral autoregulation after even relatively minor injury may persist for some time after a patient has been stabilized, with a corresponding potential for heightened susceptibility to secondary cerebral insults (class II and class III data).[8–10]

Pearl

Impairment of cerebral autoregulation may persist for quite some time after even minor brain injury.

For these reasons, aggressive resuscitation of patients with traumatic brain injury (TBI) and the need for meticulous monitoring in the ICU to prevent and promptly treat secondary cerebral insults often conflict with plans to take these patients to early surgery for repair of long bone fractures. Confounding this issue further is the fact that different studies of the effects of timing of fracture fixation have used different surgical techniques for fixation and different methods of assessing the effect of timing of surgery. Orthopedic and systemic injuries of different types and severities have often been lumped together, as have injuries to different bones.

This chapter evaluates the published literature in an attempt to formulate a recommendation about the optimal timing of surgical fixation of long bone fractures in TBI patients. All studies cited in this chapter report class III data unless otherwise specified.

Literature Review

Benefits of Early Fixation

In 1977, Riska et al[11] retrospectively reviewed 47 multiply injured patients with at least two long bone fractures that were treated by "early" fixation, defined as fixation within 2 weeks of injury. They concluded that surgery was preferable to conservative treatment.

In a report of a larger series published in 1982, Riska and Myllynen[3] concluded that early surgery is helpful in reducing the frequency of clinical fat embolism syndrome. However, the time period of "early" operation was not specified.

Seibel et al[12] analyzed the effects of early versus delayed internal fixation of femur or acetabular fractures in retrospective analyses of prospectively collected data from 56 severely injured multiple trauma patients (class II data). Patients who underwent immediate surgery (time not specified) were compared with two groups who had surgery either 10 or 30 days after injury. Immediate fixation was more beneficial than delayed surgery in terms of a constellation of findings associated with what the authors call the pulmonary failure-septic state: pulmonary function, white blood cell counts, fevers, positive blood cultures, etc.

Lozman et al[13] prospectively randomized 18 multiply injured patients with tibia or femur fractures to either immediate fixation (time not specified) or conservative treatment with plaster casts or skeletal traction (class II data). During the 4 days of the study period, cardiac index was higher and pulmonary shunt was lower in the immediate fixation group. The frequency of detection of fat macroglobules in pulmonary blood did not differ between groups.

Bone et al[14] prospectively randomized 178 patients with femur fractures to either early (within 24 hours) or late (beyond 48 hours) stabilization of their fractures. The number of patients with severe TBI is not specified but is apparently small. Among patients with isolated femur fractures, late stabilization was associated with a longer and more expensive hospital stay, but pulmonary complications were infrequent in both groups. In multiply injured patients, delayed stabilization was associated with a higher incidence of pulmonary complications [adult respiratory distress syndrome (ARDS), fat embolism, and pneumonia] and with longer and more expensive hospital stays than early stabilization. Statistical significance of the results is not reported. Long-term functional assessments were not performed. The retrospective nature of the data analyses and group assignments makes this a class II study.

Drawbacks of Early Fixation

Some reviews have suggested that early fracture fixation may have some drawbacks. Pape et al[15] reported that intramedullary femoral nailing within 24 hours of trauma in patients with preexisting pulmonary injury was associated with a higher mortality rate (21% versus 4%) and a higher incidence of ARDS (33% versus 7.7%) than delayed nailing, but in patients without pulmonary injury, duration of intubation and ICU stay were lower when early surgery was performed. Along the same lines, Poole et al[1] concluded that the risk of pulmonary complications was not related to the timing of fracture fixation but was strongly related to the severity of head and chest injuries.

Fakhry et al[16] reviewed 2805 patients with femoral shaft fractures in a statewide hospital discharge database. Although the mortality rate was higher for the 31% of patients treated nonsurgically, reasons for the choice of nonoperative management were not specified and may reflect overall worse prognoses in these patients. Among the more severely injured patients (Injury Severity Scale scores ≥15), surgery between 2 and 4 days was associated with the lowest mortality rates and shortest hospitalizations. A trend toward higher mortality and longer hospitalizations was seen when these patients underwent surgery within 1 day. The authors suggested that further study and individualized management were warranted in the more severely injured patients.

Early Fixation in Traumatic Brain Injury Patients

Benefits

Many reports that attempt to demonstrate the benefits (or lack of harm) of early fracture fixation in TBI patients suffer from major methodologic flaws.[17–20] For example, these reports are often based on retrospective reviews of patient charts or hospital trauma registries. In many of these studies, severity of head injury is assessed not on a functional scale like the Glasgow Coma Scale (GCS), but rather on an anatomic scale like the Abbreviated Injury Scale. These studies often include a large number of patients with mild TBI who might be more physiologically capable of undergoing major orthopedic surgery and who might also be able to "conceal" any subtle but still important deficits suffered as a result of surgery. Another common weakness of these retrospective studies is that long-term functional outcomes—both neurologic and orthopedic—are not determined at standardized time points (if even reported at all); instead, GCS scores at discharge are reported, perhaps because such information is often the only data available to the retrospective reviewer. An important drawback to the use of GCS scores as an outcome tool is that patients who are severely disabled or even vegetative (who would be regarded as having unfavorable outcomes by most investigators) can have relatively high GCS scores. Furthermore, the number of days postinjury at which patients are discharged can vary widely, as can their neurologic status at hospital discharge. Thus, use of time of hospital discharge as a standard reference point is not nearly as valid as use of a fixed number of weeks or months after injury.

Pearl

Many reports that describe either benefits or risks of early fracture fixation in TBI patients suffer from major methodologic flaws, including retrospective design, suboptimal methods of assessing the presence and severity of brain injury, consolidation of different severities of injury, and inadequate methods and timing of outcome assessment.

McKee et al[21] performed a retrospective case-control study comparing 46 multiply injured TBI patients with femur fractures to 99 matched multiply injured TBI patients without femur fractures (class II data). Most of the fracture patients underwent reamed femoral intramedullary nailing within 24 hours of injury. Neuropsychological assessment consisting of the Category, Trails A, and Trails B tests was performed in 10 study patients and 24 control patients, or roughly a third of the surviving patients in each group. Overall, no significant differences were found between the groups. Three patients in the fracture group had significant postoperative neurologic complications, two of which were fatal. These included cerebral infarction, intracerebral hemorrhage from coagulopathy secondary to massive transfusions, and internal carotid artery dissection with cerebral infarction.

Drawbacks

The deleterious effects of secondary insults like hypotension and hypoxia on outcome from TBI have been well documented.[22] Pietropaoli et al[23] described the frequent occurrence and devastating effects on long-term neurologic outcome of intraoperative hypotension in severe TBI patients who required any type of surgical intervention within 72 hours of injury. Such reports indicate that, if early surgical fixation of long bone fractures is to be performed in severe TBI patients, its benefits must outweigh the high risk of permanent neurologic harm from intraoperative secondary insults.

Several published studies have concluded that early fixation of long bone fractures may be harmful in head-injured patients, but these studies suffer from many of the same drawbacks as those that attempt to justify early fixation in these patients. Jaicks et al[24] compared 19 TBI patients who underwent fixation within 24 hours of injury to 14 similar patients who underwent surgery beyond 24 hours. The early group received more intraoperative crystalloid and tended to have more intraoperative hypotension and hypoxia, more units of blood transfused, and a lower average discharge GCS score.

Townsend et al[25] analyzed 61 patients with femur fractures and severe TBI (GCS score <9). Those who underwent operative fixation of their fractures within 2 hours of hospital admission were eight times more likely to become hypotensive (systolic blood pressure ≤90 mmHg) during femur repair than patients undergoing fixation more than 24 hours after admission. Overall, operation within 24 hours had twice the rate of intraoperative hypotension as surgery after 24 hours. However, some of the data presentation in this article seems incorrect; for example, the mean time to surgery for the 24- to 244-hour group is listed as 17.4 hours.

Townsend et al[25] also reported the frequent occurrence of elevation of intracranial pressure (ICP) above 20 mmHg in their patients who received such monitoring. Anglen et al[26] also found that ICP, mean arterial pressure, and cerebral perfusion pressure commonly changed in potentially deleterious directions during reamed intramedullary nailing of femur fractures in severe TBI patients. Although not explicitly stated, the timing of fracture fixation in that report seemed to be at least several days after injury, raising the question of whether earlier surgery would have been associated with even greater adverse effects on cerebral hemodynamics.

Other Approaches

Other approaches to femur fractures besides the extremes of "early" or "delayed" internal fixation are possible. In multiply injured patients with femur fractures, external fixation of the fracture may be used as a temporary means of rigid stabilization until intramedullary nailing can be performed after the patient stabilizes.[15,27] Treatment may also be individualized for each patient. Rogers et al[28] suggested that fixation of femur fractures 24 to 72 hours after injury was no more deleterious than fixation within 24 hours, indicating that a reasonable delay to ensure that patients have been adequately stabilized and resuscitated does not cause harm. A similar conclusion was reached by Reynolds et al.[2]

Pearl

One possible approach is to use external fixation of a fracture as a temporary means of rigid stabilization until intramedullary nailing can be performed after the patient stabilizes.

Conclusions

Almost all studies of this issue have been retrospective and consequently suffer from many inconsistencies that hamper comparisons. These differences include definition of head injury, for example, based on GCS score versus computed tomography (CT) appearance; use of intraoperative cerebral monitoring; and the definitions of "early" and "late" surgery. Outcome assessments generally focus on such measures as worsening of CT scan appearance, length of stay in the hospital or ICU, development of pneumonia, etc. Long-term neurologic, neuropsychological, and ambulatory outcomes are reported only rarely. Reasons why some patients undergo delayed fixation of their fractures are often not specified, even though such information may be vital for assessing the comparability of groups.

The fact that long-term ambulatory function is almost never reported is curious. Presumably, the modern practice of surgical fixation of these fractures at some time point, as opposed to treating them nonsurgically, results in a very high rate of restoration of normal or near-normal ambulation. The original debate about whether surgery was appropriate has evolved into discussions about how quickly one should rush into such surgery and about the ramifications for pulmonary and neurologic function, but generally not for orthopedic function.

Despite these limitations, several principles seem apparent. Patients who are not adequately resuscitated should not undergo any operations that can be safely postponed; patients who are otherwise stable appear to benefit if long bone fractures are treated with early surgery; and secondary cerebral insults must be avoided in brain-injured patients for at least several days after injury and possibly longer.

In 2001, the Eastern Association for the Surgery of Trauma published guidelines for the optimal timing of stabilization of long bone fractures in multiply injured patients.[29] The authors offered a level II recommendation that polytrauma patients should generally undergo stabilization of long bone fractures within 48 hours because some patients may have fewer complications (even though mortality rate is not improved) and because stabilization within that time window does not appear to cause harm. However, in brain-injured patients, a level II recommendation stated that early fixation neither improved nor worsened outcome and that timing of fracture fixation should be individualized for each patient. Recommendations for patients with chest injuries were the same as those for patients with brain injury.

Recommendation

Level III: Surgical fixation of long bone fractures in brain-injured patients may be safely delayed for several days to ensure that patients have been adequately resuscitated and stabilized. Such a delay does not appear to worsen systemic or orthopedic outcomes, but it may prevent potentially catastrophic secondary insults to the injured brain.

References

1. Poole GV, Miller JD, Agnew SG, et al. Lower extremity fracture fixation in head-injured patients. J Trauma 1992;32:654–659.
2. Reynolds MA, Richardson JD, Spain DA, et al. Is the timing of fracture fixation important for the patient with multiple trauma? Ann Surg 1995;222:470–478.
3. Riska EB, Myllynen P. Fat embolism in patients with multiple injuries. J Trauma 1982;22:891–894.
4. Garland DE, Rothi B, Waters RL. Femoral fractures in head-injured adults. Clin Orthop 1982;166:219–225.
5. Behrman SW, Fabian TC, Kudsk KA, et al. Improved outcome with femur fractures: early vs. delayed fixation. J Trauma 1990;30:792–797.
6. Johnson KD, Cadambi A, Seibert GB. Incidence of adult respiratory distress syndrome in patients with multiple musculoskeletal injuries: effect of early operative stabilization of fractures. J Trauma 1985;25:375–384.
7. Charash WE, Fabian TC, Croce MA. Delayed surgical fixation of femur fractures is a risk factor for pulmonary failure independent of thoracic trauma. J Trauma 1994;37:667–672.
8. Junger EC, Newell DW, Grant GA, et al. Cerebral autoregulation following minor head injury. J Neurosurg 1997;86: 425–432.
9. Strebel S, Lam AM, Matta BF, et al. Impaired cerebral autoregulation after mild brain injury. Surg Neurol 1997;47:128–131.
10. Hlatky R, Furuya Y, Valadka AB, et al. Dynamic autoregulatory response after severe head injury. J Neurosurg 2002;97: 1054–1061.
11. Riska EB, von Bonsdorff H, Hakkinen S, et al. Primary operative fixation of long bone fractures in patients with multiple injuries. J Trauma 1977;17:111–121.
12. Seibel R, LaDuca J, Hassett JM, et al. Blunt multiple trauma (ISS 36), femur traction, and the pulmonary failure-septic state. Ann Surg 1985;202:283–295.
13. Lozman J, Deno DC, Feustel PJ, et al. Pulmonary and cardiovascular consequences of immediate fixation or conservative management of long-bone fractures. Arch Surg 1986;121:992–999.
14. Bone LB, Johnson KD, Weigelt J, et al. Early versus delayed stabilization of femoral fractures: a prospective randomized study. J Bone Joint Surg Am 1989;71:336–340.
15. Pape HC, Auf'm'Kolk M, Paffrath T, et al. Primary intramedullary femur fixation in multiple trauma patients with associated lung contusion: a cause of posttraumatic ARDS? J Trauma 1993;34:540–547.
16. Fakhry SM, Rutledge R, Dahners LE, et al. Incidence, management, and outcome of femoral shaft fracture: a statewide population-based analysis of 2805 adult patients in a rural state. J Trauma 1994;37:255–260.
17. Brundage SI, McGhan R, Jurkovich GJ, et al. Timing of femur fracture fixation: effect on outcome in patients with thoracic and head injuries. J Trauma 2002;52:299–307.
18. Malisano LP, Stevens D, Hunter GA. The management of long bone fractures in the head-injured polytrauma patient. J Orthop Trauma 1994;8:1–5.
19. Scalea TM, Scott JD, Brumback RJ, et al. Early fracture fixation may be "just fine" after head injury: no difference in central nervous system outcomes. J Trauma 1999;46:839–846.
20. Starr AJ, Hunt JL, Chason DP, et al. Treatment of femur fracture with associated head injury. J Orthop Trauma 1998;12: 38–45.
21. McKee MD, Schemitsch EH, Vincent LO, et al. The effect of a femoral fracture on concomitant closed head injury in patients with multiple injuries. J Trauma 1997;42:1041–1045.
22. Chesnut RM, Marshall LF, Klauber MR, et al. The role of secondary brain injury in determining outcome from severe head injury. J Trauma 1993;34:216–222.
23. Pietropaoli JA, Rogers FB, Shackford SR, et al. The deleterious effects of intraoperative hypotension on outcome in patients with severe head injuries. J Trauma 1992;33:403–407.
24. Jaicks RR, Cohn SM, Moller BA. Early fracture fixation may be deleterious after head injury. J Trauma 1997;42:1–5.
25. Townsend RN, Lheureau T, Protech J, et al. Timing fracture repair in patients with severe brain injury (Glasgow Coma Scale score <9). J Trauma 1998;44:977–982.
26. Anglen JO, Luber K, Park T. The effect of femoral nailing on cerebral perfusion pressure in head-injured patients. J Trauma 2003;54:1166–1170.
27. Scalea TM, Boswell SA, Scott JD, et al. External fixation as a bridge to intramedullary nailing for patients with multiple injuries and with femur fractures: damage control orthopedics. J Trauma 2000;48:613–621.
28. Rogers FB, Shackford SR, Vane DW, et al. Prompt fixation of isolated femur fractures in a rural trauma center: a study examining the timing of fixation and resource allocation. J Trauma 1994;36:774–777.
29. Dunham CM, Bosse MJ, Clancy TV, et al. Practice management guidelines for the optimal timing of long-bone fracture stabilization in polytrauma patients: the EAST Practice Management Guidelines Work Group. J Trauma 2001;50:958–967.

♦ 33 ♦

When Should I Suspect Child Abuse in Head-Injured Children?

Ann-Christine Duhaime

Brief Answer

Child abuse, or inflicted injury, may be suspected if several characteristic features are present. Most patients are less than 3 years of age, with the majority in the first year of life. The caregiver may deny any history of trauma in the child or may report only minimal trauma, such as a fall from a short height. Although inflicted injuries have been reported in all socioeconomic groups, most series report an association with such factors as unstable family situation, young parental age, low socioeconomic status, and preexisting medical problems of the child, such as prematurity. The most common perpetrators are fathers and the mother's boyfriend. These children often present with lethargy, seizures, breathing difficulties, unresponsiveness, and similar signs and symptoms that belie the mildness of the history that is given. Computed tomography (CT) scanning may reveal subdural hematoma, subarachnoid hemorrhage, patchy hypodensity, and/or unilateral or bilateral diffuse brain swelling. Extracerebral injuries, especially of different time periods, are often present. Retinal hemorrhages are strongly suggestive of inflicted injury, but they are not pathognomonic.

Background

Inflicted head injury is the most common cause of trauma-related death during infancy. It results in at least 1000 deaths/year in the United States, more than the annual mortality of all pediatric brain tumors combined.[1,2] Furthermore, it has been theorized that the number of fatalities is far exceeded by the number of children who are permanently injured or disabled by this type of trauma (class III data).[3] The risk that a child will sustain a nonaccidental injury during the first year of life has been estimated to be one in 4065, or 0.025% (class III data).[4] Countless families are affected in profound ways by proven or suspected nonaccidental injury. Both false-negative and false-positive diagnoses can have disastrous consequences. Often, the diagnosis rests on the word of the neurosurgeon, and because of its uncertainty and potential implications, many clinicians approach this subject with reluctance.

An evidence-based approach to the diagnosis, management, and outcome of inflicted head injuries in infancy is problematic. Child abuse is by nature cloaked in guesswork and judgment because the facts on which the clinician generally relies for an accurate evaluation of a problem are usually missing. Also, in these cases, the patients cannot speak for themselves. Thus, the diagnosis must be made by inference. Management options and prognostic guidelines are similarly lacking in firm data on which to base decisions.

Despite these difficulties, some data are available to help guide the clinician, and ongoing efforts to collect more solid data may add to the degree of certainty with which opinions are rendered and decisions made. This chapter reviews some of the available studies that are relevant to making the diagnosis of inflicted injury in infants.

Literature Review

Evidence that aids in the diagnosis of an injury comes from several sources. First are case series of patients in whom the determination has been made in some manner that inflicted injury has occurred. These series provide profiles of typical presentations of patients with this type of injury. Second are series of patients with known accidental trauma. Such series provide a data set of the types of injuries that typically occur from known mechanisms, and such mechanisms may be described in cases that raise suspicion for nonaccidental injury. Third, animal experiments have attempted to model various injury types to characterize injuries resulting from various mechanisms. Fourth, anthropomorphic modeling uses surrogates to answer similar questions. More recently, mathematical modeling has attempted to combine some of these data sets to predict the specific injuries that might be expected from a given mechanism.

Case Series: Nonaccidental Injuries

Almost all series of this type are retrospective, and the vast majority suffer to a greater or lesser degree from poorly defined inclusion criteria for the diagnosis of abuse (class III data).[3,5–7] Thus, most of this information falls into the category of class III data and must be viewed accordingly. Nonetheless, certain common characteristics can be found in most descriptions of inflicted injury, as outlined below.

Patient Characteristics

The vast majority of patients with inflicted head injuries of infancy and early childhood are under 3 years of age, with most being under 1 year (class III data).[2,8,9] In series of children under 2 years of age, 24 to 32% of patients admitted because of head injury have inflicted injuries (class II and class III data).[8,10]

History and Presentation

The most commonly provided histories for patients with inflicted head injuries describe a fall from a short height or no history of trauma at all. Commonly described symptoms include lethargy, irritability, vomiting, seizure, breathing difficulty, or unresponsiveness (class III data).[6,7,11] One half of the patients in one series exhibited impairment of mental status at presentation (class III data).[11] Seizures have been reported in 40 to 71% of patients, and apnea in ~50% (class III data).[6,12]

Intracranial Injury Characteristics

Classic intracranial findings associated with inflicted head injury in infancy include acute subdural hemorrhage with or without unilateral or bilateral diffuse brain swelling. The hemorrhage may be thin and may be located over one or both cerebral convexities and may also occur in the posterior interhemispheric space. Larger acute subdural hemorrhages that require surgical evacuation are sometimes seen, particularly in older children. Subarachnoid blood and diffuse axonal injury have also been reported. One of the striking features of this syndrome is the association of holohemispheric or bilateral supratentorial loss of gray-white differentiation with brain swelling, which is seen in the most severely affected patients. During the acute phase, CT scanning may reveal a "reversal sign"; that is, a diffuse decrease in density of cortical gray and white matter with attenuation of the gray/white interface, or reversal of the usual gray/white densities and relative increase in density of the thalami, brainstem, and cerebellum (class III data).[13] In survivors, this radiologic picture may progress to one of profound atrophy. In other children, CT scans may show patchy areas of hypodensity that have the appearance of infarcts or other types of pathophysiologic perfusion/metabolic mismatch (class III data),[13–18] an assumption that is supported by the results of neuropathological studies.[19] It should be noted that these findings are suggestive of, but not absolutely specific for, inflicted injuries.

> **Pearl**
>
> The most commonly provided histories for patients with inflicted injuries deny any history of trauma or describe a fall from only a short height.

> **Pearl**
>
> The classic intracranial findings of inflicted head injury in infancy include acute subdural hemorrhage with or without brain swelling. On CT scanning, the densities of cortical gray and white matter may be reversed or decreased, making the brainstem, thalami, and cerebellum seem more prominent.

Chronic subdural hematomas have also been associated with inflicted injuries in infancy (class III data).[20] However, this pattern is less typical, and its association with a mechanism of inflicted injury rests largely on the presence of additional associated findings suggestive of nonaccidental trauma (class II data).[21]

Associated Findings

Although skull fractures, scalp swelling, subgaleal hemorrhages, and other signs of head impact are reported in variable percentages of infants with nonaccidental injuries, such signs are generally present in the majority of patients. Skull fractures are seen most often in the occipital and/or parietal regions (class III data).[7,11] Skeletal surveys and/or bone scans reveal that 30 to 70% of patients sustained extracranial bony injuries, including rib fractures and metaphyseal fractures (class III data).[15,22,23] Other injuries commonly associated with physical abuse include frenulum tears and pattern bruising or pattern burns, that is, bruises or burns that occur in a pattern suggesting that they may have been caused by identifiable objects.

Retinal hemorrhages have been reported in an average of 75% of patients with inflicted injuries. Their severity may range from severe and bilateral to relatively sparse. Folds, detachments, and other retinal pathology may be seen (class III data).[24,25] Retinal hemorrhages have been reported in accidental trauma, but except in the setting of severe head injury, these tend to be less profuse and are often unilateral (class III data).[26]

Pearl

Retinal hemorrhages are seen in most, but not all, patients with inflicted injury. They have been reported to occur after accidental trauma, but in such cases the hemorrhage tends to be less severe and is often unilateral.

Injuries of the cervicomedullary junction and upper cervical spine have been reported at autopsy (class III data).[27,28] Such injuries are rarely detected by magnetic resonance imaging (MRI) prior to death or in survivors. It has been suggested that injury at this location may play a role in contributing to such symptoms as apnea and resultant cerebral hypoxic-ischemic changes, but this hypothesis has not yet been investigated fully (class III data).[18,19]

Social Factors

Although inflicted injuries have been reported in all socioeconomic groups, most series report an association with such factors as unstable family situation, young parental age, low socioeconomic status, and preexisting medical problems of the child, such as prematurity (class III data).[29,30] Perpetrators are most likely to be fathers, followed by mothers' boyfriends, female baby-sitters, and mothers, in descending order (class III data).[31]

Case Series: Known Accidental Injuries

The most commonly considered alternative diagnosis in a child suspected of having an inflicted injury is accidental injury. Analyses of cases of known accidental injury may help to elucidate the relationship between specific mechanisms of trauma and the types of injury that they produce in infants and young children.

Several series have concluded that, with the exception of epidural hematoma, head-injury-related death or major neurologic injury after a short-distance fall is extremely rare (class III data).[32–37] Even falls from greater heights are often tolerated reasonably well (class II and class III data).[38–40] For this reason, fatal or near-fatal injuries (other than epidural hematomas in young children) that are reported to result from falls from a low height (<3–4 feet) are usually considered to be suspicious for inflicted injury. This is particularly true when subdural hematoma is present.

Pearl

Other than epidural hematomas in young children, fatal or near-fatal injuries that are claimed to result from falls from a low height are usually considered to be suspicious for inflicted injury, especially when a subdural hematoma is present.

Some case series have attempted to address the question of how quickly symptoms develop in the setting of head injuries resulting in death. One such series demonstrated that, with the exception of epidural hematoma, essentially all children with fatal head injuries had immediate onset of symptoms at the time of injury (class III data).[41] Other series analyzing particular injury types have shown that most subdural hematomas result from vehicular trauma, falls from significant heights, or abuse (class II data).[10,21] In contrast, epidural hematomas are much more likely to be caused by accidental mechanisms that are often relatively minor (class III data).[42,43] Skull fractures can occur from both accidental and nonaccidental mechanisms. Small focal extraaxial hemorrhages, often in association with skull fractures, may be seen on CT in infants who appear to be doing well after falls from low heights, but they are usually clinically insignificant (class II and class III data).[44,45]

Pearl

Because symptoms develop immediately after a severe brain injury, stories that describe a delay between injury and development of symptoms should be viewed suspiciously. Exceptions to this principle may occur when epidural hematomas are present.

Experimental Data

Several experimental approaches have been used to investigate the mechanisms that cause particular types of injuries. All of these approaches have some limitations regarding their applicability to trauma in human infants and young children. Studies in skulls from cadavers and immature animals have attempted to determine fracture tolerances of the skull.[46,47] The results indicate that the skull varies in its fracture tolerance and that the site of impact cannot be extrapolated from the fracture location. In addition, the immature skull is much more deformable than the adult skull, and more extensive inbending during impact can lead to more brain distortion in children than in adults.[47]

Primate and porcine models have been used to evaluate the input variables responsible for diffuse axonal injury and subdural hemorrhage caused by bridging vein rupture.[48–50] Such studies have shown that both of these types of injury are caused by angular acceleration of the head, but differences in direction and in duration and rate of acceleration strongly influence the predominant type of resultant pathology. In general, diffuse axonal injury is most often associated with vehicular trauma, whereas subdural hemorrhage in adults is also associated with nonvehicular trauma, especially significant falls.[48] Studies on brain tissue from neonatal swine have shown that the immature brain is stiffer than the more mature brain and is more resistant to deformation, properties that are likely related to higher water content.[51]

Anthropomorphic Modeling

Anthropomorphic modeling uses surrogates to reproduce injury mechanisms and provide input variables for mathematical models that can incorporate tissue injury thresholds. However, such studies are limited by issues of biofidelity, particularly with respect to infant neck characteristics. Studies using this methodology have shown that short-height falls are associated with forces below the threshold for primate or porcine primary brain injury, whereas falls from greater heights and onto harder surfaces can be predicted to have the potential to cause injury. Shaking produces relatively low angular decelerations that are well below values for injury thresholds. On the other hand, inflicted impacts produce significant forces that are well into threshold ranges for concussion, subdural hematoma, and diffuse axonal injury (class III data).[7,52]

Pearl

Most inflicted head injuries appear to be caused not by shaking alone, but rather by head impact.

No experimental data are presently available to answer important questions regarding repeated injuries, cervical injury thresholds in infants, or forces and other conditions necessary to cause the marked brain swelling sometimes associated with acute subdural hemorrhage in infancy.

Algorithms and Other Diagnostic Schemes

Using the data above, some authors have attempted to create diagnostic schemes by which a particular injury can be determined to be most likely inflicted, suspicious, or accidental. None of these schemes is fully validated, although some have been tested against standard methods of determination, such as the consensus of a child abuse evaluation team. They include both algorithms and lists of criteria.[10,21]

Summary

Inflicted head injury is at present a puzzle in which various pieces have become available, whereas others are still missing. In the era of evidence-based medicine, increasing attention will be paid to collecting data that are relevant to the evaluation and management of this unfortunately all-too-common problem. In the meantime, clinicians have available a reasonable database (consisting mostly of class III evidence) from which to draw conclusions. Although some of these conclusions may be quite definite, others, at present, should be tempered by acknowledgment of their limitations.

References

1. United States Department of Health and Human Services. National Center on Child Abuse and Neglect and Child Maltreatment 1993: Reports from the States to the National Center on Child Abuse and Neglect. Washington, DC: U.S. Government Printing Office, 1995.
2. Reece RM, Sege R. Childhood head injuries: accidental or inflicted? Arch Pediatr Adolesc Med 2000;154:11–15.
3. Caffey J. On the theory and practice of shaking infants: its potential residual effects of permanent brain damage and mental retardation. Am J Dis Child 1972;124:161–169.
4. Barlow KM, Minns RA. Annual incidence of shaken impact syndrome in young children. Lancet 2000;356:1571–1572.
5. Kempe CH, Silverman FN, Steele BF, et al. The battered-child syndrome. JAMA 1962;181:17–24.
6. Ludwig S, Warman M. Shaken baby syndrome: a review of 20 cases. Ann Emerg Med 1984;13:104–107.
7. Duhaime AC, Gennarelli TA, Thibault LE, et al. The shaken baby syndrome: a clinical, pathological, and biomechanical study. J Neurosurg 1987;66:409–415.
8. Dashti SR, Decker DD, Razzaq A, et al. Current patterns of inflicted head injury in children. Pediatr Neurosurg 1999;31: 302–306.
9. Barlow KM, Milne S, Aitken K, et al. A retrospective epidemiological analysis of non-accidental head injury in children in Scotland over a 15 year period. Scott Med J 1998;43:112–114.
10. Duhaime AC, Alario AJ, Lewander WJ, et al. Head injury in very young children: mechanisms, injury types, and ophthalmologic findings in 100 hospitalized patients younger than 2 years of age. Pediatrics 1992;90:179–185.

11. Hahn YS, Raimondi AJ, McLone DG, et al. Traumatic mechanisms of head injury in child abuse. Childs Brain 1983;10:229–241.
12. Johnson DL, Boal D, Baule R. Role of apnea in nonaccidental head injury. Pediatr Neurosurg 1995;23:305–310.
13. Han BK, Towbin RB, Courten-Myers GD, et al. Reversal sign on CT: effect of anoxic/ischemic cerebral injury in children. AJNR Am J Neuroradiol 1989;10:1191–1198.
14. Zimmerman RA, Bilaniuk LT, Bruce D, et al. Interhemispheric acute subdural hematoma: a computed tomographic manifestation of child abuse by shaking. Neuroradiology 1978;16:39–40.
15. Merten DF, Osborne DRS, Radkowski MA, et al. Craniocerebral trauma in the child abuse syndrome: radiologic observations. Pediatr Radiol 1984;14:272–277.
16. Dias MS, Backstrom J, Falk M, et al. Serial radiography in the infant shaken impact syndrome. Pediatr Neurosurg 1998;29:77–85.
17. Gilles EE, Nelson MD Jr. Cerebral complications of nonaccidental head injury in childhood. Pediatr Neurol 1998;19:119–128.
18. Duhaime AC, Christian CW, Rorke LB, et al. Nonaccidental head injury in infants—the "shaken-baby" syndrome. N Engl J Med 1998;338:1822–1829.
19. Geddes JF, Hackshaw AK, Vowles GH, et al. Neuropathology of inflicted head injury in children, I: Patterns of brain damage. Brain 2001;124:1290–1298.
20. Parent AD. Pediatric chronic subdural hematoma: a retrospective comparative analysis. Pediatr Neurosurg 1992;18:266–271.
21. Feldman KW, Bethel R, Shugerman RP, et al. The cause of infant and toddler subdural hemorrhage: a prospective study. Pediatrics 2001;108:636–646.
22. Lazoritz S, Baldwin S, Kini N. The whiplash shaken infant syndrome: has Caffey's syndrome changed or have we changed his syndrome? Child Abuse Negl 1997;21:1009–1014.
23. Kleinman PK. Diagnostic imaging in infant abuse. AJR Am J Roentengol 1990;155:703–712.
24. Greenwald MJ, Weiss A, Oesterle CS, et al. Traumatic retinoschisis in battered babies. Ophthalmology 1986;93:618–625.
25. Massicotte SJ, Folberg R, Torczynski E, et al. Vitreoretinal traction and perimacular retinal folds in the eyes of deliberately traumatized children. Ophthalmology 1991;98:1124–1127.
26. Christian CW, Taylor AA, Hertle RW, et al. Retinal hemorrhages caused by accidental household trauma. J Pediatr 1999;135:125–127.
27. Hadley MN, Sonntag VK, Rekate HL, et al. The infant whiplash-shake injury syndrome: a clinical and pathological study. Neurosurgery 1989;24:536–540.
28. Feldman KW, Weinberger E, Milstein JM, et al. Cervical spine MRI in abused infants. Child Abuse Negl 1997;21:199–205.
29. Klein M, Stern L. Low birth weight and the battered child syndrome. Am J Dis Child 1971;122:15–18.
30. Sills JA, Thomas LJ, Rosenbloom L. Non-accidental injury: a two-year study in central Liverpool. Dev Med Child Neurol 1977;19:26–33.
31. Starling SP, Holden JR, Jenny C. Abusive head trauma: the relationship of perpetrators to their victims. Pediatrics 1995;95:259–262.
32. Nimityongskul P, Anderson LD. The likelihood of injuries when children fall out of bed. J Pediatr Orthop 1987;7:184–186.
33. Tarantino CA, Dowd MD, Murdock TC. Short vertical falls in infants. Pediatr Emerg Care 1999;15:5–8.
34. Helfer RE, Slovis TL, Black M. Injuries resulting when small children fall out of bed. Pediatrics 1977;60:533–535.
35. Greenes DS, Schutzman SA. Infants with isolated skull fracture: what are their clinical characteristics, and do they require hospitalization? Ann Emerg Med 1997;30:253–259.
36. Reiber GD. Fatal falls in childhood: how far must children fall to sustain fatal head injury? Report of cases and review of the literature. Am J Forensic Med Pathol 1993;14:201–207.
37. Plunkett J. Fatal pediatric head injuries caused by short-distance falls. Am J Forensic Med Pathol 2001;22:1–12.
38. Musemeche CA, Barthel M, Cosentino C, et al. Pediatric falls from heights. J Trauma 1991;31:1347–1349.
39. Chiaviello CT, Christoph RA, Bond GR. Stairway-related injuries in children. Pediatrics 1994;94:679–681.
40. Albanese CT, Gardner MJ, Adkins MA, et al. Single rope tree swing injuries among children. Pediatrics 1997;99:548–550.
41. Willman KY, Bank DE, Senac M, et al. Restricting the time of injury in fatal inflicted head injuries. Child Abuse Negl 1997;21:929–940.
42. Shugerman RP, Paez A, Grossman DC, et al. Epidural hemorrhage: is it abuse? Pediatrics 1996;97:664–668.
43. Schutzman SA, Barnes PD, Mantello M, et al. Epidural hematomas in children. Ann Emerg Med 1993;22:535–541.
44. Greenes DS, Schutzman SA. Clinical indicators of intracranial injury in head-injured infants. Pediatrics 1999;104:861–867.
45. Greenes DS, Schutzman SA. Occult intracranial injury in infants. Ann Emerg Med 1998;32:680–686.
46. Yoganandan N, Pintar FA, Sances A Jr, et al. Biomechanics of skull fracture. J Neurotrauma 1995;12:659–668.
47. Margulies SS, Thibault KL. Infant skull and suture properties: measurements and implications for mechanisms of pediatric brain injury. J Biomech Eng 2000;122:364–371.
48. Gennarelli TA. Head injury in man and experimental animals: clinical aspects. Acta Neurochir Suppl (Wien) 1983;32:1–13.
49. Gennarelli TA. Animate models of human head injury. J Neurotrauma 1994;11:357–368.
50. Smith DH, Chen XH, Xu BN, et al. Characterization of diffuse axonal pathology and selective hippocampal damage following inertial brain trauma in the pig. J Neuropathol Exp Neurol 1997;56:822–834.
51. Thibault KL, Margulies S. Age-dependent material properties of the porcine cerebrum: effect on pediatric inertial head injury criteria. J Biomech 1998;31:1119–1126.
52. Prange MT, Coats B, Duhaime AC, et al. Anthropomorphic simulations of falls, shakes, and inflicted impacts in infants. J Neurosurg 2003;99:143–150.

◆ 34 ◆

Can I Say "No" If a Family Wants to Support a Vegetative Patient Indefinitely?

John M. Luce

Brief Answer

Most American courts allow surrogate decision makers to withdraw or withhold treatment for certain incompetent patients. However, the exact circumstances under which such actions are permitted may vary in different courts. When surrogate decision makers and physicians disagree about continuing therapy in apparently futile cases, courts have almost always ordered continuation of treatment. At the same time, however, courts have been reluctant to punish physicians who refused treatment when the decision seemed reasonable. Despite such cases, unilateral action by physicians is discouraged for at least two reasons. First, there exists the potential for legal action (which is burdensome even if successfully defended). Second, and more important, such actions conflict with the basic ethical principle of autonomy, even if incompetent patients must exercise that principle through surrogates. Fortunately, almost all disputes can be resolved through negotiation.

Because no clinical trials are possible in this area, designations of levels of evidence and strengths of recommendations are not used in this chapter.

Background

Patients with head injury may become severely disabled, vegetative, or brain dead. Because considerable data are available about the outcomes of such patients, neurosurgeons and other physicians who care for them are in an excellent position to provide prognostic information to family members and other surrogates who may have to make medical decisions for patients when they are incompetent; that is, unable to make decisions for themselves.[1] In the case of patients who are severely disabled, vegetative, or brain dead, physicians may accompany the prognostic information they provide with recommendations to withhold or withdraw life-sustaining therapy. Alternatively, families may request from physicians that life support be withdrawn before recommendations are made.

A study we conducted in the medical-surgical intensive care unit (ICU) at San Francisco General Hospital demonstrated that the families of 22 out of 24 patients who were severely disabled, vegetative, or brain dead concurred with the prognoses of neurosurgeons and agreed with their recommendations to withhold or withdraw treatment.[2] In some cases, the patients were dependent on mechanical ventilation and died shortly after their ventilators were removed either in the ICU or in the operating room (the latter involved brain dead patients who were organ donors). In other cases, the patients were not ventilator-dependent and died after transfer from the ICU to the neurosurgery ward nearby, where they were not given antibiotics or other medications.

Although the majority of patients with poor prognoses had life support withheld or withdrawn in this study, the families of two patients, both of whom were vegetative, insisted that treatment be continued in the ICU, on the ward, and in chronic care facilities. Both families disagreed with the neurosurgeons' opinions that the patients would not regain cortical function. They expressed a belief in miracles and stated that the patients would have asked for continued support if they were able to do so. At the same time, the physicians felt that further treatment could not restore the patients to a sentient existence and was wasteful of health care resources. They were tempted to refuse further treatment on the grounds of medical futility.

The infrequent physician–family conflicts documented in this study from San Francisco General Hospital occur from time to time in other hospitals in the United States, although they have not been formally described. They raise an important question: Can neurosurgeons and other physicians say "no" to families that want to support vegetative patients indefinitely? This chapter addresses this question while reviewing American biomedical ethics and law.

Ethical and Legal Considerations

In the United States, the primary legal justification for withholding and withdrawal of life support is found in the principles of informed consent and informed refusal. Both principles have strong roots in the common law, which reflects the American regard for self-determination as expressed in the ethical concept of autonomy. These principles hold that treatment may not be initiated without the approval of patients or their surrogates except in emergency situations and also that patients or surrogates may refuse any or all therapies. Currently, all American courts recognize a competent adult's right to refuse life-sustaining treatment, although the constitutional, statutory, and common-law bases of the right may vary from jurisdiction to jurisdiction. Most of the cases concerning that right have arisen, however, from situations involving incompetent patients.[3]

Pearl

All American courts recognize a competent adult's right to refuse life-sustaining treatment. Application of this principle to incompetent critically ill patients began in the *Quinlan* case.

The application of the principles of informed consent and informed refusal to the care of incompetent critically ill patients began in the *Quinlan* case.[4] In this case, the Supreme Court of New Jersey held that a patient had the right to refuse mechanical ventilation, and that because she was vegetative and could not exercise that right directly, her parents could act as surrogates and make a "substituted judgment" for her. The California Court of Appeal took a similar approach in the *Barber* case,[5] in which it held that physicians charged with murder had not committed an unlawful act when, with permission from a patient's family, they removed nutrition and hydration from a comatose patient. In *Barber*, the court approved of the principle of substituted judgment, as advanced in *Quinlan*. It also noted that medical interventions ranging from mechanical ventilation to nutrition and hydration should not be distinguished by terms such as "extraordinary" and "ordinary" that had been used previously. Rather, the court stated, they should be evaluated by the benefits and burdens they offer patients; if the burdens of a particular treatment outweigh the benefits it confers, the treatment can be forgone.

Pearl

Medical interventions ranging from mechanical ventilation to nutrition and hydration should not be distinguished by terms such as "extraordinary" and "ordinary."

In contrast to New Jersey and California, some states require a high level of certainty before a surrogate may refuse life-sustaining treatment. For example, in the *O'Connor* case,[6] a New York court ruled that treatment is obligatory unless evidence shows that the incompetent patient would almost certainly have refused it. Missouri also requires "clear and convincing evidence" of an incompetent patient's wishes, a position that was contested in the *Cruzan* case,[7] in which the United States Supreme Court allowed the states to impose such a requirement while also acknowledging that competent patients have a right to refuse life-sustaining treatment. In most other states, however, surrogates may consider other factors, such as the general balance between the burdens and benefits of treatment, when a patient has not expressed a prior unequivocal preference.

Pearl

Some states require a high level of certainty before a surrogate may refuse life-sustaining treatment. Others allow surrogates to consider other factors.

Although the Supreme Court approved the withholding and withdrawal of life support under the principle of informed refusal, it did not address the concept of futility in *Cruzan*. The word *futility* comes from a Greek term meaning "useless" or "incapable of being achieved." The most limited form of futility is physiologic futility, which is present when a certain treatment, such as a vasoactive medication, cannot achieve a desired physiologic effect, such as raising or lowering the blood pressure. By virtue of their training and experience, physicians are especially knowledgeable about what constitutes physiologic futility. They are not obligated to provide care they consider physiologically futile even if a patient or family insists.[8] Physicians' professional discretion in this area does not derive from a special law of futility but from the generic rules that govern professional conduct. If treatment cannot achieve its intended purpose, then to withhold it does not cause harm. Nor is failure to provide it a failure to meet the professional standard of care.

Physiologic futility differs from medical futility, a broader term that is difficult to quantify.[9] Using the concept of medical futility, some physicians would argue that mechanical ventilation is futile if it can only keep patients alive but cannot restore their health or return them to a sentient state. Yet the patients' surrogates may not consider staying alive futile, which illustrates that medical futility may mean different things to different people. Furthermore, some physicians would say that keeping patients alive but not restoring their health or returning them to a sentient state is medically futile because it consumes scarce health care resources. However, arguments based on the futility concept contain many value-laden assumptions and should not be confused with resource allocation strategies.

The history of legal cases involving futility is that courts have almost uniformly ordered treatment when asked to resolve disputes between families who favor treatment and physicians who oppose it.[10] Judges seem unwilling to cause the death of a patient, as was seen in the case of *Baby K*,[11] when the court was asked to approve in advance a physician decision to withhold life-sustaining treatment from an anencephalic infant over the child's mother's objections. The court refused to do so. However, judges and juries seem equally reluctant to punish physicians who act carefully and within professional standards in refusing to provide treatment they consider inappropriate. In this regard, the only clear legal rule on medically futile treatment is the traditional malpractice test, which measures a physician's treatment decisions against the appropriate standard of medical care and then requires that any substandard care cause the patient injury.

Pearl

Courts have almost uniformly ordered treatment when asked to resolve disputes between families who favor treatment and physicians who oppose it. On the other hand, courts seem reluctant to punish physicians who act carefully and within professional standards in refusing to provide treatment they consider inappropriate.

The issue of malpractice was raised in the *Gilgunn* case,[12] in which a Massachusetts jury imposed no liability on a hospital or the physicians practicing there after they removed a ventilator from a patient and issued a do-not-resuscitate order over the objections of one of her daughters. *Gilgunn* conforms to a trend in futility cases in which physicians are likely to get better legal results when they refuse to provide nonbeneficial treatment and then defend their decisions in court as being consistent with professional standards than when they seek advance permission from a court to withhold care.

Pearl

Although physicians may get better legal results when they refuse to provide nonbeneficial treatment and then defend their decisions in court than when they seek advance permission from a court to withhold care, unilateral action on the part of physicians is discouraged.

Recommendations

Despite the outcome of *Gilgunn* and the trend it represents, I recommend that physicians reject unilateral action. Such actions certainly may be considered ethically appropriate if they support professional integrity; that is, the obligation of each physician to define the moral practice of medicine. Nevertheless, autonomy remains the first ethical principle for removing life-sustaining treatment, even though most critically ill patients must exercise their autonomy through surrogates because their illness has disabled them to such an extent that they cannot make medical decisions themselves. Ethics here reflects law because informed consent and informed refusal are the primary legal principles that justify this practice. Unilateral action also can be risky: disagreements between families and physicians can increase the potential for legal action, and even an unsuccessful lawsuit imposes significant burdens. Finally, negotiation almost always works to resolve even the most contentious dispute.

When negotiation fails, as it did with the two families of vegetative patients from San Francisco General Hospital in the study cited previously, the physicians were tempted to invoke medical futility and withdraw support. Yet they did not do so, not only because they did not want to invoke a lawsuit, but also because they opted in favor of patient autonomy. They then transferred the patients to chronic care facilities. Six months after discharge from San Francisco General Hospital, the patients remained vegetative. One of the families still maintained its belief in miracles at that point, whereas the family of the other patient commented on the difficulty of dealing with the lack of neurologic improvement in their loved one.

References

1. Jennett B, Teasdale G, Braakman R, et al. Predicting outcome in individual patients after severe head injury. Lancet 1976;1: 1031–1034.
2. O'Callahan JG, Fink C, Pitts LH, et al. Withholding and withdrawing of life support from patients with severe head injury. Crit Care Med 1995;23:1567–1575.
3. Luce JM, Alpers A. Legal aspects of withholding and withdrawing life support from critically ill patients in the United States and providing palliative care to them. Am J Respir Crit Care Med 2000;162:2029–2032.
4. *In re Quinlan*, 755 A2A 647 (NJ), cert denied, 429 US 922 (1976).
5. *Barber v Superior Court*. 147 Cal. App. 3d 1006 (Cal. App. 1983).
6. *In re O'Connor*, 72 N.Y. 2d 517, 531 N.E. 2d 607, 534 N.Y.S. 2d 886 (1988).
7. *Cruzan v Director*, Missouri Department of Health, 497 DS 261 (1990).
8. Luce JM. Physicians do not have a responsibility to provide futile or unreasonable care if a patient or family insists. Crit Care Med 1995;23:760–766.
9. Schneiderman LJ, Jecker NS, Jonsen AR. Medical futility: its meaning and ethical implications. Ann Intern Med 1990;112: 949–954.
10. Johnson SH, Gibbons VP, Goldner JA, et al. Legal and institutional policy responses to medical futility. J Health Hosp Law 1997;30:21–36.
11. *In the matter of Baby K*, 16F. 3d 590 (4th cir. 1994).
12. *Gilgunn v. Massachusetts General Hospital*, No. 92–4820 (Mass. Super. Ct. Civ. Action Suffolk So. April 22, 1995).

◆ Part IV ◆

Spinal Cord Injury

General Management of Spinal Cord–Injured Patients

◆ 35 ◆

Does Methylprednisolone Help Patients with Spinal Cord Injury?

Alex B. Valadka

Brief Answer

The National Acute Spinal Cord Injury Study (NASCIS) 2 concluded that a protocol for administration of high-dose methylprednisolone (MP) improved neurologic change scores if it was initiated within 8 hours in patients with spinal cord injury (SCI). These benefits were found not when comparisons were made among all patients randomized to different arms of the study, but only when comparisons were made between patients who received either MP or placebo before the study's median time of drug administration; that is, 8 hours. A comparable analysis in NASCIS 3 led to the recommendation that MP be continued for 48 hours if treatment with MP was not initiated until 3 to 8 hours after injury.

Many criticisms of varying degrees of validity have been directed at the NASCIS trials. Perhaps the most commonly cited concern is that the clinical impact of the improvements in neurologic change scores is minimal. To assess effects on function, NASCIS 3 specifically examined changes in Functional Independence Measure (FIM) scores, but that study was unable to demonstrate significant improvement from administration of MP.

In summary, MP appears to confer some benefit after SCI, but the fact that this benefit has not been shown to improve function makes the use of MP after SCI only a level II recommendation.

Background

Since early 1990, administration of high doses of the steroid MP has been promulgated as a standard of care for patients with SCI. The studies that established the efficacy of this treatment, however, have been criticized ever since their publication, and recent years have seen the publication of several additional commentaries that have been quite strong in their criticisms of the original studies. Reviewing the attacks against (and defenses of) the NASCIS trials makes for fascinating reading. This chapter reviews the essential findings of these trials, some of the criticisms that have been directed against them, and the investigators' responses to these criticisms.

The following sections review the NASCIS trials in some detail. In general, the NASCIS studies were designed to provide class I data, although some of the data analysis and reporting of results may represent a lower class of evidence. Critical commentaries and letters to the editor generally reflect class III data. Readers who are not interested in the details may skip to the "Summary of the NASCIS Trials" that immediately follows the next section.

Literature Review

NASCIS 1[1,2]

The original NASCIS trial compared two MP dosing regimens: what was then considered standard therapy for SCI (100 mg bolus of MP followed by 25 mg every 6 hours for 10 days) versus a regimen of a 1000 mg bolus followed by 250 mg every 6 hours for 10 days. No placebo arm was used because withholding steroids was considered to be unethical at that time. The two groups did not differ in neurologic outcome at 6 weeks, 6 months, or 1 year after injury. Although this is largely considered to be a "negative" trial, it laid the groundwork for the design and analysis of subsequent NASCIS trials.

NASCIS 2: Six-Month Report[3]

As NASCIS 1 progressed, new animal data suggested that higher doses of steroids administered for shorter periods might provide efficacy with fewer complications. These modifications were incorporated into NASCIS 2, a study that used a placebo group and that also included a group that received naloxone, which had proved promising in preclinical studies.

Release of Results

The 6-month outcome data from NASCIS 2 were published in the *New England Journal of Medicine* on May 17, 1990. In an unusual move, the *Journal* agreed to lift its customary embargo concerning prepublication release of a study's findings, partly because the National Institute of Neurological Disorders and Stroke requested early release in the public interest. The results of NASCIS 2 were widely reported by the media roughly 6 weeks before their publication in the *Journal*.[4] Thus, a month and a half before the actual data were available for them to review, health care workers were told that they essentially had to administer MP to SCI patients. When the publication finally appeared in print, many physicians contested the importance of the findings, which they thought had been tremendously overstated.[5,6] This bitterness about the way the NASCIS 2 results were initially disseminated probably accounts for much of the ongoing antagonism toward these trials.

> **Pearl**
>
> The manner in which the results of NASCIS 2 were released and, in many opinions, overstated no doubt contributed to the ongoing animosity that many clinicians feel toward the NASCIS investigations.

Methodology

NASCIS 2 attempted to randomize SCI patients within 12 hours of injury to one of three groups: placebo, MP, or naloxone. MP was given as a bolus of 30 mg/kg of body weight over 15 minutes, followed 45 minutes later by a continuous infusion of 5.4 mg/kg/h for 23 hours. The naloxone dose was 5.4 mg/kg for the 15-minute bolus, followed 45 minutes later by 4.0 mg/kg/h for 23 hours.

Neurologic assessment was divided into motor function, sensation to pinprick, and sensation to light touch. For motor testing, 14 muscle segments (innervated by 14 different levels of the spinal cord from cervical to sacral) were each given one of six scores: 0 (no contraction), 1 (reduced contraction), 2 (active movement without antigravity, i.e., side-to-side but not upward), 3 (active movement against gravity), 4 (reduced function but active movement against resistance), or 5 (normal function). Possible scores ranged from 0 to 70.

For sensory testing, 29 segments of the spinal cord from C2 to S5 were evaluated bilaterally for pinprick and light touch according to the following scale: 1, absent; 2, decreased; or 3, normal. Possible scores ranged from 29 (absent at all levels) to 87 (normal at all levels).

The primary end point was the change in neurologic score between baseline assessment and follow-up evaluation. Additional preplanned analyses would analyze the effects of the protocol, of the time the MP dose was received, and of the degree of neurologic loss (complete or incomplete).

Each patient was placed into one of five motor and sensory categories. The five motor categories were quadriplegic, paraplegic, quadriparetic, paraparetic, and normal. Sensory categories were as follows: analgesic and anesthetic at or above T1, analgesic and anesthetic below T1, hypalgesic and hypesthetic at or above T1, hypalgesic and hypesthetic below T1, and normal.

The analysis of neurologic scores used only the right side of body, and to simplify the presentation of results, only data from the right side were shown in the initial publication. However, when the analyses were performed on the left side, essentially identical results were obtained.

Results

A total of 487 patients were randomized: 162 to MP, 154 to naloxone, and 171 to placebo.

Six-Week Results

At the 6-week outcome assessment of all patients in the MP and placebo groups, there was no significant difference in neurologic change scores between these groups. However, if only those patients treated within 8 hours were considered (remember that one of the a priori hypotheses was that effects of treatment would be influenced by how quickly the drug was given), the MP group showed significantly more improvement in motor and light touch scores, with a trend toward improvement in pinprick scores. The 8-hour cutoff interval was chosen because the average time from injury to bolus dose for all patients in the entire study was 8.7 hours,[3] with a median time of 8.5 hours.[7] The exact number of patients treated within 8 hours drops to 66 MP patients and 69 placebo patients (62 and 67, respectively, at 6 months) out of the 487 entered into the trial.

Another a priori hypothesis was that any treatment effects would be influenced by the severity of injury. Accordingly, patients treated within 8 hours were classified as either plegic with total sensory loss, plegic with partial sensory loss, or paretic with variable sensory loss. At 6 weeks, the first group had more improvement in motor function than placebo, with strong trends for sensory improvement. The small number of patients in the second group demonstrated no differences between MP and placebo, whereas the third group exhibited a trend toward improvement only in motor score.

Six-Month Results

At 6 months after injury, the entire MP group showed significantly more improvement than the placebo group in pinprick and light touch scores, but apparently not in motor improvement. However, among patients treated within 8 hours of injury, the MP group demonstrated significantly more improvement than placebo in all three measures: motor, pinprick, and light touch.

At 6 months postinjury, MP patients who were plegic with total sensory loss had more improvement than placebo patients in all three neurologic measures. On the other hand, patients who were plegic with partial sensory loss showed the same amount of improvement in neurologic scores regardless of group. Among those who were paretic with variable sensory loss, only the amount of motor improvement was significantly greater in the MP group than in the placebo group.

Among patients who were treated after 8 hours, there were no differences in neurologic change scores related to treatment. Likewise, patients treated with naloxone demonstrated no statistically significant differences in improvement.

The above analyses were done on all randomized patients; that is, "intent-to-treat analyses." If only those who received drug within the protocol's time limits are analyzed, the differences in favor of MP become larger.

If patients were classified as quadriplegic, paraplegic, quadriparetic, or paraparetic, and if they were treated within 8 hours, the odds of improving by a full category at 6 weeks tended to be higher in the MP group. The degree of such improvement was less evident at 6 months and was not seen if drug was given after 8 hours.

For MP, naloxone, and placebo patients, wound infections occurred in 7.1%, 3.3%, and 3.6% of patients, respectively, and gastrointestinal bleeding occurred in 4.5%, 2.0%, and 3.0%, respectively. These differences were not significantly different.

NASCIS 2: One-Year Report[8]

The numbers of patients who received study drug within 8 hours of injury and who were assessed 1 year after injury were 62 for MP, 56 for naloxone, and 65 for placebo.

There were no significant differences in neurologic function by treatment group. However, if only those patients who received their drug bolus within 8 hours were considered, those in the MP group demonstrated significantly greater motor recovery (17.2 versus 12.0; $p = .03$). Improvements in pinprick and light touch were not statistically significant.

Among all patients who were randomized more than 8 hours from injury, there were strong but statistically nonsignificant trends for the MP and naloxone groups to recover less neurologic function than the placebo group.

Pearl

NASCIS 2 demonstrated that MP was associated with more motor recovery than placebo, but only if given within 8 hours of injury. Beyond 8 hours, administration of MP was associated with a nonsignificant trend toward recovery of less neurologic function than that seen in the placebo group.

Analysis of changes in neurologic function scores 1 year after injury in patients who received the study drug within 8 hours demonstrated significant improvement in motor scores for patients who were plegic with total sensory loss or paretic with variable sensory loss, but not in the small group of patients who were plegic with partial sensory loss. When patients were analyzed for improvement from an abnormal neurologic category (quadriplegic, paraplegic, quadriparetic, or paraparetic) to a higher level, there was a nonsignificant trend for more improvement with MP.

The groups did not differ significantly for any of 13 complications, most of which were reported at the 6-week follow-up. For all follow-up periods, only three complications approached statistical significance, and all occurred in comparisons of the naloxone group to the placebo group. The authors note that complications, even if related to the MP treatment, were manageable and were clearly outweighed by the potential benefits of improved recovery from SCI.

NASCIS 3: Six-Month Report[9]

Methodology

NASCIS 3 randomized patients into three groups: 24 hours of MP (24MP), 48 hours of MP (48MP), or 48 hours of the free radical scavenger tirilazad mesylate (TM). Because of the presumed importance of ongoing lipid peroxidation and hydrolysis as deleterious pathophysiologic sequelae of SCI, it was thought that extension of the duration of MP therapy beyond 48 hours might confer more benefit than a 24-hour period of administration. In addition, it was thought that administration of the lipid peroxidation inhibitor TM might facilitate neurologic recovery in a manner comparable to that of MP, but with fewer complications.

Two preplanned subgroup analyses were early versus late initiation of treatment within the 8-hour window and the effect of treatment in patients with complete versus incomplete neurologic function.

Patients in all three groups received a bolus of 30 mg/kg of MP, followed by randomization to one of the three arms of the study. Neurologic assessment was the same as that used in the previous NASCIS trials, with the addition of deep pain and pressure responses in the wrist, thumb, little finger, knee, ankle, and great toe. These responses were scored as 1 (absent), 2 (decreased), or 3 (normal).

Patients were also assessed with the FIM, which assesses self-care, sphincter control, mobility, locomotion, communication, and social cognition. Overall scores range from 18 (needing assistance in all areas) to 126 (completely independent). The four outcome categories of the FIM are complete dependence, modified dependence, modified independence, and complete independence.

Analysis of results included summaries by degree of neurologic loss (complete or incomplete) and by time of drug bolus. Time of bolus was divided according to administration less than or equal to 3 hours versus greater than 3 hours from injury; 3 hours was used because it was the mean and modal interval from injury to bolus dose.

Results

A total of 499 patients was evenly distributed across the three groups. Although the TM group had significantly worse motor function than the two MP groups, the average motor function was not significantly different between the 24MP and 48MP groups.

Six-Week Results

By intent-to-treat analysis at 6 weeks, the 48MP group demonstrated a nonsignificant trend toward more motor improvement than the 24MP and TM groups. The difference between 24MP and 48MP became significant if 38 noncompliers were excluded from the analysis.

Intent-to-treat analysis of the effect of timing of drug bolus revealed significantly more motor improvement at 6 weeks among the 48MP group compared with the 24MP group, a difference that became more significant if only compliers were analyzed. When patients were analyzed by presence of complete or incomplete injuries, there were no significant differences at 6 weeks between 24MP and 48MP patients, but statistical significance was reached for both complete and incomplete groups if only compliers were analyzed.

Six-Month Results

At 6 months, neither intent-to-treat analysis nor compliers' analysis revealed significant differences in motor or sensory function between the entire 24MP and 48MP groups. There were no differences among patients who received the bolus within 3 hours, but among those bolused between 3 and 8 hours, both intent-to-treat and compliers' analysis revealed significantly greater change scores in the 48MP group compared with the 24MP group.

When 6-month improvement in completely and incompletely injured patients was compared in 24MP versus 48MP groups, the patients with complete injuries demonstrated more improvement in the 48MP group, a difference that just reached statistical significance. This statistical significance was not seen among incompletely injured patients. The same pattern was seen in a compliers' analysis: patients with complete injuries did better in the 48MP group, but the difference in improvement was not statistically significant among those with incomplete injuries.

There were no significant differences in improvement of sensory function among the three groups.

When 6-month FIM scores were analyzed, intent-to-treat analyses demonstrated significantly better scores in the 48MP group (compared with the 24MP group) in self-care and sphincter control, and these differences remained significant when a compliers' analysis was performed. Total FIM scores were not significantly better by intent-to-treat analysis, but they did reach a p value of .05 when a compliers' analysis was performed.

Finally, improvement in neurologic recovery from one of the four abnormal categories (quadriplegic, paraplegic, quadriparetic, or paraparetic) to a higher category was examined. Six-month intent-to-treat analysis revealed a strong trend toward such improvement in 48MP patients versus 24MP patients. When only those who began treatment between 3 and 8 hours were analyzed, the differences in improvement became statistically significant.

Improvements in the TM group did not reach statistical significance. However, the comparability of motor recovery rates in the TM and 24MP protocols was stressed by the authors.

Complications

There were no differences in survival in the three groups. Thirty-two categories of potential complications occurred with essentially the same frequencies in all groups. An exception was severe pneumonia, which occurred in 5.8% of 48MP patients, 0.6% of TM patients, and 2.6% of 24MP patients ($p = .02$).

Pearl

In NASCIS 3, severe pneumonia was significantly more common in the 48MP group than in the 24 MP group. Overall mortality rates did not differ, but the 48MP group tended to have more deaths from pneumonia, respiratory distress syndrome, and respiratory failure than the 24MP group (six patients vs. one patient).

NASCIS 3: One-Year Report[10]

At 1 year, there were no differences in mortality rates among the three groups. However, in terms of causes of death, the 48MP group exhibited a strong trend toward more deaths from pneumonia, respiratory distress syndrome, and respiratory failure than the 24MP group, although the numbers of patients are small (six patients versus one patient; $p = .056$).

By intent-to-treat analysis, there was a strong trend for the 48MP group to have a better motor change score than the 24MP group if treatment was initiated between 3 and 8 hours (19.0 versus 12.6; $p = .053$). This difference became significant if the analysis included only compliers (change score 19.4 versus 13.3; $p = .032$).

Intent-to-treat analysis revealed no significant differences in sensory change scores, and analysis based on the completeness of injury found no significant differences between groups with different degrees of baseline neurological function. By compliers' analysis, patients with incomplete injuries and variable sensory loss demonstrated a strong trend toward greater motor improvement in the 48MP group compared with the 24MP group (31.4 versus 27.1; $p = .054$).

Improvement from one of the four abnormal categories (quadriplegic, paraplegic, quadriparetic, or paraparetic) to a higher category or to normal was not significantly different between groups. One-year FIM scores were not significantly different between groups.

New complications reported for the first time between 6 months and 1 year occurred with essentially equal frequency in the three groups.

The authors conclude that these findings are of benefit to the approximately half of SCI patients who are admitted in the 3- to 8-hour window after injury. However, the significantly greater incidence of pneumonia at 6 weeks and the possible increase in mortality rate from pulmonary problems mandate caution and suggest that patients be treated with the 24-hour protocol whenever possible.

Summary of the NASCIS Trials

The above review may seem complex and confusing, and many who attempt to review the NASCIS literature often end up feeling the same way. The essential findings are summarized below.

NASCIS 2

Outcomes at 1 year did not differ between MP and placebo groups when all patients in each group were compared. When only patients treated within 8 hours were analyzed, the MP group had significantly greater motor change scores (17.2 versus 12.0; $p = .03$), but no significant difference was seen in pinprick and light touch scores.

NASCIS 3

The 48MP group had a better motor change score than the 24 MP group at 1 year only if patients bolused between 3 and 8 hours were compared (19.0 versus 13.7); this difference was of borderline statistical significance ($p = .053$). If only patients who complied with the protocol were included, this difference becomes more significant (19.4 versus 13.3; $p = .032$). There were no significant differences in sensory change scores. FIM scores did not differ significantly between groups.

Severe pneumonia occurred significantly more often in 48MP patients (5.8%) than in 24MP patients (2.6%) and TM patients (0.6%) ($p = .02$). Overall mortality rates did not differ among the three groups, but in terms of causes of death, the 48MP group exhibited a strong trend toward having more deaths from pneumonia, respiratory distress syndrome, and respiratory failure than the 24 MP group ($p = .056$).

Some Criticisms and Defenses of the NASCIS Trials

Space does not permit a comprehensive review of all the published critiques of the NASCIS trials. Additional discussion is readily available in the literature.[4–7,11–21] Some of the more frequently voiced criticisms are discussed below, along with possible responses that might be offered by the NASCIS investigators. Readers may judge for themselves both the validity of the criticisms and the soundness of the responses.

1. Criticism: It is not clear how the reported gains in motor recovery associated with MP relate to actual functional benefit because no measure of functional outcome was included in NASCIS 2.[17,19,21,22] Is an improvement of five or six points in motor change score due to marked improvement in an important muscle group or only to meaningless twitches in two or three muscle groups below the level of injury?[18,20]

Response: NASCIS 2 was designed to measure only neurologic status, not total functioning of the patient.[14] At the time that NASCIS 2 was being planned, no generally accepted, validated, and reliable scales existed to measure activities of daily living, urinary function, catheterization, or ambulation. Neurologic function was used because those data have high interobserver reliability and relate to the function of specific spinal tracts. "The NASCIS group prefers to interpret the results of NASCIS 2 as showing that *neurological* recovery can be influenced by pharmacological interventions early in the injury process . . ."[15] [italics present in original document].

The subsequent NASCIS 3 trial did use the FIM. Subsequently, the relationship between motor and 1-year FIM scores in NASCIS 3 was analyzed, and the results were used to estimate the degree of improvement in FIM scores that would be expected from the motor recovery observed in NASCIS 2. Overall, almost 10% of patients could be expected to show at least a 10% improvement in the modified FIM scores used in this analysis, an improvement that would be expected to represent a clinically important degree of recovery (class II data).[23]

Pearl

NASCIS 2 measured only neurologic status (not total functioning of a patient) because no generally accepted functional scales existed at the time that NASCIS 2 was being planned. NASCIS 3 did use the FIM, but no differences between groups were seen.

Moreover, it must be remembered that mean scores are obtained in an entire population of patients. Some patients may not benefit at all, but others may demonstrate a great deal more recovery than the mean.[15] The likelihood of recovery is significantly improved in patients who receive MP after SCI, but this is not the same as saying that all patients will recover by the mean value.[12]

2. Criticism: The 8-hour time limit was not specified as a hypothesis prior to commencement of NASCIS 2, and the division into less than 3 hours versus 3 to 8 hours in NASCIS 3 was not specified in advance.[5,16,18,22]

Response: Stratification of data into patients who were treated "early" versus "late" was planned from the beginning. The cut-off time of 8 hours in NASCIS 2 was chosen because that was closest to the median time of 8.5 hours for bolus dose of the entire population, thus permitting adequate statistical power for testing the effects of "early" versus "late" administration of MP.[7,13,24] In NASCIS 3, 3 hours was chosen for the same reason; that is, it was the median and mean time between injury and bolus.[7,9,24] No time points other than the ones presented were analyzed.[7,24]

3. Criticism: Why are results presented only as "change scores"? Absolute scores should demonstrate the same trends if the data are reliable.[5]

Response: Change scores are less variable than absolute neurologic scores and therefore permit more robust tests of the study hypotheses. Also, because neurologic change was the clinical outcome of interest in the trials, change scores were the most appropriate method of assessing treatment effect.[13]

4. Criticism: For the subset of patients who improved, no baseline epidemiologic, neurologic, or physiologic data are provided, even though these are the patients of greatest interest and the patients upon whom the conclusions of the studies are based.[5]

Response: Randomization ensured that severity of initial injury (as well as other factors) was distributed equally among groups, and any residual variability in neurologic injury was controlled for in the statistical analyses. This study was analyzed by well-accepted statistical techniques that withstood the process of peer review.[13] "After-the-fact" analyses of only patients who demonstrated more improvement are scientifically invalid; stratification analyses based on response rather than on treatment violate fundamental principles of analysis of clinical trial data.[15] Also, when analyses suggested that other patient characteristics might be influencing treatment effects (which occurred infrequently), they were controlled in multivariate analyses.[12]

5. Criticism: Why was there no improvement in sensory function in the MP group?[19]

Response: Sensory scores tended to improve more in MP patients, but the improvement was not statistically significant. Reasons may include the greater variability of measuring pinprick and light touch as compared with motor function, the lower resolution of a three-point sensory scale (as opposed to a six-point motor scale), and the possibility that MP does not have as much effect on sensory function as on motor function.[15]

6. Criticism: Motor scores are reported only for the right side, but sensory scores are reported bilaterally.[16,22]

Response: All three NASCIS investigations analyzed only data from the right side.[1,3,9] Neurologic function between the two sides was highly correlated, and summing both sides would amount to measuring the same phenomenon twice. This practice would be anticonservative with respect to detection of therapeutic effects.[7,25] In other words, using data from only one side actually made it harder to demonstrate that any improvement that occurred was associated with use of MP.[26]

7. Criticism: A placebo arm was not used in NASCIS 3.[18,22]

Response: Randomizing patients to placebo when an effective therapy is available is unethical.[7,25] Based on their findings in NASCIS 2, the NASCIS neurosurgeons felt it would be unethical to include a placebo group in NASCIS 3.

8. Criticism: In NASCIS 3, the two steroid arms were not equivalent: 24.7% of patients in the 24MP group had normal motor function versus 13.9% in the 48MP group ($p = .012$). Because the treatment arms are unbalanced, the small gains attributed to 48 hours of MP treatment are questionable.[18]

Response: Normal patients are uninformative because they have no room for improvement and thus do not contribute to a change score (unless they worsen, which was very rare). Also, a correct baseline analysis would account for all levels of severity, and such an analysis reveals much greater equivalence between the MP groups in NASCIS 3.[12]

9. Criticism: The detailed neurologic examination must take an hour (by conservative estimate). Pain, anxiety, distractions, fractures and other accompanying injuries, etc. must have prevented many patients from completing the entire assessment.[18]

Response: In NASCIS 3, only 2.5% of exams were incomplete, and in these cases data from the other side of the body were used. For NASCIS 2, retrospective analysis suggests an incompletion rate of 4.8 per 10,000 required parameters.[12]

10. Criticism: NASCIS 2 has not been replicated. The authors cite a Japanese article in a journal not indexed on Medline as a description of a study that replicates NASCIS 2,[7,12,24,25] but the study described in that article did not utilize blinding, did not use a placebo, compared groups with different baseline motor and functional scores, and gave MP to approximately a fifth of the control group.[18] The NASCIS investigators also refer to a relatively small French study in a manner that implies that the results of that study are supportive of the NASCIS results,[7,12,24,25] but the abstract of that study (which is available in English on Medline) concludes that there is no evidence of benefit of medical treatment in SCI (class II data?).[27]

Response: A meta-analysis that includes these trials (supplemented as needed with additional data obtained from the authors of the studies) confirms the efficacy of MP in SCI.[11] Other studies on whiplash and microdiskectomy also support the use of MP.[12]

11. Criticism: MP treatment is associated with a very high complication rate.[16,18,22]

Response: In NASCIS 2, frequency rates for 18 complications were comparable in MP and placebo groups.[12] In NASCIS 3, 31 and 50 patients, respectively, would have to be treated with 48 hours of MP in order for a single case of severe pneumonia or severe sepsis attributable to therapy to occur.[7] The availability of effective treatments for these conditions compared with the lack of effective treatment (other than MP) for SCI suggests that the risk:benefit ratio favors MP. Review of all deaths in NASCIS 2 and NASCIS 3 revealed no direct association of any individual patient's death with his or her drug therapy, and overall mortality was essentially the same in all treatment groups.[7] A recent meta-analysis of 51 trials of administration of a high dose of MP in elective and trauma surgery found no significantly increased risk of gastrointestinal bleeding, wound complications, pulmonary complications, or death (class III data).[28] In fact, MP was associated with a significantly lower rate of pulmonary complications, primarily in trauma patients.

12. Criticism: A "compliers' analysis" is not valid in NASCIS 3, and the fact that dropping the small number of noncompliers has such a dramatic effect on P values in NASCIS 3 indicates that the data are "unstable."[16]

Response: Although the primary analysis in the NASCIS trials was intent-to-treat, a compliers' analysis is also of interest because it more likely reflects the effects of a therapy in ideal circumstances. Furthermore, one cannot infer anything about the direction of effect of individual patients in a trial.[7]

13. Criticism: In NASCIS 3, analysis of 1-year motor change scores in the 48MP versus 24MP groups (19.0 versus 13.7, respectively) yields a p value of .053, which is not significant.[16,22]

Response: The p value is quite close to the significance threshold of .05, and compliers' analysis reveals that the difference between groups becomes significant (19.4 versus 13.3, $p = .032$).[10] The potential for improvement in these patients with otherwise untreatable injuries outweighs the low risk of MP associated complications, which are usually minor.

14. Criticism: Statistical analysis in the NASCIS trials is inappropriate because of multiple comparisons. So many comparisons were performed among different subgroups that there is a good likelihood that several comparisons would be statistically significant by chance alone.[16,18] Correction of analyses to minimize random associations from appearing statistically significant just by chance should have been used.[16]

Response: Many statisticians consider such types of statistical correction to be overly simplistic and even inappropriate for analysis of related aspects of a common clinical phenomenon; for example, motor function, pinprick sensation, and touch sensation.[7] Furthermore, of the 54 comparisons in NASCIS 2, statistical significance was reached for nine of them, whereas statistical significance would be expected for only two or three by using the statistical correction technique suggested by some critics. The probability that nine comparisons would be significant by chance alone is .0013. Four additional comparisons had α levels between .06 and .08, further strengthening the evidence supporting the use of MP.[7]

15. Criticism: The second a priori hypothesis of NASCIS 2—that treatment effect would be influenced by the severity of injury—was not addressed for the entire population of study patients, but only for patients who had been already stratified according to the first hypothesis, that is, time of MP administration.[22]

Response: This technique is a perfectly valid analytical strategy that documents the effects of recovery while, at the same time, analyzing the comparisons of principal interest: drug effects within severity groups.[25] Randomization within subgroups is unnecessary because of the risk of unblinding when randomization is conducted within smaller groups and because a patient may belong to several groups, making randomization within all of them impossible. Thus, postrandomization stratification, which was performed in the NASCIS investigations, is the most common analytic strategy. Importantly, such stratifications must be part of the original proposal, which was the case in the NASCIS trials.[12]

16. Criticism: No standardized medical or surgical management protocol was used, and possible effects of aggressive medical or surgical management on outcome were not addressed.[22]

Response: Standardization of treatment regimens is not common in clinical trials, not possible in this type of study, and not necessary. Randomization allows for control of variability of concurrent therapies by distributing any variations in management evenly between groups. Moreover, when other treatments are provided in accordance with local practices, generalizability of trial results is enhanced. Finally, published analyses have reported on the timing of surgery in NASCIS 2 and have documented that surgery did not affect the results regarding use of MP (class II data).[25,29]

Other Reviews

Fehlings[30] has analyzed the NASCIS data and has concluded that they represent class II evidence because, although the NASCIS investigations were conducted in a prospective, randomized, blinded fashion, both NASCIS 2 and NASCIS 3 were "negative trials" with respect to their primary outcome analyses. According to this review, the benefits of MP were established only via post hoc analyses, making the conclusions of the NASCIS trials most consistent with class II data. Despite the modest nature of the clinical benefits of MP, the devastating impact of SCI should prompt clinicians to consider its use in these patients.[30] However, it must also be remembered that initiation of MP treatment more than 8 hours after injury is not beneficial and may be harmful.

Use of MP in patients with gunshot wounds to the spine confers no benefits and may contribute to the development of complications (class III data).[31] Other common uses of MP, such as for pediatric SCI, prophylaxis during high-risk spine surgeries, etc., were not addressed in the NASCIS trials[30] and should be considered to be level III recommendations at best.

Pearl

Use of MP in patients with gunshot wounds to the spine was not studied in the NASCIS trials. Other investigators have suggested that it confers no benefits and may contribute to the development of complications (class III data). Other common uses of MP, for example, pediatric SCI, prophylaxis during high-risk spine surgeries, etc., were not addressed in the NASCIS trials and should be considered to be level III recommendations at best.

Conclusions

NASCIS 2 demonstrated that 24MP treatment is associated with more neurologic improvement than placebo. Unfortunately, despite a great deal of hype and hoopla that preceded the actual publication of the study, the average amount of improvement is modest. The manner in which the results were released and, in many opinions, overstated no doubt contributed to the ongoing animosity that many clinicians feel toward the NASCIS investigations. Furthermore, in NASCIS 3, the motor benefits of 48 versus 24 hours of MP were, at best, of borderline statistical significance ($p = .053$).

Many criticisms focus on the clinical relevance (or lack thereof) of the relatively minor amount of average neurologic improvement. Nevertheless, this improvement (however slight it may appear) was significantly greater in the MP group. The overall lack of major side effects indicates that the risk:benefit ratio is acceptable.

Other criticisms focus on the analytic and statistical methods of the studies. The NASCIS authors generally do a good job of refuting these criticisms. However, the NASCIS authors also use some weak arguments and irrelevant references to defend their studies; for example, citing trials of MP efficacy in whiplash and lumbar diskectomy.[12] Such arguments make the NASCIS authors appear almost desperate to find any kind of support for the use of high-dose steroids.

In their responses to various critics, the NASCIS authors also tend to put too much favorable spin on results that are not significant, and they gloss over major negative results of the NASCIS trials. These tendencies may perpetuate confusion and, in some cases, contribute to a perceived lack of credibility of the results. It would be better if the authors did not try so hard to "sell" their studies and, instead, let the results (both strong and weak) speak for themselves.

Recommendations

High-dose methylprednisolone after SCI does appear to improve neurologic function more than placebo. However, the improvement in neurologic change scores has not been shown to translate into improved function in SCI patients. For these reasons, use of MP as recommended in the NASCIS trials should be viewed as a level II recommendation.

Acknowledgment

This chapter is based in part on material presented at the meeting "Trauma and Critical Care—2001," Las Vegas, Nevada, March 2001.

References

1. Bracken MB, Collins WF, Freeman DF, et al. Efficacy of methylprednisolone in acute spinal cord injury. JAMA 1984;251:45–52.
2. Bracken MB, Shepard MJ, Hellenbrand KG, et al. Methylprednisolone and neurological function 1 year after spinal cord injury. Results of the National Acute Spinal Cord Injury Study. J Neurosurg 1985;63:704–713.
3. Bracken MB, Shepard MJ, Collins WF Jr, et al. A randomized, controlled trial of methylprednisolone or naloxone in the treatment of acute spinal-cord injury. Results of the Second National Acute Spinal Cord Injury Study. N Engl J Med 1990;322:1405–1411.
4. Ducker TB, Zeidman SM. Spinal cord injury. Role of steroid therapy. Spine 1994;19:2281–2287.
5. Rosner MJ. National Acute Spinal Cord Injury Study of methylprednisolone or naloxone. Neurosurgery 1991;28:628.
6. Senegor M. A randomized, controlled trial of methylprednisolone or naloxone in the treatment of acute spinal cord injury. N Engl J Med 1990;323:1208.
7. Bracken MB. Methylprednisolone and spinal cord injury [letter]. J Neurosurg (Spine 1) 2000;93:175–178.
8. Bracken MB, Shepard MJ, Collins WF Jr, et al. Methylprednisolone or naloxone treatment after acute spinal cord injury: 1-year follow-up data. Results of the second National Acute Spinal Cord Injury Study. J Neurosurg 1992;76:23–31.
9. Bracken MB, Shepard MJ, Holford TR, et al. Administration of methylprednisolone for 24 or 48 hours or tirilazad mesylate for 48 hours in the treatment of acute spinal cord injury. Results of the Third National Acute Spinal Cord Injury Randomized Controlled Trial. JAMA 1997;277:1597–1604.
10. Bracken MB, Shepard MJ, Holford TR, et al. Methylprednisolone or tirilazad mesylate administration after acute spinal cord injury: 1-year follow up. Results of the third National Acute Spinal Cord Injury randomized controlled trial. J Neurosurg 1998;89:699–706.
11. Bracken MB. Pharmacological interventions for acute spinal cord injury (Cochrane Review). In: The Cochrane Library, Issue 4. Oxford: Update Software; 2000.
12. Bracken MB, Aldrich EF, Herr DL, et al. Clinical measurement, statistical analysis, and risk-benefit: controversies from trials of spinal injury. J Trauma 2000;48:558–561.
13. Bracken MB. National Acute Spinal Cord Injury Study of methylprednisolone or naloxone. Neurosurgery 1991;28:628–629.
14. Bracken MB, Shepard MJ, Collins WF, et al. A randomized, controlled trial of methylprednisolone or naloxone in the treatment of acute spinal-cord injury. N Engl J Med 1990;323:1209.
15. Bracken MB, Shepard MJ, Collins WF Jr, et al. Methylprednisolone for spinal cord injury. J Neurosurg 1992;77:325–327.
16. Hurlbert RJ. Methylprednisolone for acute spinal cord injury: an inappropriate standard of care. J Neurosurg (Spine 1) 2000;93:1–7.
17. Lyons MK, Partington MD, Meyer FB. A randomized, controlled trial of methylprednisolone or naloxone in the treatment of acute spinal-cord injury. N Engl J Med 1990;323:1207–1208.
18. Nesathurai S. Steroids and spinal cord injury: revisiting the NASCIS 2 and NASCIS 3 trials. J Trauma 1998;45:1088–1093.
19. Rosner MJ. Methylprednisolone for spinal cord injury. J Neurosurg 1992;77:324–325.
20. Shapiro SA. Methylprednisolone for spinal cord injury. J Neurosurg 1992;77:324.
21. Yarkony GM, Roth EJ. A randomized, controlled trial of methylprednisolone or naloxone in the treatment of acute spinal cord injury. N Engl J Med 1990;323:1208.
22. Guidelines for management of acute cervical spinal cord injuries. Chapter 9: Pharmacological therapy after acute cervical spinal cord injury. Neurosurgery 2002;50(suppl 3):S63–S72.
23. Bracken MB, Holford TR. Neurological and functional status 1 year after acute spinal cord injury: estimates of functional recovery in National Acute Spinal Cord Injury Study II from results modeled in National Acute Spinal Cord Injury Study III. J Neurosurg 2002;96:259–266.
24. Bracken MB. Methylprednisolone and acute spinal cord injury: an update of the randomized evidence. Spine 2001;26:S47–S54.
25. Bracken MB. Comment on "Guidelines for Management of Acute Cervical Spinal Injuries. Chapter 9: Pharmacological therapy after acute cervical spinal cord injury." Neurosurgery 2002;50(suppl 3):S-xiv—S-xix.
26. Bullock MR, Valadka AB. Comment on "Guidelines for Management of Acute Cervical Spinal Injuries. Chapter 9: Pharmacological therapy after acute cervical spinal cord injury." Neurosurgery 2002;50(suppl 3):S-v–S-viii.
27. Petitjean ME, Pointillart V, Dixmerias F, et al. Medical treatment of spinal cord injury in the acute stage. Ann Fr Anesth Reanim 1998;17:114–122.
28. Sauerland S, Nagelschmidt M, Mallmann P, et al. Risks and benefits of preoperative high dose methylprednisolone in surgical patients: a systematic review. Drug Saf 2000;23:449–461.
29. Duh MS, Shepard MJ, Wilberger JE, et al. The effectiveness of surgery on the treatment of acute spinal cord injury and its relation to pharmacological treatment. Neurosurgery 1994;35:240–248.
30. Fehlings MG. Editorial: recommendations regarding the use of methylprednisolone in acute spinal cord injury: making sense out of the controversy. Spine 2001;26:S56–S57.
31. Heary RF, Vaccaro AR, Mesa JJ, et al. Steroids and gunshot wounds to the spine. Neurosurgery 1997;41:576–583.

◆ 36 ◆

Are There New Therapies That Improve Outcome in Spinal Cord–Injured Patients?

Fred H. Geisler

Brief Answer

Despite a report of beneficial effects of GM_1 ganglioside in a small study of spinal cord-injured patients, a larger trial found no significant effect according to the main outcome measure. Secondary analyses in that trial suggested some benefit from administration of GM_1 ganglioside, including a more rapid rate of recovery. In terms of other therapies, clinical trials have failed to demonstrate benefit from thyrotropin-releasing hormone (TRH) or from nimodipine, but the small numbers of patients in those studies may have contributed to a masking of any beneficial effects.

Background

Although prevention remains the most effective intervention for spinal cord injury (SCI), attempts to diminish and/or reverse damage to the injured spinal cord have been proceeding for decades. The many different research approaches that have been explored include pharmacologic therapies and, more recently, transplantation of fetal neural tissue. Several pharmacologic treatments have been tested in large clinical studies.

Literature Review

Prehospital Care

With the development of the 19-center National Spinal Cord Injury Database between 1973 and 1985, national data on SCI were collected in a central data repository for the first time.[1] This effort catalyzed the creation of regional centers for the treatment of SCI. Such projects also provided impetus for protocol-driven prehospital care and for triage systems that directly transported patients with SCI to definitive care facilities specializing in the treatment of these patients.

Improvements in prehospital diagnosis, initial fluid and airway management, immobilization, and rapid transportation could well be responsible for most of the improvement in outcomes of SCI patients during the last decade. For example, a recently conducted multicenter trial that enrolled patients with a significant SCI documented that 61.7% were taken to a local emergency room for stabilization and initial medical assessment before transfer to a definitive spinal care facility (class II data).[2] This process necessitates a second transport, prolonged immobilization, and consequent delay of such treatments as traction and spinal stabilization (which are often not performed at the initial hospital). Working with local prehospital care providers to improve the percentage of SCI patients who are initially transported to a definitive facility could be a big step toward improving the ultimate outcome of many patients.

Pearl

Improvements in prehospital care could well be responsible for most of the improvement in outcomes of SCI patients in recent years.

Pharmacologic Therapy

To date, at least eight prospective drug trials have investigated pharmacologic therapies for acute SCI in humans.[3–11] These trials can be divided into three groups: those investigating methylprednisolone sodium succinate (MPSS),[3–6] those evaluating Sygen (GM_1 ganglioside),[7–9] and the smaller pilot studies of TRH[10] and nimodipine.[11]

Studies that enrolled patients in the 1980s include the first National Acute Spinal Cord Injury Study (NASCIS 1),[3] NASCIS 2,[4] and the Maryland GM_1 Ganglioside Study.[7,8] These studies were followed by two additional studies in the 1990s: NASCIS 3[5] and the multicenter Sygen (GM_1 ganglioside) study.[9] (The NASCIS studies are discussed in Chapter 35.)

The Maryland GM_1 Ganglioside Study

Gangliosides are complex acidic glycolipids located in cell membranes of mammals. They are especially abundant in the membranes of central nervous system cells. Acute neuroprotective and longer-term regenerative effects have been reported in multiple experimental studies of ischemia and injury. Clinical trials have investigated the efficacy of gangliosides in stroke, Parkinson's disease, and other entities. Proposed mechanisms of action include antiexcitotoxic effects, prevention of apoptosis, and enhancement of neuroreintegration. In terms of SCI, one possible mechanism of recovery may be enhancement of function or potency of the damaged white matter passing through the level of the injury, thus facilitating increased function at caudal neurologic levels. Another possibility is that gangliosides may increase the survival of axons at the injury site or augment the response of neurons in the conus to decreased input from the damaged white matter tracts passing through the injury site.[9,12,13]

A single-center trial of monosialotetrahexosylganglioside (GM_1 ganglioside) in acute SCI enrolled patients from January 1986 to May 1987 at the Maryland Institute for Emergency Medical Services Systems in Baltimore, Maryland. Results were reported in 1991.[7,8] This prospective double-blind study randomized 37 patients, 34 of whom (23 with cervical injuries and 11 with thoracic injuries) completed the investigational protocol of either placebo or 100 mg of intravenous GM_1 ganglioside daily for a planned 30-day treatment period, with the first dose administered within 72 hours of injury. All patients received a course of methylprednisolone therapy at a dose of approximately one-tenth the NASCIS 2 dose recommendation. (The results of NASCIS 2 were not reported until after the completion of patient entry into the Maryland study.)

The American Spinal Injury Association (ASIA) motor score[7] and the Frankel scale[7,14] were used to assess neurologic status at baseline and at follow-up. The results of the Maryland study demonstrated a significant treatment effect on the distribution of improvement of Frankel grades from baseline to 1-year follow-up ($p = .034$) (class I data). However, differences in improvement in ASIA motor score were not statistically significant. (The original article reported significance in this measure, but a subsequent clarification[8] reported that the previously described significant improvement in total ASIA motor score actually referred to the motor score for the lower extremities alone.) This small study provided the foundation for the subsequent multicenter study of GM_1 ganglioside in acute SCI.

Pearl

The Maryland study demonstrated a significant effect of ganglioside treatment in terms of Frankel grades, but improvement in ASIA motor scores was not statistically significant.

Sygen Acute Spinal Cord Injury Study

Sygen is a proprietary name for GM_1 ganglioside produced by the Fidia Pharmaceutical Corporation, Washington, D.C., which sponsored the study. The Sygen Multicenter Acute Spinal Cord Injury Study[2,9,15] was designed to determine the efficacy and safety of Sygen in the treatment of patients with acute SCI following standard treatment with MPSS.

Study Design

Patients in this prospective, double-blind, randomized trial were stratified into six groups by level (cervical or thoracic) and by baseline severity [ASIA Impairment Scale (AIS) grade of A, B, or combined C+D] and randomized into three parallel treatment groups: placebo, low-dose Sygen, or high-dose Sygen. All groups received a bolus dose followed by 56 days of study treatment. The low-dose Sygen group received a 300-mg loading dose followed by 100 mg/day for 56 days, and the high-dose group received a 600-mg loading dose followed by 200 mg/day for 56 days. The placebo group received placebo both for the loading dose and for the subsequent 56 doses. At the first planned interim analysis by the Extramural Monitoring Committee, the high-dose Sygen group was dropped (while the investigators remained blinded as to which group was dropped), and an additional stratification was added for age above or below 30 years.

The primary efficacy end point was specified as the proportion of patients with "marked recovery," defined as a two-grade improvement between baseline AIS grade and 26-week modified Benzel grade. Secondary efficacy assessments included the time course of marked

Table 36-1 ASIA Impairment Scale (AIS) Used in the Baseline Evaluation

AIS Grade	Description	Equivalent MBC Grade(s)
A	No motor or sensory function is preserved in the sacral segments S4-S5	I
B	Sensory but no motor function is preserved below the neurologic level and extends through the sacral segments S4-S5	II
C	Motor function is preserved below the neurologic level, and the majority of key muscles below the level have a muscle grade less than 3	III
D	Motor function is preserved below the neurologic level, and the majority of key muscles below the level have a muscle grade greater than or equal to 3	IV, V, VI
E	Motor and sensory function are normal	VII

MBC: modified Benzel classification.

Table 36-2 Modified Benzel Classification (MBC) with Equivalent ASIA Impairment Scale (AIS) Grade(s)

MBC Grade	Description	Equivalent AIS Grade(s)
I	No motor or sensory function is preserved in the sacral segments S4-S5	A
II	Sensory but no motor function is preserved in the sacral segments S4-S5	B
III	Motor function is preserved below the neurologic level, and the majority of key muscles below the neurologic level have a muscle grade less than 3; unable to walk	C
IV	Unable to walk; some functional motor control below the level of injury that is significantly useful (assist in transfers, etc.) but that is not sufficient for independent walking.	(C*), D
V	Limited walking; motor function allows walking with assistance or unassisted, but significant problems secondary to lack of endurance or fear of falling limit patient mobility (must be able to ambulate at least 25 feet)	D
VI	Unlimited walking; ambulatory without assistance and without significant limitations other than one or both of the following: difficulties with micturition; slightly discoordinated gait (must be able to ambulate at least 150 feet without a helper)	D
VII	Neurologically intact with the exception of minimal deficits that cause no functional difficulties (must have a neurologically normal gait and be able to walk without assistance or assistive devices)	(D*), E

*Only a few patients fit this AIS description

recovery, ASIA motor and sensory scores, relative and absolute sensory levels of impairment, and assessments of bowel and bladder function.

Patients were eligible for this study if they had a major SCI, defined as an injury rostral to the T10 bony level resulting in a neurologic deficit in at least one lower limb that had an ASIA motor score of less than 15 out of a possible 25 points. Patients had to have the potential for recovery from their SCI. Thus, patients with spinal cord transection or penetration were excluded. Patients with significant cauda equina, plexus, or peripheral nerve injury were also excluded. All patients received the NASCIS 2–recommended dose regimen of MPSS within 8 hours of injury. The study medication was initiated within 72 hours of the SCI, but only after completion of the MPSS therapy to avoid possible drug–drug interaction between MPSS and Sygen.

All patients received a baseline evaluation after emergency room assessment and administration of MPSS. The baseline assessment was performed just prior to the first dose of study medication. Thus, the baseline examination to which all subsequent examinations were compared was recorded after the 24-hour MPSS had been administered and after performance of hemodynamic resuscitation, mechanical decompression, and multiple neurologic examinations. Any increase in neurologic function between the emergency room exam and the baseline examination was thus not included in the documentation of change in neurologic function between baseline and follow-up evaluations, which were performed at 4, 8, 16, 26, and 52 weeks.

The pretreatment neurologic assessment utilized both the AIS (Table 36-1) and a detailed ASIA motor and sensory examination. The modified Benzel classification (Table 36-2) and detailed ASIA motor and sensory examinations were performed at 4, 8, 16, 26, and 52 weeks. A follow-up scale different from the baseline measurement scale was used because it included walking ability and also expanded the D classification in

Table 36-3 Presence of Major Improvement: Two-Grade Change Between Baseline ASIA Impairment Scale (AIS) Category and Modified Benzel Classification Category on Follow-Up

Baseline	Modified Benzel Classification at 6 Months						
AIS	I	II	III	IV	V	VI	VII
A	No	No	Yes	Yes	Yes	Yes	Yes
B	No	No	No	Yes	Yes	Yes	Yes
C	No	No	No	No	Yes	Yes	Yes
D	No	No	No	No	No	Yes	Yes

All deaths and all losses to follow-up were counted as "No Major Recovery" in accordance with intent-to-treat analysis.

Table 36-4 Distribution of the 760 Eligible Patients by Baseline Severity and Spinal Level

	Baseline AIS			
	A	B	C+D	TOTAL
Cervical	332 (57.3%)	113 (19.5%)	134 (23.1%)	579
Thoracic	150 (82.9%)	18 (9.9%)	13 (7.2%)	181
Total	482 (63.4%)	131 (17.2%)	147 (19.3%)	760

$p < .001$, 2×3 Fisher-Freeman-Halton exact test.

the AIS. Because most patients had an unstable spinal fracture at baseline, it was not possible to assess walking ability at that time, thus necessitating the use of different baseline and follow-up scales.

The definitions of Benzel grades I, II, and III are essentially the same as those of AIS grades A, B, and C, respectively. The higher functional grades of the Benzel scale expand the AIS to include degrees of walking and hence provide information on the patient's level of function. Major improvement (Table 36-3) was defined as an improvement of at least two grades in the Benzel equivalent of the baseline AIS. For example, in a patient with a baseline AIS grade of A, improvement to at least Benzel category III would be needed to qualify as a major improvement. This definition of major recovery allows the use of a single outcome measure for populations of different injury severities at baseline.

Study Data Description

This was the largest prospective SCI drug trial ever conducted: 797 patients randomized during a 5-year recruitment period at 28 neurotrauma centers in North America. Collection of all 12-month follow-up data was completed in February 1998. Overall, 3165 patients were screened, but 2368 were excluded before randomization for failure to satisfy the entry criteria. The most common reason for exclusion was the presence of a spinal fracture with no or minimal neurologic deficits. Of the 797 patients randomized and entered into the study, 37 were later found to be ineligible. Thus, 760 patients are included in the efficacy analysis data.

Data about baseline injury severity and anatomic region of injury in the efficacy analysis data set are shown in Table 36-4. The largest severity group in both the cervical and thoracic region was AIS group A. Fewer patients in all AIS groups were injured in the thoracic than the cervical region. Cervical traction was used in 383 patients, and 604 patients had a spinal operation.

Pearl

The Sygen Multicenter Acute Spinal Cord Injury Study was the largest prospective SCI drug trial ever conducted.

Acute Sygen Conclusions

The Sygen 100 mg and placebo groups were comparable at baseline. No noteworthy differences in medical or surgical management existed between the groups. No clinically relevant safety issues associated with Sygen were identified.

The Sygen group did not have a significantly higher proportion of patients with marked recovery at week 26. Thus, the prospectively chosen primary efficacy analysis for this study was negative (class I data).

Several secondary analyses, however, did suggest some beneficial effects of Sygen (class II data). The

Table 36-5 Visit at Which Major Recovery Was First Obtained in Placebo, Sygen 100 mg, and Sygen 200 mg Groups

	Number of All Randomized Patients First Attaining Major Recovery				No Major	
	Week 4	Week 8	Week 16	Week 26	Recovery	Total *N*
Placebo	20 (6.1%)	27 (8.2%)	24 (7.3%)	24 (7.3%)	235 (71.2%)	330
Sygen 100 mg	32 (9.7%)	40 (12.1%)	16 (4.8%)	12 (3.6%)	231 (69.8%)	331
Sygen 200 mg	9 (9.1%)	11 (11.1%)	6 (6.1%)	2 (2.0%)	71 (71.7%)	99
Sygen 100 mg + Sygen 200 mg	41 (9.5%)	51 (11.9%)	22 (5.1%)	14 (3.3%)	302 (70.2%)	430

Recovery times differ significantly between placebo and Sygen 100 mg group ($p = .0275$, 2 × 5 Fisher Freeman-Halton exact test) and also between placebo and combined Sygen 100 mg plus Sygen 200 mg group ($p = .0128$, 2 × 5 Fisher Freeman-Halton exact test).

Pearl

The Sygen study was negative in terms of its prospectively chosen primary efficacy analysis, that is, the proportion of patients with marked recovery 26 weeks after injury. Several secondary analyses, however, did suggest some benefit, especially in terms of rate of recovery.

prespecified primary outcome measure of proportion of patients with two-grade improvement in AIS/Benzel score was significantly greater in the Sygen patients at 8 weeks, which corresponded to the end of the 56-day treatment period. Analysis using a Fisher's Exact Test of the 2 × 5 table of the time at which major recovery was first obtained (Table 36-5) yielded a *p* value of .0275, indicating that low-dose Sygen patients who attained major recovery did so earlier than placebo-treated patients. When the low-dose and high-dose Sygen groups were combined and compared with the placebo group, a *p* value of .0128 favoring Sygen treatment was obtained. These data indicate that Sygen may hasten recovery after SCI.

The Sygen group had consistently greater and earlier recovery than the placebo-treated group across all severities of injury at baseline. Patients whose baseline injury severity placed them in AIS group A demonstrated a slight trend toward greater recovery in the Sygen group at weeks 8 and 16. The magnitude of this effect may have been constrained by the generally smaller amounts of recovery in these patients. Group B patients demonstrated an earlier and more persistent drug effect. The combined group C+D also demonstrated a pattern of earlier recovery with Sygen, but a ceiling effect seemed to obscure differences in late recovery between treated and placebo patients in this group. A large drug effect was seen in the patients who did not undergo surgery. A pattern of trends toward positive drug effect was consistent across primary and secondary efficacy measures, including bowel, bladder and sensory recovery.

These results are consistent with the known pathophysiology of acute SCI, in which both effects of treatment and the potential for marked spontaneous recovery are largest in patients in Group B and also in those with spinal cord contusions. The largest treatment differences were observed in these groups. When all baseline severities were combined, the Sygen patients who achieved major recovery at week 26 obtained it roughly 2 months earlier than placebo patients.

Thyrotropin-Releasing Hormone Treatment for Acute Spinal Cord Injury

TRH has been shown to enhance outcome in animal models of acute SCI.[16,17] This evidence of recovery led to a small, randomized, placebo-controlled, double-blinded pilot study of the effectiveness of TRH versus normal saline in patients stratified by complete or incomplete SCI.[10] The patients were recruited from two centers during a 2-year period starting in July 1986. Eligible patients began receiving study drug within 12 hours of injury. TRH was administered as an intravenous bolus of 0.2 mg/kg followed by 0.2 mg/kg/h continuous intravenous infusion for 6 hours ($n = 11$); the placebo group received normal saline by an identical protocol ($n = 9$). Neurologic examination was performed at baseline and at 24 hours, 72 hours, 7 days, and 1, 4, and 12 months after injury. Assessment used motor and sensory scales similar to those used in the NASCIS studies and also used the Sunnybrook Cord Injury Scale.

Of the 20 patients entered, two patients died, one withdrew, and four were lost to follow-up, yielding an attrition rate of 35% and leaving 13 patients to complete the study. The authors reported no significant difference in neurologic outcome between the groups (class II data). In a study with such a small sample size and high dropout rate, it is nearly impossible to demonstrate a significant effect of TRH even though the enhancement of recovery might have been large enough to be clinically important (type II statistical error). Thus, this study should not be interpreted as providing negative information about the efficacy of TRH. Rather, it provided important safety information about the administration of TRH and also served as a basis for potential future studies.

Nimodipine Treatment for Acute Spinal Cord Injury

A prospective trial randomized SCI patients to treatment with MPSS, placebo, or the calcium channel blocker nimodipine.[11] The latter drug was administered as an intravenous bolus of 0.015 mg/kg over 2 hours, followed by 0.03 g/kg/h for 7 days if mean arterial blood pressure remained above 60 mm Hg. MPSS was administered as an intravenous bolus of 30 mg/kg over 1 hour followed by 5.4 mg/kg/h for 23 hours. In total, 106 patients were randomized into the following four treatment groups: (1) MPSS only, (2) nimodipine only, (3) both MPSS and nimodipine, and (4) no pharmacologic treatment. ASIA scores were determined at baseline and at 1-year follow-up. Patients were treated with early surgical decompression and stabilization.

The authors reported no difference in neurologic outcome among the treatment groups (class II data). Like the TRH study above, this trial was subject to type II statistical error because of the small number of patients enrolled. Thus, clinical benefit could have resulted from either MPSS or nimodipine, but the small sample sizes may have prevented detection of such benefit. As with the TRH study, these results could form the basis of a larger study of nimodipine for the early treatment of SCI.

Pearl

Small trials have not demonstrated beneficial effects of TRH or nimodipine in SCI, but the numbers of patients studied may have been inadequate for demonstrating an effect.

Neural Tissue Transplantation

Although some success has been reported in animal work on transplantation of fetal spinal cord cells, of stem cells derived from the spinal cord, and of embryonic stem cells, it remains unclear if these strategies will ultimately yield the hoped-for results.[18,19] Neuronal progenitor cells[20] within neural tissue may serve as endogenous raw material to aid in the repair and then recovery of spinal cord function.

In adult rats, transplantation of fetal spinal cord tissue has been shown to aid in recovery of locomotor function.[21] Similar improvement has been demonstrated in cats.[22] More recent studies by Wirth and colleagues[23] suggest that intraspinal grafting of human fetal spinal cord tissue is both feasible and safe (class III data). However, perhaps because of limited tissue contrast or spatial resolution on postoperative magnetic resonance imaging studies, postoperative images could not confirm survival of the grafted tissue because precise boundaries between donor and host tissue could not be defined.

Pearl

Intraspinal grafting of human fetal spinal cord tissue has been performed safely.

Restoration of Function

The most important type of restoration of function after SCI is not necessarily walking ability. Often, incontinence of bowel and bladder and impairment of breathing, sexual function, and hand function are more detrimental to the quality of life of SCI patients. Therapies aimed at restoration should optimize these areas as well as lower extremity motor function. Strategies targeted toward the recovery phase include limitation of apoptosis, enhancement of cell regeneration during the normal healing process, and cell transplantation. Experimental studies indicate that motor recovery and even restoration of locomotion are possible with maintenance of only 5 to 10% of the original axonal population at the injury site,[24,25] suggesting that marked clinical effectiveness may result even from treatments that produce only partial histologic or anatomic recovery.

Future treatment for SCI may well consist of an orderly sequence of several treatments. In the hyperacute phase of injury (within the first 2 hours), perhaps therapies that limit secondary injury and initiation of apoptotic cell death would be used. Promising agents include antiexcitotoxic and antiapoptotic factors and growth factors. During the acute injury phase (2 to 48 hours), therapy may focus on agents that block the natural inhibition of regeneration, prevent demyelination and conduction blocks, and initiate regeneration of damaged oligodendrocytes. Therapeutic goals for the chronic recovery phase (2 to 365 days) include axonal regeneration, preservation of distal target cells in the conus while they await axonal regeneration through the injury zone, and restoration of functional neural circuits. For the chronic phase after the natural recovery period (beyond 1 year), therapeutic goals could include optimization of remaining function (i.e., evoked electrical retraining of very weak muscles) and minimization of clinically unwanted sequelae of SCI (i.e., spasticity). In the prolonged chronic phase (beyond 2 years), preferred treatment options may include therapies to replace lost embryonic or stem cells or to replace lost neural conduits, for example, neural bridges inserted to replace functional tissue lost during the SCI.

Effective future therapy for patients with complete SCI will require axonal sprouting with organized synaptogenesis, long tract axonal regrowth through the injury site, and appropriate physiologic reconnection with target spinal interneurons that have been preserved or restored. Because myelin and oligodendrocytes seem to create a nonpermissive environment for neurite growth (and thereby regulate collateralization and nerve tract development under normal circumstances), axonal sprouting and neuronal reconnection may require antibodies or antagonists to several inhibitory factors that normally block these processes from occurring.[26] Obviously, the cure for SCI will not only be exceedingly complicated, but it will also require biotechnology that is currently in the infancy of its discovery phase or is not even in existence yet.

Potential Difficulties with Future Pharmacologic Trials

There exists little corporate sponsorship of ongoing SCI studies. The NASCIS studies were supported by the National Institutes of Health and by the Upjohn Corporation (which later became Pharmacia and Upjohn, Inc.), and the Sygen studies were funded by the Fidia Pharmaceutical Corporation. Currently, neither of these corporate sponsors is actively pursuing commercialization of the tested or analogous compounds or their approval by the United States Food and Drug Administration. The main reason for this lack of corporate interest seems to be the small number of acute SCI patients (~10,000 per year in the U.S.) and the low profit potential for even a successful treatment. Even assuming that the treatment would be reimbursed at $5,000 per patient and that 50% of all SCI patients received the treatment, only $25 million per year would be generated. Presumably, most pharmaceutical companies do not consider the development cost of $100 million to $150 million and the 10-year development period to be a worthwhile investment for such a low potential rate of return.

Pearl

In terms of developing a drug specifically for the treatment of SCI, it is likely that most pharmaceutical companies do not consider the high development costs and lengthy development period to be worthwhile investments for a low probable rate of return.

Conclusions

A small initial study suggested that GM_1 ganglioside enhanced recovery after SCI (class I data). However, when tested in a large multicenter trial, GM_1 ganglioside was not associated with a greater degree of recovery from SCI according to the primary efficacy assessment (class I data). Secondary analyses suggested some benefit from GM_1 ganglioside, including more rapid recovery (class II data) and a pattern of trends consistent with greater recovery of function after SCI (class III data). No significant adverse effects of GM_1 ganglioside were detected.

Smaller trials investigating TRH and nimodipine in SCI patients failed to demonstrate any benefit from these agents (class II data), perhaps because of insufficient numbers of patients in those trials. No significant adverse effects of TRH or nimodipine were reported in these studies.

Recommendations

Use of GM_1 ganglioside in SCI patients can be considered to be a level II recommendation.

Use of TRH and nimodipine cannot be recommended at this time because of the lack of demonstrated efficacy (level II recommendation). In the future, results of well-conducted studies with adequate numbers of patients may lead to modification of these recommendations.

References

1. Stover SL, DeLisa JA, Whiteneck GG. Spinal Cord Injury: Clinical Outcomes from the Model Systems. Gaithersburg, MD: Aspen Publications; 1995.
2. Geisler FH, Coleman WP, Grieco G, et al. Recruitment and early treatment in a multicenter study of acute spinal cord injury. Spine 2001;26(suppl 24):S58–S67.
3. Bracken MB, Collins WF, Freeman DF, et al. Efficacy of methylprednisolone in acute spinal cord injury. JAMA 1984;251:45–52.
4. Bracken MB, Shepard MJ, Collins WF, et al. A randomized, controlled trial of methylprednisolone or naloxone in the treatment of acute spinal-cord injury. Results of the Second National Acute Spinal Cord Injury Study. N Engl J Med 1990;322: 1405–1411.
5. Bracken MB, Shepard MJ, Holford TR, et al. Administration of methylprednisolone for 24 or 48 hours or tirilazad mesylate for 48 hours in the treatment of acute spinal cord injury. Results of the Third National Acute Spinal Cord Injury Randomized Controlled Trial. JAMA 1997;277:1597–1604.
6. Otani K, Abe H, Kadoya S. et. al. Beneficial effect of methylprednisolone sodium succinate in the treatment of acute spinal cord injury. Sekitsui Sekizui 1994;7:633–647.
7. Geisler FH, Dorsey FC, Coleman WP. Recovery of motor function after spinal-cord injury—a randomized, placebo-controlled trial with GM-1 ganglioside. N Engl J Med 1991;324:1829–1838.
8. Geisler FH, Dorsey FC, Coleman WP. Correction: recovery of motor function after spinal-cord injury—a randomized, placebo-controlled trial with GM-1 ganglioside (letter). N Engl J Med 1991;325:1659–1660.

9. Geisler FH, Coleman WP, Grieco G, et al. The Sygen multicenter acute spinal cord injury study. Spine 2001;26(suppl 24):S87–S98.
10. Pitts LH, Ross A, Chase GA, et al. Treatment with thyrotropin-releasing hormone (TRH) in patients with traumatic spinal cord injuries. J Neurotrauma 1995;12:235–243.
11. Petitjean ME, Pointillart V, Dixmerias F, et al. Medical treatment of spinal cord injury in the acute stage. Ann Fr Anesth Reanim 1998;17:114–122.
12. Geisler FH, Dorsey FC, Coleman WP. GM-1 ganglioside in human spinal cord injury. J Neurotrauma 1992;9(suppl 2): S517–S530.
13. Geisler FH. Clinical trials of pharmacotherapy for spinal cord injury. Ann NY Acad Sci 1998;845:374–381.
14. Frankel HL, Hancock DO, Hyslop G, et al. The value of postural reduction in the initial management of closed injuries of the spine with paraplegia and tetraplegia. Paraplegia 1969;7: 179–192.
15. Geisler FH, Coleman WP, Grieco G, et al. Measurement and recovery patterns in a multicenter study of acute spinal cord injury. Spine 2001;26(suppl 24):S68–S86.
16. Faden AI, Jacobs TP, Smith MT. Thyrotropin-releasing hormone in experimental spinal injury: dose response and late treatment. Neurology 1984;34:1280–1284.
17. Faden AI, Yum SW, Lemke M, et al. Effects of TRH-analog treatment on tissue cations, phospholipids and energy metabolism after spinal cord injury. J Pharmacol Exp Ther 1990;255: 608–614.
18. McDonald JW, Sadowsky C. Spinal-cord injury. Lancet 2002; 359:417–425.
19. McDonald JW and the Research Consortium of the Christopher Reeve Paralysis Foundation. Repairing the damaged spinal cord. Sci Am 1999;281:64–73.
20. Kempermann G, Gage FH. New nerve cells for the adult brain. Sci Am 1999;280:48–53.
21. Bernstein JJ, Goldberg WJ. Fetal spinal cord homographs ameliorate the severity of lesion-induced hind limb behavioral deficits. Exp Neurol 1987;98:633–644.
22. Howland DR, Bregman BS, Tessler A, et al. Transplants enhance locomotion in neonatal kittens whose spinal cords are transected: a behavioral and anatomical study. Exp Neurol 1995; 135:123–145.
23. Wirth ED III, Reier PJ, Fessler RG, et al. Feasibility and safety of neural tissue transplantation in patients with syringomyelia. J Neurotrauma 2001;18:911–929.
24. Young W. Recovery mechanisms in spinal cord injury: implications for regenerative therapy. In: Seil FJ, ed. Neural Regeneration and Transplantation. Frontier of Clinical Neuroscience, vol. 6. New York: Alan R. Liss; 1989:157–169.
25. Blight AR. Cellular morphology of chronic spinal cord injury in the cat: analysis of myelinated axons by line-sampling. Neuroscience 1983;10:521–543.
26. Schwab ME, Bartholdi D. Degeneration and regeneration of axons in the lesioned spinal cord. Physiol Rev 1996;76: 319–370.

◆ 37 ◆

When Is It Safe to Extubate a Newly Quadriplegic Patient? When Is Early Tracheostomy Appropriate?

Christopher N. Faber and Antonios Zikos

Brief Answer

There exist no criteria that reliably predict the success of weaning and extubation in the tetraplegic patient. Therefore, the decision to extubate relies almost exclusively on clinical judgment. Patients considered for extubation should have a neurologic level below C3 and should be free of copious secretions or pneumonia (level III recommendation).

Weaning by progressively prolonged periods of spontaneous breathing is a level II recommendation. The use of high tidal volumes during mechanical ventilation and resistive training of the respiratory muscles are both level III recommendations.

Patients with a complete injury above C3 should be considered for early tracheostomy since ventilator independence is unlikely (level II recommendation). Early tracheostomy is supported as a level III recommendation in patients who have extensive facial trauma, difficult airways, or multiple weaning failures, or in whom prolonged duration of mechanical ventilation is anticipated.

Background

When to wean and when to perform tracheostomy are controversial topics even in the general population of patients with respiratory failure. These questions are even more difficult in the tetraplegic patient population because of the paucity of data specific to this unique clinical situation. Most management decisions in tetraplegic patients are based on data from studies in the general patient population, with varying degrees of modification for the unique clinical features of this patient population.

There are no well-validated weaning criteria for tetraplegic patients. Poor cough and diaphragm mobility increase the frequency of secretion-related complications (such as atelectasis and pneumonia) in these patients. Even patients with normal diaphragm function at the time of injury, who have a lower incidence of respiratory complications, have impaired clearance of secretions that necessitates meticulous respiratory hygiene to avoid later respiratory complications. Patients with paralyzed diaphragms require more time to recover independent breathing and are more prone to develop respiratory complications. Therefore, standard weaning and extubation criteria may not apply to tetraplegic patients.

Airway control, secretion clearance, and expected duration of respiratory muscle paralysis are key factors influencing the decision for the necessity and timing of tracheostomy in tetraplegic patients. Unfortunately, these parameters are not easily quantified. Therefore, the decision for tracheostomy, like that for extubation, relies heavily on clinical judgment.

Literature Review

Respiratory complications are common in the spinal cord–injured patient and are the major cause of postinjury mortality, with pneumonia being the leading cause of respiratory death.[1] These complications frequently make the use of mechanical ventilation necessary. Respiratory failure complicating tetraplegia is due not only to impairment of the diaphragm's bellows function by the neurologic injury, but also to the added ventilatory burdens imposed by the associated injury complex, subsequent infectious complications, and the systemic inflammatory response. Risk factors for the need for mechanical ventilation include neurologic level above C5, complete cord lesions, copious secretions, pneumonia, and atelectasis (class III data).[2]

Weaning new quadriplegics from the ventilator is a complex process requiring optimal management of the associated injury complex followed by intensive respiratory rehabilitation. Frequently, rehabilitation of respiratory muscle function is the limiting factor in liberating spinal cord–injured patients from the ventilator. The recovery of this function may take months, even in patients who have a reasonable expectation of eventual ventilator independence.[3]

Respiratory Physiology in Tetraplegia

The bellows function of the lung requires inspiratory and expiratory muscles. The inspiratory muscles are the diaphragm (innervation from C3 to C5); the accessory muscles, consisting of sternocleidomastoids (accessory nerve, C1 and C2), trapezius (C1 to C4), scalene, and pectoralis (C4 to C8) muscles; and the intercostal muscles (T1 to T12). During inspiration, the diaphragm descends. The intercostal muscles elevate the sternum and move the ribs upward and outward. They also stabilize the chest wall. Maximal inspiration requires use of the accessory muscles. The expiratory muscles are the internal and external oblique muscles (T7 to T12), the transverses abdominus (T7 to L1), the rectus abdominus (T7 to L1), and the lateral intercostal muscles (T1 to T12).[4,5]

Cervical spine injury below C5 results in impaired expiratory function and a weakened cough. Patients with injuries from C3 to C5 have, in addition, variably diminished inspiratory function resulting in reduced vital capacity. Patients with injuries above C3 have complete loss of inspiratory and expiratory capacity; however, using forms of glossopharyngeal breathing, they may be able to sustain short periods of spontaneous breathing.[6]

Two important concepts in the respiratory management of patients with cervical spine injury are the postural dependence of vital capacity and the late development of spasticity. In the upright position, the abdominal contents descend unrestrained by the flaccid abdominal wall. This displacement of the abdominal contents passively pulls the diaphragm downward and limits inspiratory excursion, thereby paradoxically reducing vital capacity in the upright position (class II data).[7] This adverse postural consequence can be minimized through the use of abdominal binders when a patient is in a seated position (class II data).[8]

Pearl

In the upright position, downward displacement of the abdominal contents pulls the diaphragm downward and paradoxically reduces vital capacity.

Lung function in the tetraplegic patient improves as flaccidity is replaced by spasticity.[6] Increased tone in the intercostal and abdominal wall muscles stabilizes the rib cage and allows for more effective diaphragmatic function. McMichan et al[9] demonstrated an improvement in vital capacity from 1.5 to 2.7 L and an improvement in maximal inspiratory pressure from 46 to 77 cm H_2O 18 weeks after cervical spine injury (between C4 and C8) in 22 patients (class II data). Ledsome and Sharp[10] found that vital capacity nearly doubled within 5 months of cervical spine injury (class II data).

Pearl

Lung function in the tetraplegic patient improves as flaccidity is replaced by spasticity.

Respiratory Complications in Tetraplegia

In their review of the clinical outcomes for over 2000 patients from the National Spinal Cord Injury Database, Ragnarsson et al[1] found pulmonary complications to be the most common cause of death. The major pulmonary complications of incomplete and complete tetraplegia, respectively, were aspiration (4–11%), atelectasis (16–39%), pneumonia (12–38%), and ventilatory failure (11–37%). Patients with higher and more complete cervical spine injuries, as well as older patients, had greater risk of developing these complications. Claxton et al[2] found that mortality was associated with increasing age, neurologic level above C4, and Glasgow Coma Scale score ≤13 (class III data). Independent risk factors for requiring mechanical ventilation included copious secretions in the first week and pneumonia.[2] The need for and duration of mechanical ventilation may be related to completeness of myelopathy, severity of associated injuries, and presence of cardiopulmonary comorbidities (class III data).[11] Once respiratory failure occurs, it is frequently prolonged (class II data).[12]

Weaning the Tetraplegic Patient from the Ventilator

Weaning "criteria" are not defined for the tetraplegic patient. Vital capacity (10–15 mL/kg),[13,14] respiratory rate (12–20 breaths/min),[14] and minute ventilation (<10 L/min)[13] are frequently recommended weaning parameters, but these measurements have poor predictive value in general populations[15] and have not been validated in tetraplegic patients. The frequency-tidal volume ratio ($F:V_T$), or rapid shallow breathing index, also has not been validated in tetraplegics, but it does serve as a useful indicator of readiness for extubation in the general population of intensive care unit patients (class I data for a general patient population).[15] An index of 105 breaths/minute/liter or less has a positive predictive value of 0.78.

Poor cough and clearance of secretions increase the susceptibility of tetraplegic patients to respiratory complications. Unfortunately, these airway-related comorbidities are not readily quantified by the conventional weaning parameters discussed above.[16,17] Epstein[16] showed that patients with favorable $F:V_T$ who failed extubation most often failed for reasons distinct from their original respiratory process. In over half of these patients, reintubation was made necessary by an airway complication such as aspiration or obstruction (class II data). In a prospective study assessing the predictive value of weaning criteria, Vallverdu et al[17] showed that patients with the highest frequency of extubation failure (35.7%) were those with neurologic disease (class II data). Although none of the patients in this study had tetraplegia, the study underscored the importance of poor cough and secretion clearance as causes of weaning failure in the neurologically impaired patient. In this study, maximal inspiratory (>70 cmH_2O) and expiratory pressures (>50 cmH_2O) were better predictors of extubation readiness in patients with neurologic disease.

There exist several approaches to weaning the tetraplegic patient from mechanical ventilation. Peterson et al[18] found that progressively increasing times of spontaneous respiration was twice as effective in achieving ventilator weaning in tetraplegic patients as an approach employing gradual reductions in intermittent mandatory ventilation (IMV) support (class III data). This experience mirrored that of a large prospective, randomized, multicenter study that demonstrated that once-daily spontaneous breathing allowed liberation from mechanical ventilation three times more rapidly than IMV weaning and twice as fast as pressure support weaning (class I data for a general patient population).[19] This concept of respiratory muscle training is the basis for strategies employing resistive training to achieve ventilator independence.

Pearl

Progressively increasing times of spontaneous respiration appears to be more effective in ventilator weaning in tetraplegic patients than approaches using gradual reductions in IMV support or pressure support.

Use of high tidal volumes (greater the 20 mL/kg ideal body weight) to ventilate tetraplegic patients was shown to reduce the incidence of atelectasis and shorten the time to weaning in a small, nonrandomized study by Peterson et al[20] (class III data). This technique was not associated with an increased risk of barotrauma.

Resistive training may be considered as part of the respiratory rehabilitative process.[21] Rutchik et al[22] improved vital capacity and reduced dyspnea in 10 patients after an 8-week resistive inspiratory muscle-training program (class III data). Gross et al[23] were able to improve strength and endurance of the respiratory muscles (measured both physiologically by negative inspiratory pressure, as well as electromyographically) in six chronic tetraplegic patients over a period of 16 weeks using resistance training (class III data).

Indications for Tracheostomy

The American College of Chest Physicians Consensus Conference on artificial airways[24] recommended tracheostomy for patients requiring mechanical ventilation for greater than 21 days. However, this conference emphasized that "there is no specific time at which a translaryngeal tube must be removed and a tracheotomy performed." Rodriguez et al[25] demonstrated reduced ventilator days, reduced ICU stay, and shortened hospital stays in patients who underwent tracheostomy within 7 days of intubation (class II data). In contrast, in a randomized, prospective, multicenter study, Sugerman et al[26] found no differences in ICU length of stay, pneumonia, or death in patients who received early (day 3–5) versus late (day 10–14) tracheostomy (class III data).

Pearl

"There is no specific time at which a translaryngeal tube must be removed and a tracheotomy performed."[24]

For tetraplegic patients, Lanig and Peterson[5] recommended intubation and tracheostomy for those with an injury above C3. Neurologically injured patients with associated facial injuries or difficult airways (inability to get three fingers in the mouth; inability to get three fingers between thyroid cartilage and mandible; impaired neck extension; rheumatoid arthritis; or morbid obesity) should be carefully considered for early tracheostomy.[27] For tetraplegic patients who should wean but who have sustained pulmonary complications, there is no clear consensus regarding the timing of tracheostomy.

However, superimposed upon the respiratory burdens incurred by their injury, spinal cord-injured patients have the added disadvantages of a limited respiratory capacity and a predictable potential for further respiratory complications. Therefore, many authors support performance of a tracheostomy after no more than 7 to 14 days of intubation if the patient fails to wean.[5,6,28,29] Tracheostomy has the advantage of reducing anatomic dead space. In addition, the shorter tracheostomy tube has the added benefit of lower resistance to airflow. These latter potential benefits, although not universally acknowledged, may be significant in the tetraplegic patient with limited respiratory reserve.[30]

Pearl

Tracheostomy reduces anatomic dead space and resistance to airflow.

Recommendations

1. Tetraplegic patients may be considered for weaning if they have injuries below C3 and are free of copious secretions and pneumonia (level III). The decision to extubate relies almost exclusively on clinical judgment. Weaning criteria such as vital capacity, negative inspiratory force, minute ventilation, and $F{:}V_T$ are useful tools but are not reliable predictors for success of weaning and extubation. The potential for complications such as atelectasis, pneumonia, and aspiration must be considered prior to extubation (level III).
2. Tetraplegic patients with injuries above C3 should receive early tracheostomy after they have stabilized from the initial injury complex (level II) based on expectation for prolonged or permanent ventilator dependence.
3. Patients who have difficult airways or who have had extensive facial trauma should receive careful consideration for early tracheostomy (level III).
4. If the patient has diaphragmatic paralysis at the time of injury, the duration of mechanical ventilation will be prolonged and early tracheostomy should be considered (level III).
5. Tetraplegic patients who are expected to require prolonged mechanical ventilation (greater than 14–21 days) should be considered for early tracheostomy (level III). If a patient has a persistently paralyzed diaphragm or develops additional respiratory complications such as a pneumonia or lobar atelectasis, our practice has been to proceed with early tracheostomy because prolonged mechanical ventilation is expected (level III).
6. Ventilation with high tidal volumes may reduce the incidence of atelectasis and shorten the duration of mechanical ventilation (level III).
7. Weaning by progressively prolonged periods of spontaneous respiration may result in more rapid liberation from mechanical ventilation (level II).
8. Resistive training may improve strength and endurance of the respiratory muscles (level III).

References

1. Ragnarsson KT, Hall KM, Wilmot CB, et al. Management of pulmonary, cardiovascular, and metabolic conditions after spinal cord injury. In: Stover SL, DeLisa JA, Whiteneck GG, eds. Spinal Cord Injury. Clinical Outcomes from the Model Systems. Gaithersberg, MD: Aspen Publishers; 1995:79–97.
2. Claxton AR, Wong DT, Chung F, et al. Predictors of hospital mortality and mechanical ventilation in patients with cervical spinal cord injury. Can J Anaesth 1998;45:144–149.
3. Oo T, Watt JW, Soni BM, et al. Delayed diaphragm recovery in 12 patients after high cervical spinal cord injury: a retrospective review of the diaphragm status of 107 patients ventilated after acute spinal cord injury. Spinal Cord 1999;37: 117–122.
4. Aldrich TK, Rochester DF. The Lungs and Neuromuscular Diseases. In: Murray JK, Nadel JA, Mason RJ, Boushey HA, eds. Textbook of Respiratory Medicine, 3rd ed. Philadelphia: WB Saunders; 2000:2329–2356.
5. Lanig IS, Peterson WP. The respiratory system in spinal cord injury. Phys Med Rehabil Clin North Am 2000;11:29–41.
6. Mansel JK, Norman JR. Respiratory complications and management of spinal cord injuries. Chest 1990;97:1446–1452.
7. Estenne M, De Troyer A. Mechanism of the postural dependence of vital capacity in tetraplegic subjects. Am Rev Respir Dis 1987;135:367–371.
8. Goldman JM, Rose LS, Williams SJ, et al. Effect of abdominal binders on breathing in tetraplegic patients. Thorax 1986;41: 940–945.
9. McMichan JC, Michel L, Westbrook PR. Pulmonary dysfunction following traumatic quadriplegia: recognition, prevention, and treatment. JAMA 1980;243:528–531.
10. Ledsome JR, Sharp JM. Pulmonary function in acute cervical cord injury. Am Rev Respir Dis 1981;124:41–44.
11. Lemons VR, Wagner FC Jr. Respiratory complications after cervical spinal cord injury. Spine 1994;19:2315–2320.
12. Jackson AB, Groomes TE. Incidence of respiratory complications following spinal cord injury. Arch Phys Med Rehabil 1994;75:270–275.
13. Lamid S, Ragalie GF, Welter K. Respirator-dependent quadriplegics: problems during the weaning period. J Am Paraplegia Soc 1985;8:33–37.
14. Hanak M, Scott A. Spinal Cord Injury: An Illustrated Guide for Health Care Professionals. New York: Springer; 1993:47–55.
15. Yang KL, Tobin MJ. A prospective study of indexes predicting the outcome of trials of weaning from mechanical ventilation. N Engl J Med 1991;324:1445–1450.
16. Epstein SK. Etiology of extubation failure and the predictive value of the rapid shallow breathing index. Am J Respir Crit Care Med 1995;152:545–549.
17. Vallverdu I, Calaf N, Subirana M, et al. Clinical characteristics, respiratory functional parameters, and outcome of a two-hour T-piece trial in patients weaning from mechanical ventilation. Am J Respir Crit Care Med 1998;158:1855–1862.
18. Peterson W, Charlifue W, Gerhart A, et al. Two methods of weaning persons with quadriplegia from mechanical ventilators. Paraplegia 1994;32:98–103.
19. Esteban A, Frutos F, Tobin MJ, et al. A comparison of four methods of weaning patients from mechanical ventilation.

Spanish Lung Failure Collaborative Group. N Engl J Med 1995;332:345–350.
20. Peterson WP, Barbalata L, Brooks CA, et al. The effect of tidal volumes on the time to wean persons with high tetraplegia from ventilators. Spinal Cord 1999;37:284–288.
21. Viroslav J, Rosenblatt R, Tomazevic SM. Respiratory management, survival, and quality of life for high-level traumatic tetraplegics. Respir Care Clin North Am 1996;2:313–322.
22. Rutchik A, Weissman AR, Almenoff PL, et al. Resistive inspiratory muscle training in subjects with chronic cervical spinal cord injury. Arch Phys Med Rehabil 1998;79:293–297.
23. Gross D, Ladd HW, Riley EJ, et al. The effect of training on strength and endurance of the diaphragm in quadriplegia. Am J Med 1980;68:27–35.
24. Plummer AL, Gracey DR. Consensus conference on artificial airways in patients receiving mechanical ventilation. Chest 1989; 96:178–180.
25. Rodriguez JL, Steinberg SM, Luchetti FA, et al. Early tracheostomy for primary airway management in the surgical critical care setting. Surgery 1990;108:655–659.
26. Sugerman HJ, Wolfe L, Pasquale MD, et al. Multicenter, randomized, prospective trial of early tracheostomy. J Trauma 1997;43:741–747.
27. Wijdicks EF, Borel CO. Respiratory management in acute neurologic illness. Neurology 1998;50:11–20.
28. Fromm B, Hundt G, Gerner HJ, et al. Management of respiratory problems unique to high tetraplegia. Spinal Cord 1999;37: 239–244.
29. Wicks AB, Menter RR. Long-term outlook in quadriplegic patients with initial ventilator dependency. Chest 1986;90: 406–410.
30. O'Connor MF, Keamy M, Hall JB. Airway Management. In: Hall JB, Schmidt GA, Wood LD, eds. Principles of Critical Care, 2nd ed. New York: McGraw-Hill; 1999:111–120.

◆ 38 ◆

How Do I Diagnose and Manage SCIWORA?

Jack E. Wilberger

Brief Answer

Neurologic complaints that develop in a child after apparently trivial spine trauma should be taken seriously. Even seemingly minor injuries may make the spinal cord more susceptible to a subsequent insult, which can precipitate the ultimate neurologic manifestations of SCIWORA (spinal cord injury without radiographic abnormality). Appropriate workup may include spine x-rays, computed tomography (CT) scans of inadequately visualized or suspicious areas, and flexion/extension views of lateral cervical spine x-rays. Magnetic resonance imaging (MRI) is indicated if all of the above studies are normal. Somatosensory evoked potentials (SEPs) may be useful in documenting and following any subclinical electrophysiologic spinal cord dysfunction. Immobilization for 2 to 3 months with intensive education of both child and parents is advisable. Repeat flexion/extension films should be obtained 2 to 3 weeks after the initial injury and before immobilization is discontinued.

Background

The term *SCIWORA* was coined in 1982 by Pang and Wilberger[1] to describe the entity of traumatic myelopathy in the absence of any abnormality on plain spine x-rays, flexion/extension radiographs, CT, or myelography. Since the introduction of MRI, SCIWORA has become a misnomer because only rarely is MRI normal in such situations. Nevertheless, SCIWORA is a distinct clinical entity in the spectrum of spinal cord injury (SCI) and warrants elucidation of its presentation, pathophysiology, and treatment.

Pearl

Since the introduction of MRI, SCIWORA has become a misnomer because only rarely is MRI normal in these cases.

Literature Review

A Medline search of the literature from 1980 to 2001 was conducted with the following key words: SCIWORA, Spinal Cord Injury Without Radiographic Abnormality, and MRI in Spinal Cord Injury. One hundred twenty-two articles were found. All represented case reports, retrospective studies, and reviews; that is, only class III data were available for review. Only articles from which specific patient information could be gleaned were reviewed.

A total of 364 cases were identified, with all but 15 occurring in individuals over 15 years of age.[2–14] The cervical spine was affected more than twice as frequently as the thoracolumbar spine: 68% versus 32%, respectively.

Even though pediatric spinal cord injury is a rare entity that makes up no more than 10 to 12% of all spinal cord injury,[15] SCIWORA is the most common cause of pediatric SCI; up to 60% of such cases may fall into the category of SCIWORA.[16,17]

Age was a significant determinant not only of location but also of injury severity. Virtually all reported cases of SCIWORA involving the upper cervical spine occurred in children under 8 years of age, as did the most severe neurologic syndromes and sequelae.[1,12,13]

> **Pearl**
>
> SCIWORA is the most common cause of pediatric SCI.

Pathophysiology

The suspected pathophysiology of SCIWORA as first postulated by Pang and Wilberger has not been challenged. These injuries are thought to occur as a result of flexion, hyperextension, longitudinal distraction, and ischemia.

> **Pearl**
>
> These injuries are thought to occur as a result of flexion, hyperextension, longitudinal distraction, and ischemia.

The pediatric population is particularly susceptible to excessive flexion and hyperextension because of the inherent ligamentous laxity of this age group and because of the more horizontal orientation of the cervical facet joints, which permits excessive translational movement.[3,18] In addition, the relatively larger size of the head in relation to the weak cervical musculature predisposes the cervical spine to undergo a fulcrum-like movement. With extreme hyperextension, the spinal canal can narrow by up to 50% because of buckling of the ligamentum flavum, with possible transient obstruction of one or both vertebral arteries.[3]

Longitudinal distraction occurs most commonly in neonatal injuries. Once again, because of ligamentous laxity, the spine can "stretch" up to 2 inches without suffering apparent damage. Spinal cord disruption, however, occurs after approximately $\frac{1}{4}$-inch of distraction.[19]

In the few adult cases reported, 50% were thought to be due to a concussive injury to the bone, with subsequent transmission to the spinal cord.[20]

The literature contains 29 reported cases of SCIWORA due to traumatic disk herniations. In each case, the patient returned to normal neurologic function after treatment. Also, Bondurant and Oro[4] suggested an association between Arnold-Chiari malformation type I and SCIWORA in four children.

Clinical Presentation

Virtually all reported SCIWORA cases describe a transient, often nonspecific neurologic syndrome followed within hours to days by the onset of more severe symptoms, up to and including quadriplegia. In most instances, no "secondary injury" could be identified.[1,12,13] The reported incidence of this type of delayed onset of SCIWORA varies, exceeding 50% in some series.[1,6,12–14] Although the underlying mechanism is far from clear, it is suspected that the pathophysiologic factors previously described play a significant role in making the spine/spinal cord more susceptible to a seemingly trivial and perhaps unperceived second insult, which precipitates the ultimate neurologic manifestations.

Pollack et al[13] studied a further variation of the delayed presentation of SCIWORA. Eight children suffered further neurologic injury in spite of 2 months of immobilization with collars and restrictions on activity. There was a clear inciting traumatic incident in seven of the eight children and, in many cases, activity limitations were ignored and collars were discarded. This, however, suggests that healing of the spinal ligamentous injuries may be prolonged, even in a young population.

Magnetic Resonance Imaging in SCIWORA

MRI findings have been reported in 45 reported cases of SCIWORA (15 adults and 30 children).[2,20–22] The incidence of MRI abnormalities appears to be greater in adults (14 out of 15) than in children (19 out of 30).

Grabb and Pang[22] reviewed MRIs in seven children with SCIWORA and found no extraaxial compressive lesions. They concluded that MRI in SCIWORA "probably influences its acute management infrequently." However, these same authors did identify two significant ligamentous injuries on MRIs in this small series of patients.

SCIWORA Management

Virtually all authors on this subject recommend a complete workup in any child presenting with transient neurologic deficits after suspected spine trauma. This workup includes adequate spine x-rays, CT scans of any inadequately visualized area or any area that is suspicious for injury, and flexion/extension views. It must be recognized, however, that "normal" flexion/extension films may not rule out SCIWORA because, when muscle spasm is present, suboptimal studies may be obtained. Additionally, flexion/extension films are generally accomplished in a gentle fashion in a supervised setting, which in no way simulates real-life situations. MRI is indicated if all of the above studies are normal. SEPs may be useful in documenting and following any subclinical electrophysiologic spinal cord dysfunction.

If SCIWORA is diagnosed, a period of supervised immobilization, appropriate restriction of activity, and follow-up radiographic investigation is necessary. Immobilization for 2 to 3 months with intensive child and parental education is advisable. Repeat flexion/extension films should be obtained 2 to 3 weeks after the initial injury and before immobilization is discontinued.

Pearl

If SCIWORA is diagnosed, a period of supervised immobilization, appropriate restriction of activity, and follow-up radiographic investigation is necessary.

Recommendations (Level III)

1. Trivial spinal trauma with accompanying neurologic complaints in a child must be taken seriously.
2. SCIWORA is a diagnosis of exclusion requiring careful and complete workup, frequently including MRI and SEPs.
3. Treatment of SCIWORA requires appropriate patient and family education, especially about the importance of maintaining spinal immobilization. Adequate immobilization for 2 to 3 months is advisable. Confirmation of either healing or lack of stability with appropriate postinjury radiographic investigations should be considered.

References

1. Pang D, Wilberger JE Jr. Spinal cord injury without radiographic abnormalities in children. J Neurosurg 1982;57:114–129.
2. Beck A, Gebhard F, Kinzl L. Spinal cord injury without radiographic abnormalities in children and adolescents: case report of a severe cervical spine lesion and review of the literature. Knee Surg Sports Traumatol Arthrosc 2000;8:186–189.
3. Burke DC. Traumatic spinal paralysis in children. Paraplegia 1974;11:268–276.
4. Bondurant CP, Oro JJ. Spinal cord injury without radiographic abnormality and Chiari malformation. J Neurosurg 1993;79: 833–838.
5. Cheshire DJ. The pediatric syndrome of traumatic myelopathy without demonstrable vertebral injury. Paraplegia 1977;15: 74–85.
6. Dickman CA, Rekate HL, Sonntag VK, et al. Pediatric spinal trauma: vertebral column and spinal cord injuries in children. Pediatr Neurosci 1989;15:237–256.
7. Dickman CA, Zabramski JM, Hadley MN, et al. Pediatric spinal cord injury without radiographic abnormalities: report of 26 cases and review of the literature. J Spinal Disord 1991;4:296–305.
8. Kriss VM, Kriss TC. SCIWORA (spinal cord injury without radiographic abnormality) in infants and children. Clin Pediatr (Phila) 1996;35:119–124.
9. MacMillan M, Stauffer ES. Transient neurologic deficits associated with thoracic and lumbar spine trauma without fracture or dislocation. Spine 1990;15:466–469.
10. Melzak J. Paraplegia among children. Lancet 1969;2:45–48.
11. Osenbach RK, Menezes AH. Spinal cord injury without radiographic abnormality in children. Pediatr Neurosci 1989;15: 168–175.
12. Pang D, Pollack IF. Spinal cord injury without radiographic abnormality in children—the SCIWORA syndrome. J Trauma 1989;29:654–664.
13. Pollack IF, Pang D, Sclabassi R. Recurrent spinal cord injury without radiographic abnormality in children. J Neurosurg 1988;69:177–182.
14. Walsh JW, Stevens DB, Young AB. Traumatic paraplegia in children without contiguous spinal fracture or dislocation. Neurosurgery 1983;12:439–445.
15. Aufdermaur M. Spinal injuries in juveniles: necropsy findings in twelve cases. J Bone Joint Surg Br 1974;56B:513–519.
16. Kewalramani LS, Tori JA. Spinal cord trauma in children: neurologic patterns, radiologic features, and pathomechanics of injury. Spine 1980;5:11–18.
17. Kewalramani LS, Kraus JF, Sterling HM. Acute spinal cord lesions in the pediatric population: epidemiological and clinical features. Paraplegia 1980;18:206–219.
18. Bailey DK. The normal cervical spine in infants and children. Radiology 1952;59:712–719.
19. Leventhal HR. Birth injuries of the spinal cord. J Pediatr 1960;56:447–453.
20. Gupta SK, Rajeev K, Khosla VK, et al. Spinal cord injury without radiographic abnormality in adults. Spinal Cord 1999;37: 726–729.
21. Felsberg GJ, Tein RD, Osumi AK, et al. Utility of MR imaging in pediatric spinal cord injury. Pediatr Radiol 1995;25:131–135.
22. Grabb PA, Pang D. Magnetic resonance imaging in the evaluation of spinal cord injury without radiographic abnormality in children. Neurosurgery 1994;35:406–414.

Spinal Cord Injury

Surgical Treatment

39

Do I Need to Decompress Patients with Spinal Cord Injury Right Away?

Lali H.S. Sekhon and Michael G. Fehlings

Brief Answer

Despite strong experimental evidence that early decompression after acute spinal cord injury (SCI) improves outcome in animal models, no class I or class II evidence indicates that decompression, either early or late, improves outcome in patients. However, numerous retrospective studies, anecdotes, and case reports document the benefit of surgery (both acute and even many months after injury) for spinal cord decompression. It is quite possible that the prospective studies that have investigated the timing of decompression did not use a sufficiently short time window; that is, they did not perform "early decompression" soon enough. No level I or level II recommendations regarding this intervention can be made. Early decompression can thus be viewed only as a treatment option. Clinical experience, however, suggests that early intervention should be considered in patients with bilaterally jumped facets and in patients with incomplete SCI who demonstrate neurologic deterioration.

Background

Despite the widespread use of operative intervention in patients with acute SCI in North America, the role of surgery in enhancing neurologic recovery remains controversial because of the lack of well-designed and well-executed randomized controlled trials. Experimental evidence from animal models suggests that early decompression of the spinal cord improves recovery after SCI.[1] However, using these animal models to determine the time window for the effective application of decompression in the clinical setting is difficult. So far, clinical studies that have examined the role of surgical decompression in SCI are limited to class II and class III evidence.

Literature Review

The Role of Conservative Management

Prior to evaluating the role of surgery in the management of SCI, one must, for comparative purposes, examine the results of conservative, nonoperative treatment. The nonoperative approach has been advocated by those who adhere to the tenets of Sir Ludwig Guttmann, founder of the Stoke-Mandeville Hospital in England. Guttmann used postural techniques combined with bed rest to achieve reduction and spontaneous fusion of the spine. Operative approaches were used only rarely because of a higher incidence of neurologic complications and poor recovery with laminectomy (class III data).[2,3]

Spontaneous improvement in neurologic status with conservative therapy alone has been demonstrated in several more recent studies (class III data).[4,5] Accordingly, any beneficial results of surgical treatment need to be weighed against any spontaneous recovery that might occur after SCI. Indeed, some authors have reported that neither spinal surgery nor anatomic realignment of the spinal column improves neurologic outcome in patients with acute SCI, with the possible exception of those with bilateral locked facets (class III data).[6,7]

Pearl

Spontaneous improvement in neurologic status often occurs with conservative therapy alone. This phenomenon makes it important to include a control group in any surgical study.

To date, studies of nonoperative management have been limited to noncontrolled, retrospective analyses of clinical databases and accordingly provide class III evidence. Furthermore, it is now well recognized that laminectomy as the sole surgical technique is contraindicated in most cases of acute SCI because it usually fails to produce adequate decompression of the cord and often causes spinal instability, which in and of itself may lead to neurologic deterioration.

The Role and Timing of Decompressive Surgery

Although meticulous conservative care remains the cornerstone of SCI management, surgical techniques have evolved considerably since the era of Guttmann. Furthermore, use of a policy of exclusively nonoperative treatment of SCI would have major limitations. Up to 10% of patients with incomplete cervical SCI who undergo an exclusively conservative management protocol may neurologically deteriorate (class III data).[8] For such reasons, the role of prompt surgical management has been revisited. With a few notable exceptions, most studies consist of retrospective case series, sometimes with historical controls (i.e., class III evidence). These studies offer no clear consensus as to the appropriate timing of surgical intervention, and they provide no compelling evidence that decompression influences the neurologic outcome after SCI.[8,9]

The benefits of early reduction of dislocations of the spine by either open or closed techniques are difficult to evaluate in the absence of randomization (class III studies).[9,10] Accounts of impressive neurologic recovery in cervical injuries decompressed early by traction must be considered anecdotal (class III data).[11] Moreover, some studies have not found any neurologic benefit to reduction (class III data),[6,7] with the possible exception of patients with bilateral facet dislocation (class III data).[12] Aebi et al[9] retrospectively examined the records of 100 patients with cervical spine injuries and attempted to relate neurologic recovery to the timing of the reduction by closed manual traction or open surgical reduction (class III data). A manual or surgical reduction was performed within the first 6 hours after the accident in only 25% of the cases and within the first 24 hours in 57%. Overall, 31% of the 100 patients demonstrated neurologic improvement, and 75% of the recoveries were in patients reduced manually or surgically within the first 6 hours. Mirza et al[10] retrospectively reviewed 30 patients who sustained cervical spine injuries and underwent surgical decompression and stabilization either within or beyond 72 hours (class III data). They suggested that the group that underwent early surgery exhibited immediate postoperative neurologic improvement without an increased complication rate.

Pearl

Strong consideration should be given to reducing bilaterally jumped facets with cord compression as soon as possible.

In contrast to the aforementioned studies of early decompression, Larson and coworkers[13] advocated delaying surgery for a week or more after SCI to allow medical and neurologic stabilization of the injured patient (class III data). This remains the practice in many institutions, particularly in light of reports suggesting an increased risk of neurologic deterioration with early surgery, that is, less than 6 days after SCI (class II data).[14] Interestingly, several authors have documented recovery of neurologic function after delayed decompression of the spinal cord even months to years after the injury (class III data).[15–17] Although these studies are retrospective in design, the reported improvement in neurologic function after delayed decompression in patients with cervical or thoracolumbar SCI who have plateaued in their recovery is noteworthy and suggests that ongoing compression of the cord may be an important contributing cause of persistent neurologic deficits.

Although many studies have described the effects of surgical decompression in SCI patients,[9,10,13,15–36] relatively few investigations into the optimal timing of decompression have been conducted in a prospective or controlled manner. In a retrospective analysis of prospectively collected data on 208 patients with acute spinal cord or cauda equina injury, Tator and colleagues[30] compared the results after surgery (56% of patients) to those of nonoperative management (44%). Operative management was associated with a lower overall mortality rate (6.1%) than nonoperative treatment (15.2%) despite a higher rate of thromboembolic complications in the surgical group. Overall, however, there was no difference between operated and nonoperated patients in length of stay or in neurologic recovery.

In an analysis of the National Acute Spinal Cord Injury Study (NASCIS) II database (class II evidence), Duh et al[24] reported that patients undergoing acute surgery (within 25 hours of injury) exhibited a nonsignificant trend toward better outcomes when compared with those treated nonoperatively. Interestingly, results of surgery were similar in the early (within 25 hours) and delayed (beyond 200 hours) groups. In other class II studies, Vaccaro et al[31] and Waters et al[34] could not document a beneficial effect of surgical decompression. It is noteworthy, however, that all patients underwent delayed operative management (average time >14 days after injury) in the study by Waters et al,[34] and in the study of Vaccaro et al,[31] "early" surgery was defined as that occurring as late as 72 hours after SCI. Moreover, although the study by Vaccaro et al was a prospective, randomized trial, 20 of the 62 patients (32%) were lost to follow-up. It is this high rate of patient attrition that leads us to classify the study by Vaccaro et al as class II evidence.

The Effect of Surgery on Complication Rate and Length of Stay after Spinal Cord Injury

Considerable controversy has surrounded the question of whether surgery, especially early surgery, increases the rate of complications in patients with SCI. Many SCI patients with complete high cervical injuries or significant associated injuries to the limbs or viscera are critically ill due to hemodynamic or respiratory difficulties. However, there is no compelling evidence that early surgery increases the rate of complications.

Pearl

Surgical intervention does not increase the rate of complications or the length of hospital stay.

The debate about early decompression has been reviewed in detail by Fehlings and Tator,[37] and the reader is referred to that publication for more in-depth analysis. Clearly, to better define the role of surgery in the management of acute SCI, randomized, controlled, prospective trials are required.

Conclusions

Strong experimental evidence suggests that decompression of the spinal cord improves recovery after SCI. However, it is difficult to use these results to determine the time window within which decompression may be effective in the clinical setting. Studies of secondary injury mechanisms, including ischemia, free radical–mediated lipid peroxidation, and calcium-mediated cytotoxicity, suggest that early intervention within hours of SCI is critical if a neuroprotective effect is to occur. Whether the same time window applies to surgical treatment is as yet unclear. So far, the clinical studies that have examined the role of surgical decompression in SCI provide only class II and class III evidence. Surgery remains a valid practice option, although there exist no conclusive data showing a benefit of surgery over conservative management. Limited class II evidence suggests that both early (within 25 hours) or delayed (beyond 200 hours) surgical intervention may be equally safe and effective. Randomized, controlled, prospective trials are required to better define the role of surgery in the management of acute SCI.

Recommendations

Level III: To date, the efficacy of decompression in patients with SCI is supported only by class III evidence. The literature does not allow definite conclusions to be drawn regarding appropriate timing of intervention.

References

1. Dimar JR II, Glassman SD, Raque GH, et al. The influence of spinal canal narrowing and timing of decompression on neurologic recovery after spinal cord contusion in a rat model. Spine 1999;24:1623–1633.
2. Guttmann L. Initial treatment of traumatic paraplegia and tetraplegia. In: Harris P, ed. Spinal Injuries Symposium. Edinburgh: Morrison & Gibb, Royal College of Surgeons; 1963: 80–92.
3. Guttmann L. Spinal Cord Injuries. Comprehensive Management and Research, 2nd ed. Philadelphia: JB Lippincott; 1976.
4. Tator CH, Duncan EG, Edmonds VE, et al. Neurological recovery, mortality and length of stay after acute spinal cord injury associated with changes in management. Paraplegia 1995;33: 254–262.
5. Wu L, Marino RJ, Herbison GJ, et al. Recovery of zero-grade muscles in the zone of partial preservation in motor complete quadriplegia. Arch Phys Med Rehabil 1992;73:40–43.
6. Dall DM. Injuries of the cervical spine, II: Does anatomical reduction of the bony injuries improve the prognosis for spinal cord recovery? S Afr Med J 1972;46:1083–1090.
7. Harris P, Karmi MZ, McClemont E, et al. The prognosis of patients sustaining severe cervical spine injury (C2–C7 inclusive). Paraplegia 1980;18:324–330.
8. Katoh S, El Masry WS, Jaffray D, et al. Neurologic outcome in conservatively treated patients with incomplete closed traumatic cervical spinal cord injuries. Spine 1996;21:2345–2351.
9. Aebi M, Mohler J, Zach GA, et al. Indication, surgical technique, and results of 100 surgically-treated fractures and fracture-dislocations of the cervical spine. Clin Orthop 1986;203:244–257.
10. Mirza SK, Krengel WF III, Chapman JR, et al. Early versus delayed surgery for acute cervical spinal cord injury. Clin Orthop 1999;359:104–114.
11. Brunette DD, Rockswold GL. Neurologic recovery following rapid spinal realignment for complete cervical spinal cord injury. J Trauma 1987;27:445–447.
12. Bedbrook GM. Spinal injuries with tetraplegia and paraplegia. J Bone Joint Surg Br 1979;61:267–284.
13. Larson SJ, Holst RA, Hemmy DC, et al. Lateral extracavitary approach to traumatic lesions of the thoracic and lumbar spine. J Neurosurg 1976;45:628–637.
14. Marshall LF, Knowlton S, Garfin SR, et al. Deterioration following spinal cord injury: a multicenter study. J Neurosurg 1987;66:400–404.
15. Anderson PA, Bohlman HH. Anterior decompression and arthrodesis of the cervical spine: long-term motor improvement, II: Improvement in complete traumatic quadriplegia. J Bone Joint Surg Am 1992;74:683–692.

16. Bohlman HH, Kirkpatrick JS, Delamarter RB, et al. Anterior decompression for late pain and paralysis after fractures of the thoracolumbar spine. Clin Orthop 1994;300:24–29.
17. Transfeldt EE, White D, Bradford DS, et al. Delayed anterior decompression in patients with spinal cord and cauda equina injuries of the thoracolumbar spine. Spine 1990;15:953–957.
18. Benzel EC, Larson SJ. Recovery of nerve root function after complete quadriplegia from cervical spine fractures. Neurosurgery 1986;19:809–812.
19. Benzel EC, Larson SJ. Functional recovery after decompressive spine operation for cervical spine fractures. Neurosurgery 1987;20:742–746.
20. Bohlman HH, Freehafer A, Dejak J. The results of treatment of acute injuries of the upper thoracic spine with paralysis. J Bone Joint Surg Am 1985;67:360–369.
21. Botel U, Glaser E, Niedeggen A. The surgical treatment of acute spinal paralysed patients. Spinal Cord 1997;35:420–428.
22. Chen TY, Dickman CA, Eleraky M, et al. The role of decompression for acute incomplete cervical spinal cord injury in cervical spondylosis. Spine 1998;23:2398–2403.
23. Donovan WH, Kopaniky D, Stolzmann E, et al. The neurological and skeletal outcome in patients with closed cervical spinal cord injury. J Neurosurg 1987;66:690–694.
24. Duh MS, Shepard MJ, Wilberger JE, et al. The effectiveness of surgery on the treatment of acute spinal cord injury and its relation to pharmacological treatment. Neurosurgery 1994;35: 240–248.
25. Krengel WF III, Anderson PA, Henley MB. Early stabilization and decompression for incomplete paraplegia due to a thoracic-level spinal cord injury. Spine 1993;18:2080–2087.
26. Levi L, Wolf A, Rigamonti D, et al. Anterior decompression in cervical spine trauma: does the timing of surgery affect the outcome? Neurosurgery 1991;29:216–222.
27. Maynard FM, Reynolds GG, Fountain S, et al. Neurological prognosis after traumatic quadriplegia. Three-year experience of California Regional Spinal Cord Injury Care System. J Neurosurg 1979;50:611–616.
28. Murphy KP, Opitz JL, Cabanela ME, et al. Cervical fractures and spinal cord injury: outcome of surgical and nonsurgical management. Mayo Clin Proc 1990;65:949–959.
29. Petitjean ME, Pointillard V, Daverat P, et al. Administration of methylprednisolone or nimodipine or both versus placebo at the acute phase of spinal cord injury. J Neurotrauma 1995;12: 456.
30. Tator CH, Duncan EG, Edmonds VE, et al. Comparison of surgical and conservative management in 208 patients with acute spinal cord injury. Can J Neurol Sci 1987;14:60–69.
31. Vaccaro AR, Daugherty RJ, Sheehan TP, et al. Neurologic outcome of early versus late surgery for cervical spinal cord injury. Spine 1997;22:2609–2613.
32. Vale FL, Burns J, Jackson AB, et al. Combined medical and surgical treatment after acute spinal cord injury: results of a prospective pilot study to assess the merits of aggressive medical resuscitation and blood pressure management. J Neurosurg 1997;87:239–246.
33. Wagner FC Jr, Chehrazi B. Early decompression and neurological outcome in acute cervical spinal cord injuries. J Neurosurg 1982;56:699–705.
34. Waters RL, Adkins RH, Yakura JS, et al. Effect of surgery on motor recovery following traumatic spinal cord injury. Spinal Cord 1996;34:188–192.
35. Weinshel SS, Maiman DJ, Baek P, et al. Neurologic recovery in quadriplegia following operative treatment. J Spinal Disord 1990;3:244–249.
36. Wolf A, Levi L, Mirvis S, et al. Operative management of bilateral facet dislocation. J Neurosurg 1991;75:883–890.
37. Fehlings MG, Tator CH. An evidence-based review of decompressive surgery in acute spinal cord injury: rationale, indications, and timing based on experimental and clinical studies. J Neurosurg 1999;91:1–11.

40

When Is Surgery Indicated for Patients with Gunshot Wounds to the Spine?

Robert F. Heary and Christopher M. Bono

Brief Answer

The role of surgery in the management of a gunshot wound to the spine (GSWS) is limited. In general, surgical decompression does not improve neurologic recovery after spinal cord injury (SCI) from a GSWS, but evidence suggests better motor recovery with operative decompression than with nonoperative treatment of gunshot wounds of the lumbar spine when the bullet is lodged in the spinal canal. At all levels, a progressive neurologic deficit associated with an intracanalicular bullet, bony fragment, or expanding hematoma is an indication for urgent surgical intervention. Surgery is rarely required for stabilization of fractures from gunshot wounds because the majority are stable injuries. If clinical suspicion warrants, dynamic flexion–extension views can be used to assess mechanical instability, which may require instrumentation and fusion. Surgical debridement is not indicated after transcolonic GSWSs because the lowest infection rates have been documented with 7 to 14 days of antibiotics without operative intervention. For persistent cutaneous cerebrospinal fluid (CSF) leak through bullet entry or exit sites, surgery should be considered to reduce the risk of meningitis.

Question 1: Does Spinal Decompression Improve Neurologic Recovery After Gunshot Wound to the Spine?

Background

GSWSs often result in SCI. More than half of these cases result in paraplegia or tetraplegia (class III data).[1] Compared with blunt trauma, gunshot injuries to the spine are more likely to produce complete injuries and are usually associated with stable fracture patterns that do not require surgical stabilization (class III data).[2–4]

Controversy

Although the beneficial effect of neural decompression for canal compromise after blunt spinal trauma is becoming increasingly accepted, the effectiveness of decompression after gunshot wounds is less clear. Both class II (prospective, nonrandomized) and class III (retrospective) evidence suggests that surgical decompression of cervical and thoracic gunshot wounds has no beneficial effect on the likelihood of neurologic recovery. However, class II evidence supports operative decompression for gunshot wounds at the T12 to L4 levels when a bullet remains in the spinal canal. No class I studies have investigated the surgical treatment of gunshot wounds to the spine.

Literature

Stauffer et al[2] retrospectively reviewed 185 cases of GSWS, half of which were treated with laminectomy and half with observation only (class III data). For complete lesions, the authors documented no appreciable return of neurologic function after either surgery or nonoperative management. With incomplete injuries, 71% of the decompressed spines and 76% of the nonoperated spines improved neurologically. Injuries near the thoracolumbar junction, which tended to be incomplete, were associated with better neurologic recovery than injuries to more cranial levels, which were more likely to be complete. Although the antibiotic regimen was not documented, four wound infections, six CSF fistulas, and six cases of late spinal instability were reported in the operative group. There were no cases of infection, CSF fistula, or spinal instability in the patients treated without surgery. Both groups had a high incidence of causalgia (19% and 13% for operative and nonoperative groups, respectively).

Further support of a nonoperative approach was provided by Robertson and Simpson,[5] who reported no increase in neurologic improvement after lumbar laminectomy versus nonsurgical treatment in 33 patients with gunshot wounds to the cauda equina region (class III data). They documented a high rate of postoperative complications. In no case did the authors report a bullet within the spinal canal.

In a prospective study, Waters and Adkins[6] demonstrated statistically significant motor improvement after surgical decompression between the T12 and L4 levels compared with nonoperatively treated GSWSs (class II data). Importantly, only patients with bullets lodged within the spinal canal were included. At more rostral sites in the thoracic and cervical regions, surgical removal of the bullet and decompression of the neural elements were not found to have a significant effect. No infections were reported in either group.

An important consideration is the timing of surgery. Cybulski et al[7] reported rates of occult abscess and arachnoiditis of 17% and 15%, respectively, if decompressive laminectomy of the lumbar spine was performed more than 2 weeks from the time of injury (class III data). In other reports, however, the majority of reported cutaneous CSF fistulas and spine infections have occurred after early surgical exploration (class III data).[2,8] Regardless of the level of injury, most authors agree that documented progression of a neurologic deficit, although quite rare, is an indication for urgent surgical decompression and possibly removal of the bullet. In the acute setting, a progressive neurologic deficit can result from an expanding subdural or extradural hematoma (class III data).[9]

Late bullet migration can cause neurologic deficits months to years after the initial injury. Kuijlen and associates[10] reported a case of neurogenic claudication 11 years after a gunshot wound to the abdomen (class III data). The bullet had migrated from the paraspinal muscles at the L3 level into the spinal canal, where it had disintegrated into multiple fragments that had caused a diffuse inflammatory reaction. The patient responded favorably to decompressive laminectomy and removal of the inflammatory mass. Conway et al[11] reported a case of cauda equina syndrome after a bullet previously lodged in an intervertebral disk migrated into the spinal canal 9 years after injury (class III data). Again, decompressive laminectomy and removal of the bullet and associated inflammatory mass were effective. Bullet migration within the spinal canal has been documented in numerous other cases.[12,13] However, because bullet migration or entry into the spinal canal is not always associated with neurologic deficit,[14] the advisability of bullet removal must be assessed on an individual basis.

Disk herniation after a GSWS is a rare but potentially significant cause of neurologic compromise (class III data).[15] Entry of a bullet into the intervertebral space is postulated to increase the pressure in the nucleus pulposus. If a defect exists in the posterior or posterolateral annulus, the disk material can be expelled into the canal or foramen, compressing the spinal cord or nerve root. Treatment recommendations are similar to those for other acute disk herniations. Significant and acute neurologic deficits may improve after disk excision. A disk herniation causing cauda equina syndrome is widely regarded to be a surgical emergency. Bullet removal is neither necessary nor indicated unless it can be accomplished easily, without further jeopardizing surrounding neural or bony supporting structures.

Pearl

Surgical decompression of intracanalicular bullets between T12 and L4 has been reported to produce statistically significant motor improvement.

Recommendations

For low-energy civilian GSWSs to the spine, most authors agree that surgical decompression of the cervical and thoracic spinal canal has little utility (level II). Substantial rates of postoperative complications with no demonstrable improvement in neurologic outcome lead to the general conclusion that surgery is not indicated in these regions. However, in the specific situation in which a neurologic deficit is associated with an intracanalicular bullet at the conus medullaris or cauda equina level, surgical decompression may be beneficial (level II).

Question 2: Do Spine Fractures from Gunshot Wounds Require Surgical Stabilization?

Background

In the terminology of the three-column spine model of Denis,[16] disruption of two or more columns of the spine may indicate spinal instability. In contrast to blunt trauma, two- or even three-column disruption from a GSWS is less likely to result in instability. In Denis's original work, the proposed mechanisms of injury implied an abrupt acceleration/deceleration of the body/spine in space. In the case of gunshot wounds, the body/spine can be considered stationary, and the bullet is the directional force. In the best-case scenario, a through-and-through bullet wound will only damage those structures that lie directly in its effective path. Low-energy gunshots have a narrower circumference of damage than high-energy wounds. These factors influence the amount of spinal instability after GSWSs. These concepts can be likened to a magician pulling a tablecloth from underneath a table that has been set with glasses and plates. The bullet acts as the tablecloth. If the tablecloth is pulled very quickly, the glasses and plates (i.e., the spinal elements) stay in place. If the table is pushed abruptly (i.e., motor vehicle accident), the contents will surely fall and break.

Controversy

Most spine fractures after gunshot wounds are stable injuries (class III data).[3] Interestingly, most cases of spinal instability after gunshot wounds may be associated with overly aggressive decompression (class III data).[2]

Literature

In the retrospective review by Stauffer et al,[7] 185 patients were treated either operatively or nonoperatively for GSWSs (class III data). The only cases of spinal instability occurred in the operative group (6%). These were attributed to removal of the posterior elements during laminectomy. Similarly, Kupcha and associates[3] reported no cases of instability from the GSWS itself in a retrospective review of 28 patients who sustained cervical gunshot wounds (class III data). Again, the only case of late instability occurred after decompressive laminectomy.

Recommendations

In general, the majority of gunshot wounds are stable injuries and do not require surgical stabilization (level III). If stability is questionable, careful flexion and extension radiographs of the spine can demonstrate pathologic mobility of adjacent spinal segments in an awake, cooperative, neurologically intact patient. For the cervical spine, commonly used criteria for radiographic instability are angulatory change exceeding 11 degrees or translation exceeding 3.5 mm between flexion and extension views (class III data).[17] In cases of instability, the affected segments can be stabilized with a variety of instrumentation and fusion constructs, detailed discussion of which is beyond the scope of this chapter.

Surgical decompression of spinal gunshot injuries can lead to vertebral instability (level III). Aggressive laminectomy with substantial removal of the facet joints and posterior elements can destabilize the spine. Laboratory studies suggest that instrumentation and fusion should be contemplated if total facetectomy has occurred, even if only unilateral.[18]

Pearl

The majority of spinal gunshot wounds are stable injuries that do not require surgical stabilization. Surgical decompression of these injuries can lead to spinal instability.

Question 3: Is Surgical Debridement Warranted After Transcolonic Gunshot Wounds to the Spine?

Background

Viscus perforations from gunshot wounds carry a high risk of spinal infection. The highest rates of infection (up to 88%) have been reported with colonic perforations that occur prior to the bullet entering the spine (class III data),[19] but not all authors agree with these results (class III data).[20] It is thought that the stomach and small bowel are sterile, but spinal infection has been associated with gunshot paths that violate these organs (class III data).[21]

Controversy

Because of high rates of infection, initial recommendations for transcolonic GSWSs called for careful observation and a low threshold for surgical debridement.[19] At the time of these studies, however, the role of proper antibiotic therapy was not appreciated. Subsequent authors examined the influence of the duration of broad-spectrum antibiotic administration on infection rates after transcolonic gunshot injuries. The lowest spinal infection rates after colonic perforation by GSWSs have been reported after antibiotics have been continued for at least several days (class III data)[22,23]; a reasonable average duration would seem to be at least 7 to 14 days after injury. Bullet removal and surgical debridement have been associated with higher rates of infection (class III data).[8] Barring other indications, such as neurologic deterioration or lead toxicity, bullet extraction is not advocated as a means to decrease infection risk (class III data).[24] As far as the authors are aware, no class I or II studies have investigated this issue.

Literature

Romanick et al[19] retrospectively reviewed the charts of 20 nonoperated patients who had sustained low-velocity gunshot wounds to the abdomen with associated spinal fractures or disk space disruptions (class III data). No infections occurred in eight patients without a viscus perforation. Twelve patients had a viscus injury that occurred before the projectile hit the spinal column. Spinal infection (meningitis, paraspinal abscess, or vertebral osteomyelitis) developed in seven of eight patients with a transcolonic injury. No infection developed in the four patients with associated gastric or small bowel perforations. Although the authors concluded that early surgical debridement may be indicated in transcolonic GSWSs, the antibiotic regimens that the patients received were variable. All patients received a minimum of 2 days of broad-spectrum coverage, and six of the seven infections developed in patients who received a maximum of only 5 days of antibiotic prophylaxis.

In a subsequent retrospective study, Roffi et al[23] examined outcomes in 42 patients with gunshot wounds with an associated viscus perforation that occurred prior to the spinal injury (class III data). Information about antibiotic administration was available for 21 patients. Antibiotics were continued for an average of 11 days after injury. Three patients developed spinal infections. One case of meningitis was reported after a gastric perforation. Surprisingly, that patient had been on antibiotics continuously up to the time that he developed meningitis. Two of the 14 colonic injuries resulted in paraspinal (psoas) abscesses, one in a patient who received only 6 days of prophylaxis.

Recommendations

The role of surgical debridement after transcolonic injury seems to be limited after low-velocity civilian GSWSs. The lowest documented infection rates have been demonstrated after approximately 7 to 14 days (at least) of broad-spectrum antibiotics (level III recommendation).[22,23] The authors prefer a nonoperative approach to gunshot wounds that pierce a hollow viscus prior to lodging in the spine (level II recommendation). To the authors' knowledge, there are no prospective investigations comparing the effects of antibiotic prophylaxis with or without surgical debridement. Because of the substantially greater rate of infection in surgically versus nonsurgically managed patients after gunshot wounds in general (class III data),[8] as well as the relatively low risk associated with leaving retained bullets in situ (class III data),[25] it would be difficult to justify such a study. Nonetheless, a prospective investigation of a standardized antibiotic protocol for transabdominal gunshot wounds to the spine could be informative. Importantly, these recommendations are applicable only to low-energy injuries because high-energy wounds (AK-47, M-16, military assault weapons, etc.) may more often require surgical intervention for extensive soft tissue loss and for life-threatening systemic injuries (class III data).[26,27]

Pearl

Surgical debridement of the spine has only a limited role in transcolonic injuries from low-velocity civilian gunshot wounds. The lowest infection rates have been associated with approximately 1 to 2 weeks of broad-spectrum antibiotics.

Question 4: Should Bullets Be Removed from the Spine to Prevent Lead Toxicity?

Background

Lead intoxication is a recognized complication that may arise from retained bullets (class III data).[28,29] Among other complications, lead toxicity may cause anemia and progressive motor neuropathy. Because synovial fluid appears to be an effective solvent (class III data),[30] bullet removal from appendicular joints has been recommended. On the other hand, lead elution from bullets bathed in CSF seems to be rare. Accordingly, bullets in close proximity to facet joints (i.e., synovial joints) may be more likely to cause lead intoxication (class III data).[31] Of interest, plumbism has also been reported in association with a bullet lodged in an intervertebral disk.

Controversy

Lead intoxication is a rarely reported complication of spinal gunshot wounds (class III data).[8,28,31,32] If it occurs, however, removal of the bullet should be considered in addition to appropriate drug therapy.

Literature

Lead toxicity after GSWSs has been described only in case reports. Grogan and Bucholz[31] reported acute lead poisoning 12 years after an initial injury in which a bullet became lodged in an intervertebral disk (class III data).[31] Though the diagnosis was missed for more than 2 weeks, gingival biopsy definitively revealed lead particles. Preoperative treatment with chelating agents, including dimercaprol, calcium disodium edetate, and oral D-penicillamine, was followed by surgical removal of the bullet, with good results.

Another potential source of toxicity is copper-jacketed bullets in the spinal canal. In vivo experiments in monkeys have demonstrated the local necrotic effect of copper powder on brain tissue.[33] Some postulate that copper-jacketed bullets might have a similar effect on human spinal cord tissue.

Recommendations

Because the diagnosis of lead intoxication requires a high level of suspicion, it may often be missed. Blood testing can reveal abnormally high levels. When documented lead intoxication occurs, treatment with chelating agents is initiated immediately. If pharmacologic treatment alone is insufficient, it should be followed by carefully planned bullet removal (level III recommendation). Delaying surgery until a patient has received pharmacologic therapy for a sufficient period of time, for example, until blood levels of lead have decreased to less dangerous or even normal levels, may help prevent a sudden and potentially disastrous flush of lead into the bloodstream during operative manipulation. For the majority of cases, however, most authors would agree that bullet removal to prevent plumbism after GSWSs is not necessary, regardless of the location of the bullet fragments.

Some authors recommend removal of copper-containing bullets from the spinal canal to prevent progressive damage to neural tissue (level III recommendation).[34] A major clinical challenge is determining the composition of the bullet, which in many instances is not known preoperatively.

Question 5: Do All Cerebrospinal Fluid Leaks After Gunshot Wounds to the Spine Require Repair?

Background

CSF leak may occur after GSWS. Persistence of a leak can predispose to meningitis or to formation of a cutaneous CSF fistula. Accurate diagnosis of a CSF leak is crucial to making treatment decisions. CSF must be differentiated from other sources of clear wound drainage. Assay of a sample of the collected fluid for β_2-transferrin has been recommended because β_2-transferrin immunofixation is a very specific test for confirming the presence of CSF (class III data).[35]

Controversy

Surgical intervention to repair dural injuries resulting in CSF leaks after GSWSs may seem intuitively appealing. Other clinicians, however, might consider more conservative management, such as the placement of a subarachnoid drain, as a first course of treatment, reserving open dural repair for refractory cases.

Literature

Robertson and Simpson[5] reported two CSF fistulas and one pseudomeningocele in a review of 33 patients with penetrating injuries of the cauda equina (class III data). Of note, these complications occurred only in surgically treated cases. Similarly, Stauffer et al[2] documented a 6% incidence of CSF fistulas in operatively treated gunshot wounds, but no such complications in conservatively managed patients (class III data). Unfortunately, the treatment of this complication is not described in these studies. Our review did not uncover any reported series specifically focusing on CSF leaks or fistulas after GSWSs.

Recommendations

In the initial treatment of gunshot wound patients, the bullet entry site should be treated with debridement of any devitalized skin and superficial soft tissues. If a CSF leak appears to be present, a lumbar subarachnoid drain should be placed (level III recommendation). When a persistent CSF leak is present through the bullet entry or exit sites at the level of the skin, open surgery should be considered.[5,34] Because of the risk of meningitis from a persistent CSF leak, the treatment would involve a laminectomy with repair of the dural violation either primarily or by use of a dural graft (level III recommendation).[34] In these relatively rare instances, placement of a temporary lumbar subarachnoid drain after the laminectomy may help protect the dural repair.

Pearl

A lumbar subarachnoid drain should be considered as the first option for treating a CSF leak after a GSWS. Persistent CSF leakage through bullet entry or exit sites may require open surgery.

References

1. Young JA, Burns PE, Bowen AM, et al. Spinal Cord Injury Statistics: Experience of the Regional Spinal Cord Injury Systems. Phoenix: Good Samaritan Medical Center; 1982.
2. Stauffer ES, Wood RW, Kelly EG. Gunshot wounds of the spine: the effects of laminectomy. J Bone Joint Surg Am 1979;61: 389–392.

3. Kupcha PC, An HS, Cotler JM. Gunshot wounds to the cervical spine. Spine 1990;15:1058–1063.
4. Farmer JC, Vaccaro AR, Balderston RA, et al. The changing nature of admissions to a spinal cord injury center: violence on the rise. J Spinal Disord 1998;11:400–403.
5. Robertson DP, Simpson RK. Penetrating injuries restricted to the cauda equina: a retrospective review. Neurosurgery 1992;31: 265–269.
6. Waters RL, Adkins RH. The effects of removal of bullet fragment retained in the spinal canal: a collaborative study by the National Spinal Cord Injury Model Systems. Spine 1991;16: 934–939.
7. Cybulski GR, Stone JL, Kant R. Outcome of laminectomy for civilian gunshot injuries of the terminal spinal cord and cauda equina: review of 88 cases. Neurosurgery 1989;24:392–397.
8. Heary RF, Vaccaro AR, Mesa JJ, et al. Thoracolumbar infections in penetrating injuries to the spine. Orthop Clin North Am 1996;27:69–81.
9. Weinshel S, Maiman D. Spinal subdural hematoma presenting as an epidural hematoma following gunshot wound: report of a case. J Spinal Disord 1988;1:317–319.
10. Kuijlen JM, Herpers MJ, Beuls EA. Neurogenic claudication, a delayed complication of a retained bullet. Spine 1997;22: 910–914.
11. Conway JE, Crofford TW, Terry AF, et al. Cauda equina syndrome occurring nine years after a gunshot injury to the spine: a case report. J Bone Joint Surg Am 1993;75:760–763.
12. Gupta S, Senger RL. Wandering intraspinal bullet. Br J Neurosurg 1999;13:606–607.
13. Oktem IS, Selcuklu A, Kurtsoy A, et al. Migration of bullet in the spinal canal: a case report. Surg Neurol 1995;44:548–550.
14. Jeffery JA, Borgstein R. Case report of a retained bullet in the lumbar spinal canal with preservation of cauda equina function. Injury 1998;29:724–726.
15. Robertson DP, Simpson RK, Narayan RK. Lumbar disc herniation from a gunshot wound to the spine: a report of two cases. Spine 1991;16:994–995.
16. Denis F. The three column spine and its significance in the classification of acute thoracolumbar spine injuries. Spine 1983;8: 817–831.
17. White AA, Panjabi MM. Clinical Biomechanics of the Spine. Philadelphia: Lippincott; 1990.
18. Abumi K, Panjabi MM, Kramer KM, et al. Biomechanical evaluation of lumbar spinal stability after graded facetectomies. Spine 1990;15:1142–1147.
19. Romanick PC, Smith TK, Kopaniky DR, et al. Infection about the spine associated with low-velocity-missile injury to the abdomen. J Bone Joint Surg Am 1985;67:1195–1201.
20. Kihtir T, Ivatury RR, Simon R, et al. Management of transperitoneal gunshot wounds of the spine. J Trauma 1991;31: 1579–1583.
21. Hales DD, Duffy K, Dawson EG, et al. Lumbar osteomyelitis and epidural and paraspinous abscesses: case report of an unusual source of contamination from a gunshot wound to the abdomen. Spine 1991;16:380–383.
22. Kumar A, Wood GW II, Whittle AP. Low-velocity gunshot injuries of the spine with abdominal viscus trauma. J Orthop Trauma 1998;12:514–517.
23. Roffi RP, Waters RL, Adkins RH. Gunshot wounds to the spine associated with a perforated viscus. Spine 1989;14:808–811.
24. Lin SS, Vaccaro AR, Reich SM, et al. Low-velocity gunshot wounds to the spine with an associated transperitoneal injury. J Spinal Disord 1995;8:136–144.
25. Velmahos G, Demetriades D. Gunshot wounds of the spine: should retained bullets be removed to prevent infection? Ann R Coll Surg Engl 1994;76:85–87.
26. Parsons TW III, Lauerman WC, Ethier DB, et al. Spine injuries in combat troops—Panama, 1989. Mil Med 1993;158:501–502.
27. Simpson RK Jr, Venger BH, Fischer DK, et al. Shotgun injuries of the spine: neurosurgical management of five cases. Br J Neurosurg 1988;2:321–326.
28. Linden MA, Manton WI, Stewart RM, et al. Lead poisoning from retained bullets: pathogenesis, diagnosis, and management. Ann Surg 1982;195:305–313.
29. Machle W. Lead absorption from bullets lodged in tissues. JAMA 1940;115:1536–1541.
30. Leonard MH. The solution of lead by synovial fluid. Clin Orthop 1969;64:255–261.
31. Grogan DP, Bucholz RW. Acute lead intoxication from a bullet in an intervertebral disc space: a case report. J Bone Joint Surg Am 1981;63:1180–1182.
32. Cagin CR, Diloy-Puray M, Westerman MP. Bullets, lead poisoning and thyrotoxicosis. Ann Intern Med 1978;89:509–511.
33. Chusid JG, Kopeloff LM. Epileptogenic effects of metal powder implants in the motor cortex in monkeys. Int J Neuropsychiatry 1967;3:24–28.
34. Wigle RL. Treatment of asymptomatic gunshot injuries to the spine. Am Surg 1989;55:591–595.
35. Bateman N, Jones NS. Rhinorrhoea feigning cerebrospinal fluid leak: nine illustrative cases. J Laryngol Otol 2000;114:462–464.

♦ Part V ♦

Postacute Care

◆ 41 ◆

What Is the Outcome of Patients with Mild, Moderate, or Severe Traumatic Brain Injury?

Peter B. Letarte

Brief Answer

Even under the best of circumstances, severe traumatic brain injury (TBI) has a mortality rate of 30 to 36%. Approximately 5% of patients remain vegetative, 15% severely disabled, and 15 to 20% moderately disabled. Good recovery can be expected in more than 25% of patients. The following breakdown of outcomes has been reported after moderate TBI: 60% good recovery, 25% moderate disability, 7% severe disability, 1% persistent vegetative state, and 7% mortality. It must be remembered, however, that even patients with "good outcomes" after moderate or severe TBI may have significant cognitive and emotional difficulties that prevent their reintegration into society. For mild TBI, the mortality rate is quite low. Thus, outcome from these injuries is often discussed in terms of the development and duration of such complaints as headache, decreased energy, dizziness, and a host of other postconcussive symptoms. Although such symptoms are not unusual, their duration tends to be self-limited in the majority of cases.

Background

Different Perspectives on Outcome

The first step in answering the question, What is the outcome of patients with mild, moderate, and severe head injury? is consideration of what different people mean by *outcome*, and in particular by the term *good outcome*. To neurosurgeons, a good outcome might mean survival or a return of the ability to care for oneself, whereas to the patient's family it might mean a return to premorbid status. To an insurer it might mean a rapid end to the need for ongoing payments. The original International classification of Impairments, Disabilities, and Handicaps (ICIDH)[1] looked at outcome from four perspectives: pathology, impairment, disability, and handicap.

Pathology

Most neurosurgeons view outcome from the perspective of pathology. This approach focuses on clinical findings, such as a subdural hematoma, and their effect on a patient's outcome. This view of outcome is often what dominates discussions with family and other providers early in a patient's hospital course. During this time period, a focus of this type is often essential for a patient's survival. Such an emphasis, however, does not address the main concerns of families and loved ones about return to premorbid status and future lifestyle.

Impairment

The impairment view of outcome looks at the functional consequences of the underlying pathology, such as weakness, personality change, or aphasia. To patients and their families, impairments are the primary focus of concern.

Disability

Disability is the loss of function caused by an impairment. For example, an accountant and a bricklayer may have identical impairment of concentration after a frontal lobe injury. The bricklayer, however, may be able to return to his previous employment with minimum disability, whereas the accountant may no longer be able to function in her job, resulting in major disability.

Handicap

Handicap is the social disruption that results from a disability. In the above example of the bricklayer, his impairment of concentration may not result in any handicap as he resumes most of his previous life. The accountant, on the other hand, may experience significant alterations of her lifestyle because of her significant handicap.

Practical Considerations

Ideally, evidence-based studies of outcome would explore the impact of mild, moderate, and severe head injury on impairment, disability, and handicap. However, such studies are very time-consuming and expensive. For this reason, most outcomes research focuses on much simpler end points, such as death, or on simple scoring systems such as the Glasgow Outcome Scale[2] (GOS) or the Disability Rating Scale.[3]

Pearl

Good outcome means different things to different people. A broad perspective on outcome can be maintained by remembering the ICIDH model that considers outcome with respect to pathology, impairment, disability, and handicap.

Prognostication

Prognostic Variables

Many characteristics can be used as prognostic variables to predict outcome from head injury. Patient age, findings on computed tomography (CT) scan, findings on neurologic examination, the presence of fixed and dilated pupils, and the presence of hypotension have all been used to build models for the prediction of outcome from head injury. All of these models, however, are derived from studies of very specifically defined patient populations, from which attempts are often made to formulate generalizable, evidence-based recommendations.[4]

Application of the results of such studies to particular patients is often hampered by the fact that head-injured patients are not a homogeneous group. Choi et al[5] have demonstrated that predictors are population-specific; different predictors of outcome will have varying significance in different patient populations (class II data). For example, the important predictors of outcome for a 40-year-old are likely to be different from those for a 10-year-old, and patients with fixed and dilated pupils have a different order of importance for predictors of outcome than patients with normal pupils. Before clinicians use any outcome studies in their clinical practices, they need to be sure that they appreciate how their particular patients are both different from and similar to those in the outcomes studies that they are reviewing.

Glasgow Coma Scale

In reality, the question, What is the outcome of patients with mild, moderate and severe head injury? is simply asking what is known about the Glasgow Coma Scale (GCS) as a predictor of outcome from TBI, because the categories of mild, moderate, and severe head injury are usually based on the GCS score.

Without question, the GCS has become an extremely powerful tool for the initial and early assessment of TBI patients. It is easy to learn, widely disseminated, and extensively validated. However, clinicians should be aware that it may have important limitations. Many patients who present to emergency rooms cannot have their GCS score calculated. In one study, a full GCS score was not obtainable in 44% of patients, and 28% could not have their motor score assessed (class III data).[6] The principal reasons for such incompleteness are intubation in the field, which prevents assessment of the verbal score, and the early use of paralytics and sedatives in the emergency department. In addition, techniques for assigning the GCS may vary widely from institution to institution, potentially resulting in difficulties transferring results from one institution to another.

Furthermore, it appears that the predictive value of the GCS changes based on when in the patient's treatment course it is assessed. Using the initial GCS score as a basis for prediction, one study found that 68.6% of head-injured patients predicted to have a good outcome and 76.5% of those predicted to have a poor outcome actually had those outcomes at 1 year (class II data).[7] The predictive accuracy went up if a later GCS was used (obtained a mean of 7 days after injury), with 80.6% of those predicted to have a good outcome actually achieving such an outcome at 1 year. The ability to predict poor outcomes remained essentially unchanged at 78.6%.

Pearl

Resist the temptation to make definitive prognostications early in the patient's course, especially during resuscitation.

Accuracy of Prognostication

Even when the best efforts are made to apply evidence-based data to prediction of outcome from TBI, the results can be discouraging. Current methods often overestimate the likelihood of poor outcomes and underestimate the probability of good outcomes. Kaufmann et al[8] investigated the accuracy of an experienced neurosurgeon in using overall clinical assessment and initial CT scan results to predict outcome on the first day of admission (class III data). The predictive accuracy was only 56%. Because the "false pessimism rate" may be higher if predictions are based on assessments that are obtained very early in a patient's treatment, providers should be leery of making definitive predictions immediately after a patient is admitted to the hospital.

Thus, even in the best possible circumstances, outcome prediction is quite difficult in the head-injured population, especially early in a patient's course. These observations are disturbing in light of an observation made by Murray et al[9] in 1993 that physicians, when provided with models of outcome prediction after head injury, alter their care in response to these models (class III data). Use of therapies considered beneficial to the head-injured patient increased for those patients predicted to have a good outcome and decreased for those patients predicted to have a poor outcome.

Pearl

Most early evidence-based prognostications err on the side of being overly pessimistic. Be cautious with giving too firm a prognosis early in a patient's course, because such opinions really do influence the care given to patients.

Literature Review

Severe Head Injury

In 1977 Jennett et al[10] reported a 50% mortality rate from head injury in three countries (class II data). By 1987, the Traumatic Coma Data Bank (TCDB) in the United States was reporting a 36% mortality rate (class II data).[11] Although some would disagree, most people accept this difference as evidence of interval improvement in the treatment of TBI. These studies enrolled patients with severe TBI; that is, a GCS score of 3 to 8. Some investigators group patients differently. Narayan et al[12] examined the relationship between admission GCS score and outcome and found that a GCS score of 3 to 5 was associated with a poor outcome 77% of the time. A GCS score of 6 to 8 was associated with a poor outcome 26% of the time (class II data).

In terms of GOS categories, outcome of TCDB patients was as follows: 36% mortality, 5% vegetative state, 15% severe disability, 15 to 20% moderate disability, and 25% good recovery (class II data).[11] For specific GCS scores, mortality rates in the TCDB were 78.4% for an initial GCS of 3, 55.9% for a GCS of 4, and 40.2% for a GCS of 5 (class II data).[11] Patients with GCS scores of 3, 4, and 5 had good outcomes 4.1%, 6.3%, and 12.2% of the time, respectively (class II data).[11] These results are consistent with those of other studies, although further evidence suggests that particular types of pathology can affect outcomes. For example, one study showed worse outcomes at each GCS level when an acute subdural hematoma was present (class III data).[13]

Pearl

Any given predictive feature is contextual, and the relative prognostic importance of a particular feature changes with the presence or absence of other features. Beware of overgeneralizing the literature when attempting to predict outcome.

Early discussions of outcome in severe head injury tend to focus on the pathologic aspects of the injury and on patient survival rather than on the impairment, disability, and handicap issues that dominate the discussion of mild and moderate head injury. It should be noted, however, that these issues are immense for those who survive the acute posttraumatic period. Neuropsychological recovery lags well behind physical recovery in severe head injury, and cognitive and emotional sequelae that emerge after the physical recovery is complete may have a devastating and profound impact on the lives of brain injury survivors. These sequelae of severe TBI can continue to emerge months to years after severe head injury. Survivors of severe TBI often describe the immense effort it takes to continue living with these sequelae. Tate et al[14] found that only 24% of all severe head injury survivors have reasonable reintegration into society (class III data). Of those described as having good outcome or moderate disability on the GOS, less than 50% achieved good social reintegration.

Pearl

Warn families about, and be sensitive to, the difficulties with social reintegration that patients with severe, moderate, and even mild head injury may encounter.

Mild and Moderate Brain Injury

For most patients with mild or moderate brain injury, survival is generally not a major concern. The outcome focus for mild and moderate head injury is on impairment, disability, and handicap, and less on pathology. Because most patients survive and do not require dramatic resuscitative or therapeutic measures, many providers tend to inappropriately minimize the impact and importance of these injuries.

Mild Head Injury

Mild head injury has traditionally been defined in general terms as an injury caused by blunt trauma and/or sudden acceleration/deceleration that produces a period of unconsciousness for 20 minutes or less, no focal neurologic deficit, no intracranial complications, and CT findings limited to skull fracture (class III data).[15] Rimel et al[16] introduced the concept of using a GCS-based definition; that is, a GCS score of 13 to 15 (class III data). Not all discussions of mild head injury acknowledge such definitions, however, and the term *mild head injury* may be defined differently at different institutions. More recently, it has been proposed that the definition of *mild head injury* be expanded to include any patient with brief retrograde amnesia, even if loss of consciousness (LOC) has not occurred (class III data).[17] In addition, because the incidence of intracranial pathology in patients with a GCS score of 13 has been reported to be more like that of patients with GCS scores of 9 to 12 than that of patients with scores of 14 to 15 (class III data), it has been proposed that patients with head injuries resulting in a GCS score of 13 be included in the moderate head injury group, with the designation "mild traumatic brain injury" being reserved only for patients with GCS scores of 14 to 15.[18]

Pearl

Mild head injury may be characterized only by a period of posttraumatic amnesia. Loss of consciousness does not always occur after injuries that produce mild TBI.

It must be remembered that objective data about outcome after mild TBI are difficult to obtain. The magnitude of this problem should not be underestimated. Many patients with mild TBI are lost to follow-up after discharge from the emergency room. In addition, mild TBI is often not witnessed or recognized, and concomitant intoxication with alcohol or other drugs often obscures the initial presentation.

A term often used to describe a symptom complex that has been described after mild TBI is *postconcussion syndrome* (PCS). In a class II study, Levin et al[19] found that over 90% of patients complained of a wide variety of PCS symptoms within 1 week of injury, the most common being headache (71%), decreased energy (60%), and dizziness (53%). Rimel et al[16] found that, 3 months after injury, 79% of patients still complained of headaches, and 59% described memory problems (class II data). A third of the patients who had been employed before injury were unemployed 3 months postinjury. A class II study from Rutherford et al[20] showed that 51% of 131 patients complained of at least one PCS symptom 6 weeks after injury. One year after injury, 14.5% (19 patients) were still symptomatic, with six patients reporting one symptom, seven complaining of two symptoms, and six reporting more than two symptoms. Headache, irritability, and dizziness led a long list of complaints that were still present after 1 year.[21]

Pearl

Consider formal neuropsychological testing for patients who continue to experience postconcussive symptoms more than 6 weeks after mild TBI.

Pearl

A sizable percentage of patients with mild TBI still complain of at least one postconcussive symptom 1 year after injury.

In the same study, Rutherford et al[21] also addressed the question of whether de novo PCS symptoms can occur in a delayed fashion after an injury. They noticed that of the 19 patients who had symptoms at 1 year, nine had reported the same symptoms at 6 weeks, but 10 were reporting at least one new symptom that had not been present at 6 weeks. Of the second group, six patients (60%) were involved in litigation. Only two of the nine whose symptoms were not new (22%) were involved in litigation. On the other hand, Rimel et al[16] concluded that litigation and compensation have a minimal role in determining outcome in these patients. They suggested that emotional stress caused by persistent symptoms may be a significant factor in the long-term disability of patients with mild TBI.

Pearl

Postconcussion syndrome usually follows a steadily improving course. Exacerbations of symptoms or new symptoms may often be due to factors beyond the original injury.

Moderate Head Injury

The term *moderate head injury* is generally used to describe a GCS score of 9 to 12, but some authors also include patients with a GCS score of 13. Moderate head injuries constitute 7 to 28% of all head injuries (class III data).[22] In comparison to patients with mild head injuries, those with moderate head injuries have a much higher incidence of abnormalities on CT scanning, averaging ~40% in a report by Stein and Ross[18] (class III data). In many cases, repeat CT scans reveal delayed brain injury; that is, either new lesions or worsening of lesions that were seen on the initial CT scan.

Epidemiologic studies of moderate head injury reveal several characteristics of this population that may affect outcome. Among this group, 73% have a detectable blood alcohol level, 34% have a history of alcohol abuse, 42% have had a prior head injury, and 21% are chronically unemployed (class II and class III data).[22,23] The frequent presence of alcohol and other drugs may often affect the accuracy of GCS determination in these patients.[22] About one fifth of all patients presenting with an initial GCS score in the moderate range improve to the level of mild head injury within 6 hours of presentation (class II data).[23] On the other hand, perhaps 10% or more of these patients will deteriorate neurologically as evidenced by the need for intracranial pressure (ICP) monitoring and/or cranial surgery,[23] and as many as 25% of comatose head-injured patients in a large series were reported to be speaking prior to deterioration into coma.[24]

Although moderate head injuries often appear innocuous on presentation and rarely require ICP monitoring, their outcome is frequently quite unsatisfactory, and the impact of these injuries should not be minimized. Recovery from moderate head injury is much less rapid and much less complete than that from mild head injury. Only a third of patients return to work at 3 months (class III data),[23] and approximately one fourth still have not returned to their previous employment after 1 year (class III data).[25] Fully 50% have emotional or behavioral sequelae at 1 year (class III data).[22] Approximately 60% go on to make a good recovery, 26% have moderate disability, 7% are severely disabled, less than 1% remain vegetative, and almost 7% die (class III data).[22]

Pearl

Remember that 25% of all moderate head injury patients cannot return to their former jobs. Consider utilizing rehabilitation services liberally when planning follow-up for these patients.

Combining Mild and Moderate Traumatic Brain Injury

Traditionally, outcomes from mild head injury and moderate head injury have been discussed separately. A different approach was used in a class II study by van der Naalt et al,[25] who reported that for patients with a GCS score of 9 to 14, the duration of posttraumatic amnesia (PTA) outperforms the admission GCS score in terms of predicting the likelihood of developing the disabling impairments that are the focus of this injury category. One year after injury, 73% of those with a GCS score of 9 to 14 and at least 1 hour of PTA had returned to their previous jobs or study. However, 84% still reported complaints. The most common problems at 1 year included fatigue (45%), forgetfulness and poor concentration (42%), irritability (34%), and headache (32%). Although the mean GCS score of 12.6 indicates that this study population was skewed toward moderate head injury, its results demonstrate the devastating effect of these supposedly "unimportant" injuries, with 27% of the patients in the study not returning to their jobs after 1 year. These results are consistent with the findings of other studies of moderate TBI.

Conclusions

Fortunately, the vast majority of closed head injuries are mild and have few or no sequelae. However, as the severity of the injury increases, the incidence and severity of life-disrupting long-term sequelae also increase. Cognitive deficits, emotional difficulties, headache, and dizziness top the list of a wide variety of problems that may occur after closed head injury. The incidence and impact of these problems are often underestimated by practitioners. In the most severely injured patients, concern over these sequelae is generally subordinated to immediate treatment of the life-threatening aspects of the injury and to the shift of focus to the patient's survival.

Evidentiary Table

Choi 1991

Description of study: Twenty-three prognostic variables were retrospectively evaluated in 555 patients using prediction tree analysis to predict outcome.

Classification: Class II

Conclusion: The overall predictive accuracy of the technique was 77.7%.

Jennett 1977

Description of study: Collection of data on almost 700 severely head-injured patients in three countries.

Classification: Class II

Conclusion: Approximately 50% mortality observed in each center.

Kaufmann 1992

Description of study: A neurosurgeon and a neuroradiologist used data available soon after admission to predict outcome within 24 hours of injury in 100 consecutive head-injured patients.

Classification: Class III

Conclusion: The neurosurgeon tended to overestimate unfavorable outcomes, whereas the neuroradiologist overestimated favorable outcomes. The respective accuracy rates were 56% and 59%. When both predicted the same outcome, the accuracy rate was 73%.

Levin 1987

Description of study: Fifty-seven consecutive mild head injury patients at three centers underwent neurobehavioral testing within 1 week of injury and at 1 and 3 months after injury. Results were compared with those of 56 selected control subjects at three centers.

Classification: Class II

Conclusion: Although nearly all patients initially experienced symptoms, most had resolved at 3 months. Only rarely does a single mild head injury produce permanent impairment.

Marshall 1991

Description of study: Collection of data on 746 patients with severe TBI.

Classification: Class II

Conclusion: Overall mortality for all patients across the four participating centers was 36%. Mortality rate was 78.4% for an initial GCS of 3, 55.9% for a GCS of 4, and 40.2% for a GCS of 5.

Murray 1993

Description of study: Investigation of the effect that providing computer-based predictions of outcome has on clinician's management of severely head-injured patients. An increase in specific aspects of critical care was seen in patients predicted to have a good outcome, but a 39% decrease in certain aspects of care occurred in patients predicted to have the worst outcome.

Classification: Class III

Conclusion: Physicians alter their management of patients based on the provision of outcomes estimates.

Narayan 1981

Description of study: Evaluation of 133 patients with severe head injury.

Classification: Class II

Conclusion: A GCS score of 3 to 5 was associated with a poor outcome 77% of the time, whereas a score of 6 to 8 was associated with a poor outcome 26% of the time.

Phuenpathom 1993

Description of study: One hundred nine consecutive patients with acute subdural hematoma. Outcome assessed at 6 months.

Classification: Class III

Conclusion: For GCS scores between 3 and 7, the presence of an acute subdural hematoma was associated with higher mortality than that routinely reported in the literature.

Rimel 1981

Description of study: Prospective data collection on 538 hospitalized head-injured patients with GCS 13 to 15, LOC ≤20 minutes, and hospitalization <48 hours; 3-month follow-up evaluations were performed on 424 of them.

Classification: Class II

Conclusion: Rates of morbidity and unemployment after mild TBI are surprisingly high.

Rimel 1982

Description of study: Prospective data collection on 199 head-injured patients with GCS 9 to 12; 3-month follow-up evaluations were performed on 159 of them.

Classification: Class II

Conclusions: Moderate head injury results in substantial morbidity.

Rutherford 1977

Description of study: Analysis of sequelae of concussion 6 weeks after injury in 145 patients admitted to a hospital.

Classification: Class II

Conclusion: High correlation between signs and symptoms at 24 hours and symptoms at 6 weeks.

Rutherford 1979

Description of study: Analysis of sequelae of concussion 1 year after injury in 131 patients admitted to a hospital.

Classification: Class II

Conclusion: 19/131 concussion patients (14.5%) still complained of symptoms after 1 year.

Stein 1992

Description of study: A retrospective review that evaluated the incidence of abnormalities on CT in 341 patients with GCS scores of 9 to 12 and 106 patients with a GCS score of 13.

Classification: Class III

Conclusion: GCS 13 patients have an incidence of abnormalities on CT that is similar to that of GCS 9 to 12 patients. They should be included in the moderate head injury category.

Tate 1989

Description of study: One hundred consecutive patients with severe closed head injury were evaluated 6 years after head injury using the GOS and Psychosocial Disability Scale as estimates of social reintegration.

Classification: Class III

Conclusion: Of 87/100 patients evaluated, only 24% achieved good overall psychosocial reintegration.

Thatcher 1991

Description of study: One hundred sixty-two patients with closed head injury underwent encephalography (EEG) and brainstem auditory evoked potentials within 3 weeks of injury, in addition to initial and subsequent CT scanning. GCS was assessed at the time of admission and at the time of EEG and evoked potential testing. Outcome was assessed at 1 year to determine which combination of assessment tools was most predictive of outcome.

Classification: Class II

Conclusions: EEG plus delayed GCS was the best combination of predictors. Delayed GCS was superior to GCS on admission as a predictor of outcome.

van der Naalt 1999

Description of study: Prospective study of prognostic value of injury characteristics and duration of PTA in 67 patients with GCS 9 to 14, with follow-up at 1, 3, 6, and 12 months.

Classification: Class II

Conclusion: In mild and moderate head injury, duration of PTA is a better predictor of outcome than admission GCS score.

References

1. World Health Organization. International Classification of Impairments, Disabilities, and Handicaps: A Manual of Classification Relating to the Consequences of Disease. Geneva: World Health Organization; 1980.
2. Jennett B, Bond M. Assessment of outcome after severe brain damage. Lancet 1975;1:480–484.
3. Rappaport M, Hall KM, Hopkins K, et al. Disability rating scale for severe head trauma: coma to community. Arch Phys Med Rehabil 1982;63:118–123.
4. Brain Trauma Foundation, American Association of Neurological Surgeons, Joint Section on Neurotrauma and Critical Care. Management and prognosis of severe traumatic brain injury. J Neurotrauma 2000;17:449–627.
5. Choi SC, Muizelaar JP, Barnes TY, et al. Prediction tree for severely head-injured patients. J Neurosurg 1991;75:251–255.
6. The Brain Trauma Foundation, the American Association of Neurological Surgeons, and the Joint Section on Neurotrauma and Critical Care. Management and prognosis of severe traumatic brain injury. Glasgow Coma Scale score. J Neurotrauma 2000;17:563–571.
7. Thatcher RW, Cantor DS, McAlaster R, et al. Comprehensive predictions of outcome in closed head-injured patients. The development of prognostic equations. Ann NY Acad Sci 1991;620:82–101.
8. Kaufmann MA, Buchmann B, Scheidegger D, et al. Severe head injury: should expected outcome influence resuscitation and first-day decisions. Resuscitation 1992;23:199–206.
9. Murray LS, Teasdale GM, Murray GD, et al. Does prediction of outcome alter patient management? Lancet 1993;341:1487–1491.
10. Jennett B, Teasdale G, Galbraith S, et al. Severe head injuries in three countries. J Neurol Neurosurg Psychiatry 1977;40:291–298.
11. Marshall LF, Gautille T, Klauber MR, et al. The outcome of severe closed head injury. J Neurosurg 1991;75:S28–S36.
12. Narayan RK, Greenberg RP, Miller JD, et al. Improved confidence of outcome prediction in severe head injury: a comparative analysis of the clinical examination, multimodality evoked potentials, CT scanning, and intracranial pressure. J Neurosurg 1981;54:751–762.
13. Phuenpathom N, Choomuang M, Ratanalert S. Outcome and outcome prediction in acute subdural hematoma. Surg Neurol 1993;40:22–25.
14. Tate RL, Lulham JM, Broe GA, et al. Psychosocial outcome for the survivors or severe blunt head injury: the results from a consecutive series of 100 patients. J Neurol Neurosurg Psychiatry 1989;52:1128–1134.
15. Levin HS. Outcome from mild head injury. In: Narayan RK, Wilberger JE Jr, Povlishock JT, eds. Neurotrauma. New York: McGraw-Hill; 1996:749–754.
16. Rimel RW, Giordani B, Barth JT, et al. Disability caused by minor head injury. Neurosurgery 1981;9:221–228.
17. Cushman JG, Agarwal N, Fabian TC, et al. Practice management guidelines for the management of mild traumatic brain injury: the EAST Practice Management Guidelines Work Group. J Trauma 2001;51:1016–1026.
18. Stein SC, Ross SE. Moderate head injury: a guide to initial management. J Neurosurg 1992;77:562–564.

19. Levin HS, Mattis S, Ruff RM, et al. Neurobehavioral outcome following minor head injury: a three-center study. J Neurosurg 1987;66:234–243.

20. Rutherford WH, Merrett JD, McDonald JR. Sequelae of concussion caused by minor head injuries. Lancet 1977;1:1–4.

21. Rutherford WH, Merrett JD, McDonald JR. Symptoms at one year following concussion from minor head injuries. Injury 1979;10:225–230.

22. Stein SC. Outcome from moderate head injury. In: Narayan RK, Wilberger JE Jr, Povlishock JT, eds. Neurotrauma. New York: McGraw-Hill; 1996:755–765.

23. Rimel RW, Giordani B, Barth JT, et al. Moderate head injury: completing the clinical spectrum of brain trauma. Neurosurgery 1982;11:344–351.

24. Lobato RD, Rivas JJ, Gomez PA, et al. Head-injured patients who talk and deteriorate into coma: analysis of 211 cases studied with computerized tomography. J Neurosurg 1991;75: 256–261.

25. van der Naalt J, van Zomeren AH, Sluiter WJ, Minderhoud JM. One-year outcome in mild to moderate head injury: the predictive value of acute injury characteristics related to complaints and return to work. J Neurol Neurosurg Psychiatry 1999;66: 207–213.

◆ 42 ◆

How Well Can Patients Be Expected to Recover After Spinal Cord Injury?

Charles H. Tator

Brief Answer

Most patients achieve some degree of neurologic recovery after an acute spinal cord injury (SCI). Patients who present with a complete SCI have less than a 10% chance of improving even slightly, and the likelihood of a functional outcome is only 2 to 3%. In patients with preserved sensory function but no motor function below the level of injury, the probability of recovering to functional status is ~25%. This likelihood exceeds 50% in patients who present with at least some motor and sensory function. However, the extent of the neurologic recovery varies widely and depends on several factors, the most important of which is the severity of the initial neurologic deficit: patients with the least injury recover the most neurologic function. Other factors affecting neurologic recovery include age of the patient and associated injuries. Survival from SCI is dependent on these same factors. In most patients, spinal stability can be restored.

Background

Data about neurologic recovery as part of the natural history of SCI have been collected over the past several decades in many countries. These data have accrued as a result of the development of accurate measures for classifying, grading, and serially assessing the neurologic deficits associated with the acute and subsequent rehabilitative phases of care of SCI, including long-term follow-up. The inherent slowness of recovery of the central nervous system makes accurate long-term assessment an essential part of any outcome study.

Pearl

The inherent slowness of recovery of the central nervous system makes accurate long-term assessment an essential part of any outcome study.

The effort to accurately classify and record the clinical neurologic features of SCI to document the natural history began in the 1940s in England at Stoke-Mandeville Hospital under Guttman.[1] These efforts then spread to the United States, Canada, Australia, and several European countries, including France and Switzerland. In 1969, the author developed a new system of grading neurologic function to assess neurologic recovery in SCI patients and applied it retrospectively to several hundred SCI patients during the spectrum of care from the acute phase to long-term follow-up. Considerable neurologic recovery was evident in some patients (class III data).[2,3] Later, this system was applied to prospectively gathered data about SCI patients, and again, considerable neurologic recovery was seen in some patients (class III data).[4,5] In 1969, Frankel et al[6] published a similar grading method (class III data), and subsequently, many features of the two systems were combined to form the current American Spinal Injury Association (ASIA) grading and scoring system[7] that is now used in most centers (class III data).

Since the late 1980s, the ASIA system has been used in several studies that have included long-term follow-up. These reports have confirmed that a remarkable propensity for neurologic recovery exists in SCI patients. Indeed, in the author's own studies, the majority of SCI patients showed some degree of neurologic recovery (class III data).[4,8] Also, knowledge of the natural history of acute SCI has been markedly enhanced since the advent in 1979 of multicenter, randomized, prospective clinical trials of the treatment of SCI. These trials have generally utilized the ASIA system and have produced additional data about recovery. Thus, reliable information about the natural history of SCI is now available.

Pearl

The majority of SCI patients show some degree of neurologic recovery.

Literature Review

Survival after Spinal Cord Injury

Survival after SCI has improved greatly over the past several decades due to several improvements in management. Prior to 1950, SCI was characterized by mortality rates as high as 50%, whereas recent studies have shown mortality rates in the 5 to 10% range (class II data).[9] This marked decline in mortality can be attributed to many improvements in both the acute and rehabilitation phases of care. In the acute phase the important factors have included better first aid and more rapid referral to regional centers with trained staff and appropriate facilities for hemodynamic and respiratory resuscitation (class III data).[8] In the rehabilitation phase the important factor has been prevention of complications, especially urinary tract infections, decubiti, deep venous thrombosis, and pulmonary embolism. In both phases of injury, mortality is related to patient age, severity of injury, accompanying injuries, and other factors. Multiple regression analysis has demonstrated an association between higher mortality and increasing age, more rostral vertebral levels of injury, and higher injury severity scores (class III data).[8]

Pearl

Mortality after SCI has decreased from as high as 50% to 5 to 10% because of advances in prehospital care, resuscitation and stabilization, and prevention and management of complications related to long-term survival.

Recovery of Spinal Stability

Methods for reducing spinal deformity and restoring spinal stability improved dramatically during the latter half of the 20th century. Previously, such methods were limited to traction and crude forms of fusion. Currently, operative reduction and internal fixation of fractures and dislocations can be successfully performed with a variety of surgical approaches and instrumentation. Thus, the majority of SCI patients recover stability and near-normal alignment of the spine. It is likely, although not proven, that restoration of alignment and stability has a positive effect on neurologic recovery, although the magnitude of such an effect is probably small. It is also likely that restoration of alignment and stability improves quality of life and reduces costs of care because of decreased pain, increased patient mobility and independence, and decreased length of hospitalization.

Recovery of Neurologic Function

Mechanisms of Neurologic Recovery

Recovery of neurologic function after SCI is the result of recovery of various anatomic structures, including the nerve roots and the gray and white matter of the spinal cord. The propensity for neurologic recovery differs among these structures: the roots show the best ability to recover, followed by the local gray matter, and then the white matter. In addition, motor roots and tracts have increased vulnerability to injury and decreased propensity for recovery compared with sensory roots and tracts. This hierarchy is probably based on an inherent combination of increasing vulnerability to injury and decreasing ability to recover. Nerve roots at or below the site of injury are the structures that recover most frequently because the peripheral nervous system is more resistant to injury and has a greater ability to recover than the central nervous system. Indeed, local nerve root recovery probably occurs to some degree in every patient after SCI. This recovery may appear as restoration of function in muscles, dermatomes, or organs innervated by the nerve roots at the immediate vertebral level of injury or by roots traversing the level of injury to innervate structures below the vertebral level of injury. For example, a C5 burst fracture may directly compress both the C5 and C6 nerve roots because the C6 nerve roots emanate from the C6 cord level, which is slightly rostral to the site of compression at C5. Due to the increasing obliquity of the roots in the more caudal segments of the spinal cord, more caudal injuries are associated with a greater extent of possible caudal neurologic recovery due to root recovery. Such recovery of nerve roots explains why conus medullaris or cauda equina injuries demonstrate the greatest caudal extent of neurologic recovery. For example, a patient with a T12 burst fracture can obtain neurologic recovery in structures innervated by the L1-L5 roots because all of these roots emanate from the lumbar cord, which is located almost entirely opposite the T12 vertebral body.

Similarly, recovery of neurologic function at the injury level may originate from local recovery of spinal cord tissue that innervates structures at the injured level, or it may involve structures innervated one or more segments below the injured level. The extent of caudal recovery of neurologic function due to cord recovery also depends on the level of injury. For example, an injury of the cord at the T12 vertebral level could be followed by recovery of all the anterior horn cells of the lumbar cord and could result in restoration of motor function in the L1-L5 segments based on local circuit recovery rather than long tract recovery. In contrast, recovery of cord function caudal to L5 would require recovery of long white matter tracts in the cord. Thus, cord recovery can be divided into two main anatomic types: (1) local circuit recovery involving either gray matter or white matter or both; and (2) long tract recovery involving long white matter tracts.

The time course of neurologic recovery is also related to the same factors. The rate is fastest with the less severe injuries. In general, recovery begins almost immediately after injury, then accelerates between about 1 day and 6 months, and then declines rapidly over the next 6 months. The majority of the recovery occurs within 1 year of injury, although small amounts can continue for even 3 or 4 years in some patients, especially those who are relatively young.

Pearl

The majority of neurologic recovery occurs within 1 year of injury, although small amounts can continue for even 3 or 4 years in some patients.

Clinical Evidence of Neurologic Recovery

Clinical neurologic recovery has been accurately documented in studies utilizing the clinical neurologic measures outlined above. Neurophysiologic and functional outcome measures that are not as developed have also been used.

The National Spinal Cord Injury Database reported by Stover et al[10] is a rich source of information about neurologic recovery in almost 10,000 SCI patients (class III data). This database was compiled by the Model Spinal Cord Injury System Program in the United States at 19 centers during 1973 to 1985. The Frankel system of grading was used. These data showed that a small number of neurologically complete cases can recover some caudal neurologic function indicative of cord recovery. However, Stover et al found the best recovery in the B and C categories of incomplete injuries, in which 40 to 55% of patients improved at least one Frankel grade. Currently, 60% of patients with SCI have incomplete injuries (class III data).[11] These high rates of natural recovery make it mandatory to employ rigorous study methodology and accurate outcome measures in clinical trials of patients with SCI, especially for incomplete patients.

Pearl

Although a small number of patients with neurologically complete injuries can recover some neurologic function below the level of injury, the best recovery occurs in patients with incomplete injuries, roughly half of whom improve at least one Frankel or ASIA grade.

The accuracy of all systems of scoring depends on the precision and thoroughness of the clinical neurologic examination. For example, unless the examination is performed thoroughly, with careful attention to the motor and sensory functions of the sacral cord and roots, it is not possible to accurately distinguish even between complete and incomplete cases (ASIA A and B). Unfortunately, 100% accuracy is not possible if the patient is uncooperative due to head injury, hypoxia, associated injuries, inebriation, language barrier, or drugs.

In the author's study of neurologic recovery in 552 SCI patients, linear regression and multiple regression analyses pointed to several factors affecting neurologic recovery (class III).[8] As expected, less severe injuries were associated with more frequent and more extensive neurologic recovery. Patients with neurologically incomplete injuries had much more recovery than those with complete injuries. Patients with a less severe total injury burden with respect to multiple system injuries had greater neurologic recovery, and it was postulated that neurogenic or systemic shock, hemodynamic instability, and hypotension may all have accounted for reduced neurologic recovery. A more rostral location of cord injury in the spinal column was associated with greater neurologic recovery. Patients injured after 1974 had greater neurologic recovery than those injured before 1974, suggesting that newer methods of management, such as better first aid, were effective. We also documented a change in the epidemiology of SCI toward less severe cord injury in the more recent cases (class III data),[12] which is probably due to several factors such as improved first aid and greater use of seat belts. Surprisingly, we found the age of the patient, the interval from trauma to admission, and the cause of injury had no effect on recovery. It should be noted that the median time from injury to admission prior to 1974 was 13 hours, whereas after 1974 the median time was 5 hours (class III data).[8]

Hansebout[13] reviewed a large number of reports of patients with clinically complete SCI and found that the percentage of patients who recovered the ability to walk was ~1% of cervical injuries and 2% of injuries at all cord levels (class III data). However, in some of the reports in his review, the percentage of complete or incomplete patients with some degree of neurologic recovery was as high as 73% (class III data).

Several randomized, prospective clinical trials also provide good evidence for neurologic recovery in both the treatment and control groups. For example, the pharmacotherapy trials with methylprednisolone or GM_1 ganglioside have shown progressive improvement in neurologic function in both treatment and control groups as documented by the careful application of the clinical outcome measures described above. The National Acute Spinal Cord Injury Study (NASCIS) group[14,15] has been especially successful in applying the clinical measures described above. A recent meta-analysis[16] (class III data) showed that the treatment groups improve an average of 4.1 points in unilateral motor score, which is equivalent to one muscle improving from a motor score of 1 to normal (Medical Research Council scale[17]) on each side of the body. For patients with incomplete injuries, motor recovery was twice that of patients with complete injuries (7.3 versus 3.6).[16] Furthermore, the NASCIS group has been able to differentiate recovery at the level of injury from caudal recovery (class II data).[18]

The GM_1 ganglioside studies also provided a great deal of information about neurologic recovery (class II data).[9,19,20] For example, patients with complete injuries had about a 20% chance of improving one grade or more (calculated on the basis of ASIA grade at baseline to modified Benzel grade[21] at 26 weeks from injury), whereas incomplete ASIA B patients (motor complete, sensory incomplete) had roughly a 70% chance of improving one grade or more. In the placebo group, almost 29% of patients improved two or more grades. Geisler et al[9] also concluded that the prognosis for recovery had improved in their study of patients injured in the 1990s as compared with studies of patients injured in the 1980s. This conclusion parallels the present author's experience (class III data).[12]

The above-described clinical trials of pharmacotherapy have provided some evidence for improved neurologic recovery as a result of pharmacologic treatment. The best known examples are the methylprednisolone studies, although the evidence is only class II.[22] However, it should be noted that considerable debate continues about the effectiveness of methylprednisolone in SCI.[23]

Although many studies in SCI patients have examined neurologic recovery after various surgical maneuvers such as decompression (class III data)[24] or skeletal traction (class III data),[25–27] and although some authors have claimed that neurologic improvement can occur as a result of these treatments, no class I evidence supports the effectiveness of surgery or traction for enhancing neurologic recovery in SCI patients. Indeed, there has only been one prospective, controlled randomized trial of surgical decompression in patients with SCI, and this study examined the timing of surgery. This study found that there was no evidence for improved recovery in the early surgery group (mean time to surgery of 1.8 days) compared with the late surgery group (mean time of 16.8 days) (class II).[28] The evidence for surgery and traction has been thoroughly reviewed.[29]

Pearl

No class I evidence supports the effectiveness of surgery or traction for enhancing neurologic recovery in SCI patients.

Some neurophysiologic outcome measures, such as evoked potentials, have been used for assessing neurologic recovery in patients with SCI.[30] Class III evidence suggests that serially recorded evoked potentials may be useful for early prognostication because electrophysiologic recovery may precede recovery detected by the clinical neurologic exam.[31] Rarely, electrophysiologic recovery has occurred without accompanying clinical neurologic recovery. Such occurrences have led to the concept of discomplete lesions (class III data),[32] implying that recovery or regeneration of axons may not always be detectable by the clinical neurologic examination. None of the major prospective, randomized clinical trials has included neurophysiologic outcome measures to answer the primary question of efficacy, and most centers are not routinely employing them for the management of SCI. Thus, experience with such measures is quite limited. In general, they are difficult to perform in the acute stage. They can also involve considerable expense in terms of equipment and personnel. No class I evidence supports the necessity of using these tests for assessing neurologic recovery in SCI patients. However, they are often useful for intraoperative monitoring in SCI patients.

Other Measures to Assess Functional Recovery

There is a need for functional measures that relate to neurologic recovery in SCI patients. Some clinical studies such as NASCIS III[15] have used the Functional Independence Measure (FIM).[33] The FIM includes categories of function such as sphincter control, self-care, locomotion, and communication. There is some evidence that the FIM relates to the ASIA scores and to neurologic recovery (class II).[34]

Some evidence also suggests that magnetic resonance imaging (MRI) findings in the acute phase can provide some prognostic information about neurologic recovery. For example, it has been shown that hemorrhage, the extent of edema, and a more rostral location of lesions point to less neurologic recovery and lower FIM scores (class III data).[35]

Neurologic Deterioration

Very few studies have carefully examined the incidence and causes of neurologic deterioration after SCI. The natural history studies described above[3,6,10] have all shown that a small percentage of patients, ~5 to 10%, deteriorate neurologically after SCI, sometimes without any identifiable cause (class III data). Other studies have linked a particular form of management, such as traction, to the deterioration (class II and III data).[36,37] Farmer et al[38] related deterioration to sepsis, ankylosing spondylitis, and intubation (class III).

Pearl

About 5 to 10% of SCI patients demonstrate neurologic deterioration after injury, sometimes without any identifiable cause.

Conclusions

Neurologic recovery after SCI is related to many factors, the most important of which is the severity of the initial injury. Overall, there has been a reduction in severity due to many factors, such as improved first aid and more widespread use of preventive measures, including seat belts. Some degree of neurologic recovery occurs in the majority of patients. Excellent clinical measures of neurologic recovery have been developed and tested in SCI patients, although further development of functional measures is required. Unfortunately, there exists only class II evidence of the effectiveness of pharmacotherapy and only class III evidence of the effectiveness of various surgical treatments.

References

1. Guttman L. Initial treatment of traumatic paraplegia and tetraplegia. In: Harris P, ed. Spinal Injuries Symposium, Royal College of Surgeons. Edinburgh, UK: Morrison and Gibb; 1963:80–92.
2. Tator CH, Rowed DW, Schwartz ML. Sunnybrook Cord Injury Scales for assessing neurological injury and recovery. In: Tator CH, ed. Early Management of Acute Spinal Cord Injury. New York: Raven Press; 1982:7–24.
3. Tator CH. Spine-spinal cord relationships in spinal cord trauma. Clin Neurosurg 1983;30:479–494.
4. Tator CH, Duncan EG, Edmonds VE, et al. Comparison of surgical and conservative management in 208 patients with acute spinal cord injury. Can J Neurol Sci 1987;14:60–69.
5. Pitts LH, Ross A, Chase GA, et al. Treatment with thyrotropin-releasing hormone (TRH) in patients with traumatic spinal cord injuries. J Neurotrauma 1995;12:235–243.
6. Frankel HL, Hancock DO, Hyslop G, et al. The value of postural reduction in the initial management of closed injuries of the spine with paraplegia and tetraplegia. Paraplegia 1969;7:179–192.
7. Standards for Neurological and Functional Classification of Spinal Cord Injury, revised ed. Chicago: American Spinal Injury Association; 1992.
8. Tator CH, Duncan EG, Edmonds VE, et al. Neurological recovery, mortality and length of stay after acute spinal cord injury associated with changes in management. Paraplegia 1995;33:254–262.
9. Geisler FH, Coleman WP, Grieco G, et al. Measurements and recovery patterns in a multicenter study of acute spinal cord injury. Spine 2001;26:S68–S86.
10. Stover SL, DeLisa JA, Whiteneck GG. Spinal Cord Injury. Clinical Outcomes from the Model Systems. Gaithersburg, MD: Aspen Publications; 1995.
11. Tator CH. Clinical manifestations of acute spinal cord injury. In: Benzel EC, Tator CH, eds. Contemporary Management of Spinal Cord Injury. Park Ridge, IL: American Association of Neurological Surgeons; 1995:15–26.
12. Tator CH, Duncan EG, Edmonds VE, et al. Changes in epidemiology of acute spinal cord injury from 1947 to 1981. Surg Neurol 1993;40:207–215.
13. Hansebout R. Comprehensive review of methods of improving cord recovery after acute spinal cord injury. In: Tator C, ed. Early Management of Acute Spinal Cord Injury. New York: Raven Press; 1982:181–196.
14. Bracken MB. Methylprednisolone in the management of acute spinal cord injuries. Med J Aust 1990;153:368.
15. Bracken MB, Shepard MJ, Holford TR, et al. Administration of methylprednisolone for 24 or 48 hours or tirilazad mesylate for 48 hours in the treatment of acute spinal cord injury. Results of the Third National Acute Spinal Cord Injury Randomized Controlled Trial. National Acute Spinal Cord Injury Study. JAMA 1997;277:1597–1604.
16. Bracken MB. Methylprednisolone and acute spinal cord injury: an update of the randomized evidence. Spine 2001;26:S47–S54.
17. Aids to Investigation of Peripheral Nerve Injuries. Medical Research Council War Memorandum, 2nd ed., revised. London: HMSO; 1943.
18. Bracken MB, Holford TR. Effects of timing of methylprednisolone or naloxone administration on recovery of segmental and long-tract neurological function in NASCIS 2. J Neurosurg 1993;79:500–507.
19. Geisler FH, Coleman WP, Grieco G, et al. The Sygen multicenter acute spinal cord injury study. Spine 2001;26:S87–S98.
20. Geisler FH, Coleman WP, Grieco G, et al. Recruitment and early treatment in a multicenter study of acute spinal cord injury. Spine 2001;26:S58–S67.
21. Benzel EC, Larson SJ. Functional recovery after decompressive operation for thoracic and lumbar spine fractures. Neurosurgery 1986;19:772–778.
22. Fehlings MG. Editorial: recommendations regarding the use of methylprednisolone in acute spinal cord injury: making sense out of the controversy. Spine 2001;26:S56–S57.
23. Hurlbert RJ. The role of steroids in acute spinal cord injury: an evidence-based analysis. Spine 2001;26:S39–S46.
24. Wagner FC Jr, Chehrazi B. Early decompression and neurological outcome in acute cervical spinal cord injuries. J Neurosurg 1982;56:699–705.
25. Brunette DD, Rockswold GL. Neurologic recovery following rapid spinal realignment for complete cervical spinal cord injury. J Trauma 1987;27:445–447.
26. Cotler JM, Herbison GJ, Nasuti JF, et al. Closed reduction of traumatic cervical spine dislocation using traction weights up to 140 pounds. Spine 1993;18:386–390.
27. Cotler HB, Miller LS, DeLucia FA, et al. Closed reduction of cervical spine dislocations. Clin Orthop 1987;214:185–199.
28. Vaccaro AR, Daugherty RJ, Sheehan TP, et al. Neurologic outcome of early versus late surgery for cervical spinal cord injury. Spine 1997;22:2609–2613.
29. Fehlings MG, Tator CH. An evidence-based review of decompressive surgery in acute spinal cord injury: rationale,

indications, and timing based on experimental and clinical studies. J Neurosurg (Spine 1) 1999;91:1–11.
30. Rowed DW. Value of somatosensory evoked potentials for prognosis in partial cord injuries. In: Tator CH, ed. Early Management of Acute Spinal Cord Injury. New York: Raven Press, 1982:167–180.
31. Rowed DW, McLean JA, Tator CH. Somatosensory evoked potentials in acute spinal cord injury: prognostic value. Surg Neurol 1978;9:203–210.
32. Dimitrijevic MR. Residual motor functions in spinal cord injury. Adv Neurol 1988;47:138–155.
33. Keith RA, Granger CV, Hamilton BB, et al. The functional independence measure: a new tool for rehabilitation. Adv Clin Rehabil 1987;1:6–18.
34. Marino RJ, Ditunno JF Jr, Donovan WH, et al. Neurologic recovery after traumatic spinal cord injury: data from the Model Spinal Cord Injury Systems. Arch Phys Med Rehabil 1999;80:1391–1396.
35. Flanders AE, Spettell CM, Friedman DP, et al. The relationship between the functional abilities of patients with cervical spinal cord injury and the severity of damage revealed by MR imaging. AJNR Am J Neuroradiol 1999;20:926–934.
36. Tator CH, Fehlings MG, Thorpe K, Taylor W. Current use and timing of spinal surgery for management of acute spinal cord injury in North America: results of a retrospective multicenter study. J Neurosurg 1999; 91:S12–S18.
37. Marshall LF, Knowlton S, Garfin SR, et al. Deterioration following spinal cord injury: a multicenter study. J Neurosurg 1987;66:400–404.
38. Farmer J, Vaccaro A, Albert TJ, et al. Neurologic deterioration after cervical spinal cord injury. J Spinal Disord 1998;11: 192–196.

◆ 43 ◆

Does Rehabilitation Facilitate Neurologic Recovery After Spinal Cord Injury?

Justin Pik and Michael G. Fehlings

Brief Answer

No published studies have randomized patients to a "no rehabilitation" group. Thus, it is not possible to make level I recommendations about whether rehabilitation facilitates neurologic recovery after spinal cord injury (SCI).

Ideally, patients should commence rehabilitation within 2 weeks of the initial injury. Although postponing rehabilitation by more than 6 months from the time of injury may decrease the chance of satisfactory motor recovery, a properly designed and implemented rehabilitation program can still be of benefit to SCI patients who are 1 year or more postinjury.

Locomotor training, whether with body weight support, functional electrical stimulation, or both, is safe and may be useful for improving ambulation in patients with incomplete SCI. On the other hand, neurostimulation and biofeedback techniques, either alone or in combination, appear to be no more efficacious than standard physical exercise therapy for restoring function. Neurostimulation may improve the strength and electromyogram (EMG) activity of individual muscles, however, which may be important if supraspinal control eventually returns.

Background

The care of patients with SCI involves a multidisciplinary approach. In the acute phase of SCI, a team of intensive care specialists, surgeons, and acute care nursing staff management focus on preservation of remaining spinal cord function and prevention of secondary injury to the spinal cord. The emphasis is on resuscitation, treatment of immediately life-threatening injuries, and subsequent stabilization of the injured vertebral column. Once acute problems have resolved, rehabilitation specialists, physiotherapists, nurses, occupational therapists, social workers, and patients themselves all work together to maximize functional outcome following SCI.

Many patients with SCI go on to achieve significant recovery of neurologic function, particularly during the first 6 months after the injury. Since rehabilitation has become an integral part of SCI management, it is difficult to critically assess how much improvement is due to rehabilitation and how much is secondary to the natural healing process. This chapter examines the evidence regarding the timing of rehabilitation and the efficacy of some of the available modalities of facilitating neurologic recovery after SCI.

Literature Review

An Internet-based search of the National Library of Medicine (NLM) database was conducted using PubMed (*www.nlm.nih.gov*). The medical subject headings (MeSH) "spinal cord injury AND rehabilitation" were used. Only articles reporting human studies in the English language were retrieved. A total of 2513 articles were identified as fitting our selection criteria. Of the 162 retrieved articles concerning clinical trials, 42 studies involved randomized controlled trials.

Timing of Rehabilitation

Sumida et al[1] examined the effect of early rehabilitation after traumatic SCI (class III data). In their retrospective, multicenter study, 123 patients from 16 hospitals and one medical school were divided into two groups: an early rehabilitation group (beginning rehabilitation within 2 weeks of injury) and a delayed group. In each of the two groups, the patients were further subdivided according to the type of SCI: tetraplegia excluding central cord injury, central cord injury, and paraplegia. The authors found that SCI patients not receiving rehabilitation for over 6 months postinjury had a low probability of acceptable motor recovery. Also, they found early rehabilitation was more effective than delayed rehabilitation in improving the activities of daily living in all patients with SCI. However, the advantage of early rehabilitation was not apparent in the tetraplegia subgroup when the American Spinal Injury Association (ASIA) motor score was used to measure neurologic improvement.

Pearl

In one study, SCI patients not receiving rehabilitation for more than 6 months postinjury had a lower probability of acceptable motor recovery than patients receiving rehabilitation soon after the injury. Other studies, however, suggest that at least some delayed neurologic improvement is possible with training even in the chronic setting.

Celani et al[2] investigated factors influencing the length of stay in a rehabilitation center, the incidence of pressure ulcers, and the neurologic improvement of patients with traumatic and nontraumatic spinal cord injuries (class III data). In their multicenter, retrospective study of 859 consecutive adult patients, the authors found that the presence of pressure ulcers was statistically associated with a longer interval from initial injury to admission to a rehabilitation center. Furthermore, in a multiple logistic regression analysis, the model that best predicted neurologic improvement included, among other factors, absence of pressure ulcers on admission to the rehabilitation facilities. By inference, the authors of this study concluded that early admission to a rehabilitation facility is likely to facilitate clinical recovery.

The Role of Locomotor Training in Spinal Cord Injury Patients

It has been recognized that coordinated stepping movements in patients with complete paraplegia can be induced by weight support and by standing on a moving treadmill (class III data).[3] This is the basis for Laufband (treadmill) therapy in SCI patients. Wernig et al[4] studied a series of 76 patients who underwent locomotor training by Laufband therapy (class III data). This noncontrolled study found supported treadmill ambulation training to be effective for improving the walking capabilities of patients with either chronic or acute incomplete SCI. However, the measures for assessing gait performance were different at the beginning and end of the study. In addition, the patients' training regimes were variable in their duration and intensity.

Pearl

Supported treadmill ambulation training may be effective for improving the walking capabilities of patients with either chronic or acute incomplete SCI.

In an attempt to quantify the improvement in ambulation after treadmill training, Protas et al[5] studied a single group of three patients with incomplete paraplegia (class III data). The authors measured gait function (speed, endurance, walking status, use of assistive devices, and orthotics); oxygen costs of walking; brain motor control assessment; self-report indices; ASIA classification; muscle function test results; and safety. As a result of the training measures, the three subjects tripled their gait speed and endurance. Energy expenditure as measured by oxygen consumption per meter walked decreased by 32%. Interestingly, at follow-up 12 weeks after finishing the training program, two out of the three subjects had a decrease in their gait speed as compared with the speed they achieved at the end of the training period. The other outcome measures listed above did not show any significant change. The authors concluded that these ordinal measures were not sensitive enough to detect the small changes brought about by the training. The authors have begun a larger, controlled trial to examine further the benefits of supported treadmill ambulation training.

In another noncontrolled study looking at the effects of moving treadmill training on SCI patients, Wirz et al[6] obtained serial EMG recordings of the medial head of the gastrocnemius in 32 patients (class III data). The patients were equally divided between a complete and an incomplete SCI group. Both groups consisted of patients with cervical as well as thoracic lesions. The authors found that EMG activity significantly increased in both groups over the training period. This increase in EMG activity was associated with improved locomotion in the incomplete SCI group. During the follow-up period, the increase in EMG activity seen during the training period was sustained in the incomplete SCI group but not in the complete SCI group. Because this study did not have a control group, it is difficult to ascertain whether these increases in EMG activity and locomotive ability in the incomplete SCI group were secondary to the treadmill training or merely part of the natural recovery after an incomplete injury to the spinal cord.

Field-Fote[7] studied 19 subjects with incomplete SCI who had significant asymmetry in their lower limb strength (class III data). The patients all underwent 12 weeks of treadmill training that included body weight support (BWS) and functional electrical stimulation (FES) of the common peroneal nerve of the weaker leg during the swing phase of gait. All the subjects had sustained their SCI at least 1 year before enrolling in the study, thus largely negating the confounding effect of natural recovery after SCI. In this noncontrolled, before-and-after comparison, the author found that the training protocol significantly improved the walking speed of subjects over ground as well as on the treadmill. During the training period, the lower extremity motor score increased significantly for both the stimulated and nonstimulated leg. Although treadmill training with BWS and FES significantly improved ambulation in patients with incomplete SCI, the lack of a control group made it impossible to discern whether similar improvement may be seen with only BWS or FES alone or, indeed, with some other forms of training.

Usefulness of Electrical Stimulation and Electromyogram Biofeedback

To differentiate the effect of physical exercise programs from that of neuromuscular stimulation (NMS), Needham-Shropshire et al[8] studied the effects of NMS on triceps motor function in 34 patients who had sustained cervical SCI at least 1 year prior to the study (class II data). The subjects were randomized into three groups. The first group received 8 weeks of NMS-assisted arm ergometry exercise. The second group received 4 weeks of NMS-assisted arm ergometry exercise followed by 4 weeks of voluntary arm crank exercise without NMS. The last group acted as controls and underwent 8 weeks of voluntary arm exercise without NMS. A blinded assessor performed manual muscle testing at four intervals before and during the training period.

After 4 weeks of training, the authors found no significant difference in the change in ASIA motor scores between the first and second groups and between the second and control groups. However, a significant difference was detected between the first and control groups, with a higher proportion of initially weak muscles improving one or more motor grades in the NMS group. After 8 weeks of training, the significant difference persisted between the first and control groups, and a significant difference was also seen between the second and control groups. No significant difference existed between the first and second groups. An important limitation of this randomized, controlled study lies in the fact that an improvement in strength of a muscle following 8 weeks of training does not necessarily equate to significant functional recovery. Nevertheless, this report does highlight the potential of neuromuscular stimulation to improve individual muscle strength after SCI even in the chronic setting, when most of the expected neurologic recovery has already taken place.

On the other hand, other studies of functional recovery after neurostimulation and EMG biofeedback techniques have been less encouraging. Kohlmeyer et al[9] performed a randomized, controlled study to evaluate the effectiveness of electrical stimulation and biofeedback on the recovery of tenodesis grasp in 45 tetraplegic subjects (class II data). The upper limbs of these patients were treated by one of four randomly assigned methods: group 1 received conventional treatment, group 2 electrical stimulation, group 3 EMG biofeedback, and group 4 both electrical stimulation and biofeedback. Treatment was given 5 days per week for 5 to 6 weeks. A blinded assessor recorded the subjects' muscle strength and function scores at the end of the treatment period. The authors found no significant differences among the four groups in terms of change in muscle strength or level of function after treatment. The authors concluded that the addition of electrical stimulation or biofeedback did not provide any additional benefit over conventional treatment.

Pearl

The preponderance of published data suggests that electrical stimulation and biofeedback are no more efficacious than standard physical exercise therapy for improving function after SCI.

Klose et al[10] conducted a randomized study in 39 SCI patients who were at least 1 year postinjury (class II data). Patients were randomized to one of four groups. The control group received standard physical exercise therapy (PET) for 16 weeks. One group received EMG biofeedback for 8 weeks, followed by PET for 8 weeks. Another group received 8 weeks of EMG biofeedback followed by 8 weeks of NMS. The last group received NMS for 8 weeks followed by PET for 8 weeks. A comprehensive set of measurements, including manual muscle tests, self-care scores, mobility measures, and voluntary EMG activity, was assessed before training, after 8 weeks, and after 16 weeks. The authors did not find any significant difference between the different modalities or different treatment combinations. However, for all groups, scores in most outcome measures were significantly better at the end of the 16 weeks. These results once again suggest that delayed neurologic improvement is achievable with training even in the chronic setting, in this case more than a year after the initial SCI. The specific type of therapeutic modality seems to be less important.

Recommendations

Due to the absence of studies containing a "no rehabilitation" group, it is not possible to provide an evidence-based answer to the question of whether rehabilitation facilitates neurologic recovery after SCI.

Level II Recommendation

Evidence from most randomized, controlled studies suggests that neurostimulation and biofeedback techniques, used either alone or in combination, are no more efficacious than standard physical exercise therapy for improving motor function.

Level III Recommendations

1. Spinal cord rehabilitation should begin as soon as a patient is medically stable. Ideally, patients should commence rehabilitation within 2 weeks of the initial injury. Postponing rehabilitation more than 6 months from the time of injury may decrease the chance of satisfactory motor recovery, but a properly designed and implemented rehabilitation program may help even SCI patients whose injury occurred 12 or more months ago.
2. Locomotor training, whether with body weight support, functional electrical stimulation, or both, is safe and may be useful for improving ambulation in patients with incomplete SCI.
3. Neurostimulation may improve the strength and EMG activity of individual muscles. This result may not lead to significant functional improvement, but improvements in muscle strength and EMG activity may be important if supraspinal control eventually returns. Such a return may occur either spontaneously in the setting of incomplete SCI or, it is hoped, in the near future, with spinal cord regeneration.

References

1. Sumida M, Fujimoto M, Tokuhiro A, et al. Early rehabilitation effect for traumatic spinal cord injury. Arch Phys Med Rehabil 2001;82:391–395.
2. Celani MG, Spizzichino L, Ricci S, et al. Spinal cord injury in Italy: a multicenter retrospective study. Arch Phys Med Rehabil 2001;82:589–596.
3. Dietz V, Colombo G, Jensen L. Locomotor activity in spinal man. Lancet 1994;344:1260–1263.
4. Wernig A, Nanassy A, Muller S. Maintenance of locomotor abilities following Laufband (treadmill) therapy in para- and tetraplegic persons: follow-up studies. Spinal Cord 1998;36: 744–749.
5. Protas EJ, Holmes SA, Qureshy H, et al. Supported treadmill ambulation training after spinal cord injury: a pilot study. Arch Phys Med Rehabil 2001;82:825–831.
6. Wirz M, Colombo G, Dietz V. Long term effects of locomotor training in spinal humans. J Neurol Neurosurg Psychiatry 2001;71:93–96.
7. Field-Fote EC. Combined use of body weight support, functional electrical stimulation, and treadmill training to improve walking ability in individuals with chronic incomplete spinal cord injury. Arch Phys Med Rehabil 2001;82:818–824.
8. Needham-Shropshire BM, Broton JG, Cameron TL, et al. Improved motor function in tetraplegics following neuromuscular stimulation-assisted arm ergometry. J Spinal Cord Med 1997;20:49–55.
9. Kohlmeyer KM, Hill JP, Yarkony GM, et al. Electrical stimulation and biofeedback effect on recovery of tenodesis grasp: a controlled study. Arch Phys Med Rehabil 1996;77:702–706.
10. Klose KJ, Schmidt DL, Needham BM, et al. Rehabilitation therapy for patients with long-term spinal cord injuries. Arch Phys Med Rehabil 1990;71:659–662.

◆ Part VI ◆

Sports Medicine

◆ 44 ◆

How Soon After Head Injury (With or Without Craniotomy) Can Patients Resume Contact Sports?

Julian E. Bailes and Vincent J. Miele

Brief Answer

Currently accepted guidelines for return to play following a mild traumatic brain injury (MTBI) may be classified as level III recommendations (Table 44-1). There exist only limited data comparing different return-to-play guidelines in terms of outcomes. Recommendations for return to play in athletes who have suffered life-threatening head injury (LTHI) or head injury requiring craniotomy (HIRC) are also classified as level III.

Background

It has been estimated that 750,000 Americans annually sustain injuries from participation in recreational activities; 82,000 (10.9%) sustain some form of head injury.[1] The primary concern in these cases is the potential for an insult to the brain; when oculofacial and scalp injuries are excluded, concussion becomes the most frequently reported type of recreation-associated head injury. The annual number of sports-related concussions in the United States has been estimated to be as high as 300,000 (class III data).[2]

Among organized athletics in the United States, football ranks first in both the number of participants and the incidence of head injuries. Nearly 1.5 million individuals participate in contact football in the U.S. each year, and it has been variously estimated that 4 to 20% sustain an MTBI each season (class II and III data).[3] Each year, a small number suffer either cumulative MTBI or serious head injury.[3] Currently, there are approximately four deaths (range 0–7) annually in the U.S. from head injuries in organized football (class II data).[4] At the high school level, as many as 20% of football players may suffer concussions of varying severity (class II and III data).[5]

Mild Traumatic Brain Injury

Multiple recommendations have been made for allowing athletes to return to play after MTBI. These are based on expert opinion and on data of varying degrees of reliability. The time at which a player should be allowed to return to contact sports following a head injury depends on several factors. The severity of the injury, presence of residual neurologic deficits, and history of previous injuries must be taken into account. One problem with performing outcome studies for return-to-play guidelines is that there exists no universally accepted definition of concussion. This limitation substantially complicates the evaluation of epidemiologic data in the literature. Furthermore, MTBI may be classified according to the duration of loss of consciousness (LOC), persistence of retrograde/posttraumatic amnesia, or duration of neurologic/neuropsychological abnormalities. Numerous concussion classification schemes exist (Table 44-1).

Potential issues that affect a return-to-play decision in a patient who has suffered MTBI include the risk of second impact syndrome (which is discussed in further detail below), increased vulnerability to subsequent

Table 44-1 Return to Play Guidelines Following Mild Traumatic Brain Injury

System	Concussion Grade	Signs/Symptoms	1st Concussion	2nd Concussion	3rd Concussion
American Academy of Neurology[8]	I (Mild)	Transient confusion; no LOC; symptoms or abnormalities resolve in less than 15 minutes	Remove from contest; may RTP if abnormalities or symptoms clear within 15 minutes	Terminate contest; may RTP after 1 week without symptoms at rest and with exercise	
	II (Moderate)	Transient confusion; no LOC; symptoms or abnormalities last over 15 minutes	Terminate contest; may RTP after 1 week asymptomatic at rest and with exertion	Terminate contest; may RTP after at least 2 weeks asymptomatic at rest and with exertion; withdraw from play for the rest of the season if any CT/MRI abnormalities	
	III (Severe)	Any LOC, either brief (seconds) or prolonged (minutes)	Terminate contest; transport to hospital if unconscious or if there is evidence of neurological abnormality; if concussion is brief, may RTP in 1 week if no symptoms at rest and with exertion; if concussion is prolonged, RTP in 2 weeks if no symptoms	Terminate contest; may RTP after minimum of 1 month asymptomatic; withdraw from play for the rest of the season if any CT/MRI abnormalities	
Colorado Medical Society[6]	I (Mild)	Confusion without amnesia; no LOC	May RTP if without symptoms at rest and exertion for at least 20 minutes	Terminate contest/ practice; may RTP if asymptomatic for at least 1 week	Withdraw from play for remainder of season; or may RTP in 3 months if asymptomatic
	II (Moderate)	Confusion with amnesia; no LOC	Terminate contest or practice; may RTP if asymptomatic for at least 1 week	Consider with-drawing from play for remainder of season; may RTP in 1 month if asymptomatic	Withdraw from play for remainder of season; may RTP next season if asymptomatic
	III (Severe)	LOC	Terminate contest/ practice and transport to hospital; may RTP in 1 month, after 2 consecutive asymptomatic weeks	Withdraw from play for remainder of season; may RTP next season if asymptomatic	Withdraw from play for remainder of season; strongly discourage return to contact sports
Cantu[14]	I (Mild)	No LOC; posttraumatic amnesia of less than 30 minutes duration	May RTP if asymptomatic for 1 week; terminate season if CT/MRI abnormalities	RTP in 2 weeks if asymptomatic at the time for 1 week	Withdraw from play for remainder of season; may RTP next season if asymptomatic
	II (Moderate)	LOC less than 5 minutes in duration or posttraumatic amnesia longer than 30 minutes but less than 24 hours in duration	RTP after asymptomatic for 1 week; terminate season if CT/MRI abnormalities	Withdraw athlete for a minimum of 1 month; may RTP if asymptomatic for 1 week; consider withdrawing from play for the remainder of season	Withdraw athlete from play for remainder of season; may RTP next season if asymptomatic

Table 44-1 (*continued*)

System	Concussion Grade	Signs/Symptoms	1st Concussion	2nd Concussion	3rd Concussion
	III (Severe)	LOC for more than 5 minutes or posttraumatic amnesia for more than 24 hours	Withdraw for minimum of 1 month; may then RTP if asymptomatic 1 week	Withdraw from play for remainder of season; may RTP next season if asymptomatic	Consider no further contact sports

CT, computed tomography; LOC, loss of consciousness; MRI, magnetic resonance imaging; RTP, return to play.
Refer to specific reference for detailed recommendation.

Pearl

Concussions usually (90%) occur without LOC. The signs and symptoms of concussion are often confusion and amnesia, not LOC.

early head injury, and the potential for long-term cumulative effects of repetitive mild injuries. It is inarguable that any athlete who remains symptomatic should be excluded from contact sports.

Life-Threatening Head Injury and Head Injury Requiring Craniotomy

LTHI is defined as an injury that is acutely life-threatening, such as intracranial hemorrhage, malignant brain edema, or second impact syndrome. LTHIs characterized by lesions requiring craniotomy are described as HIRCs. In addition to the previously mentioned issues regarding return to play, several additional factors must be addressed in this population. It has been surmised that parenchymal injury may result in obliteration of the normal cerebrospinal fluid (CSF) pathways through scarring. Theoretically, this could affect the brain's buoyancy and result in a loss of cushioning effect, increasing susceptibility to subsequent injury. In patients who have had craniotomies, the craniotomy flap may also be vulnerable to recurrent bony injury, which may in turn cause additional brain injury.

Literature Review

Mild Traumatic Brain Injury

In 1991, guidelines for return to competition were created by the Colorado Medical Society (CMS).[6] These were reviewed and endorsed by several professional organizations, including the American Academy of Pediatrics, the American Academy of Sports Medicine, and the American College of Surgeons Committee on Trauma.[7] Partly because of a feeling among the experts that the scientific data available as a basis for constructing medical practice parameters were limited and partly because of a desire for a broader consensus of expert opinion, the Quality Standards Subcommittee of the American Academy of Neurology revisited this project several years later.[8,9] To aid in creating guidelines that were based more solidly on available evidence, this group reviewed the literature published from 1966 to 1996 and modified the guidelines based on these data and on a consensus of experts.[8] No class I studies were available. The American Academy of Neurology guidelines were reviewed by several expert organizations, including the American Association of Neurological Surgeons, American College of Emergency Physicians, American Academy of Pediatrics, American Academy of Family Physicians, National Athletic Trainers Association, and the American Academy of Neurology Member Reviewer Network.[8]

Second-impact syndrome (SIS) is the most catastrophic potential sequela of an inappropriately early return to play by an athlete. It is believed to be the result of a second MTBI occurring while the athlete is still symptomatic from a previous concussion, before the brain has had a chance to recover fully from the first injury.[10–12] Its etiology may be loss of autoregulation of the cerebral vasculature, with subsequent uncontrolled intracranial hypertension and cerebral edema. Although the evidence supporting the existence and occurrence of SIS is based only on case reports and expert opinion (class III), its existence has been widely accepted.

Pearl

In a small percentage of patients, seemingly trivial concussions can have catastrophic outcomes if they occur soon after a prior brain injury. A detailed history of recent head injuries, including those not associated with sports (such as from motor vehicle accidents or at work), should be obtained and considered when evaluating an athlete for return to play.

Several studies have suggested that a premature return to play can increase adverse outcomes from the initial injury and increase a player's risk for repeat injuries.[13,14] However, no class I studies are available to confirm or refute this premise. Perhaps the closest substitutes are studies that found that the risk of loss of consciousness is four to six times greater in football players who have a prior history of loss of consciousness (class III).[15]

Neuropsychological testing is important for identifying the extent of injury and for following its evolution. Even mild abnormalities may indicate persistent and ongoing adverse sequelae of a previous head injury. Many experts suggest that athletes undergo neuropsychological assessment before they are allowed to return to contact sports following a head injury. A controlled, prospective study (class I)[16] examined outcomes in football players suffering MTBI using standardized neuropsychological testing. The study found that the vast majority of football-related head injuries were mild and that the majority of the affected athletes had reversal of their deficits by 5 days. All demonstrated resolution of neuropsychological testing abnormalities by 10 days. A second study[17] reported similar findings in patients suffering minor head injuries that were not sports related (class I).

Pearl

Many experts suggest that athletes undergo neuropsychological assessment before they are allowed to return to contact sports following a head injury.

Life-Threatening Head Injury/Head Injury Requiring Craniotomy

To our knowledge, no studies address the safety of returning to play in these situations. The present state of knowledge is primarily anecdotal. It has been recommended that after any head injury that requires surgical correction or causes documented intracranial parenchymal injury, return to competition is to be discouraged even if the athlete is completely neurologically intact.[18] In patients who suffer epidural hematomas or other brain injuries for which surgery is not required, it has been suggested that the athlete may return to contact sports in select cases 1 year or longer following the injury if neurologic recovery is complete. Such a recommendation, however, is based only on expert opinion (class III).

Pearl

Parenchymal injury or craniotomy have been used as criteria to discourage return to play, whereas epidural lesions, nonoperative injuries, and concussions that do not cause parenchymal injury have been viewed as less severe injuries that may not necessarily prevent return to competition.

Although no studies have addressed scarring of the CSF pathways and consequent decreased buoyancy of the brain and increased susceptibility to concussive forces, other conditions believed to cause a similar problem have been investigated, such as Chiari I malformations and arachnoid cysts. It has been questioned whether the presence of Chiari I malformations may alter the normal CSF capacity for buffering the brain from forceful impacts by altering the fourth ventricular outflow tracts.[19] However, the presence of a Chiari I malformation has not been deemed an absolute contraindication for contact sports in asymptomatic athletes. No case evidence exists demonstrating that these athletes are more susceptible to head injury than those without Chiari malformations. Arachnoid cysts, which are present in ~1% of the general population, are another cause of alterations in normal CSF circulation. In addition, hemorrhage from fragile vessels in the walls of arachnoid cysts has been reported (class III data).[20] The asymptomatic athlete with this condition has ordinarily been allowed to continue participation in contact sports. To date, no significant reporting of adverse consequences from such a decision has occurred. We do not suggest that information of this type can justify the return to play of an affected athlete, but it does represent a starting point for further study.

In several known instances, athletes have returned to contact sports following LTHI/HIRC. Helmets may provide some protection to such athletes. A professional hockey player recently returned to competition less than a year after a craniotomy for a ruptured arteriovenous malformation (class III).[3] Fractures of the anterior or posterior wall of the frontal sinus may occur in ice hockey or soccer players,[21] and many of these athletes have returned to play without significant negative sequelae.

Pearl

A professional hockey player recently returned to competition less than a year after a craniotomy for a ruptured arteriovenous malformation.

In patients who are without residual cerebral parenchymal abnormality or clinical evidence indicating alterations in CSF circulation and who are neurologically intact with a normal examination, consideration may be given for return to participation in contact sports. Of course, such decisions must be made only after great deliberation and with an individualized approach.[3] We commonly use the criterion of radiographically demonstrated healing of the craniotomy bone flap as a prerequisite to return to play. Such healing commonly occurs within 1 year in nonsmokers. It has been suggested that newer cranial reconstruction plates provide more rigidity of fixation of cranial bone flaps than wire fixation.[22] No standardized studies are available to determine whether recently introduced bone matrix products contribute to more rapid and secure healing of a craniotomy flap.

Recommendations

Mild Traumatic Brain Injury

With regard to MTBI, we recommend adherence to the current guidelines for return to play constructed by the American Association of Neurologists, the Colorado Medical Society, or Cantu[14] (Table 44–1) (level III). Because of the potential for (and unknown incidence of) catastrophic outcomes in this population, erring on the side of conservative management cannot be faulted. We also agree with the recommendation of Cantu that the occurrence of three grade I concussions, two to three grade II concussions, or one or two grade III concussions in the same season are grounds for withdrawal from competition for the remainder of the season (level III).

Life-Threatening Head Injury/Head Injury Requiring Craniotomy

The advisability of allowing athletes who have had a previous craniotomy to return to contact sports remains unclear. Based solely on experience, we commonly discourage return to contact sports in athletes who have suffered parenchymal injuries that required craniotomy. More recently, however, we have considered rigid cranial fixation in an athlete with a normal neurologic exam not to be an absolute contraindication to later participation in contact sports. Serious deliberation about the pros and cons of such a decision must be carefully weighed on a case-by-case basis.

References

1. Fact Sheet. Sports and brain injury. Brain Injury Assoc., Inc., 1776 Massachusetts Ave. N.W., Suite 100, Washington, DC 20036.
2. Centers for Disease Control and Prevention. Sports-related recurrent brain injuries, United States. MMWR Morb Mortal Wkly Rep 1997;46:224–227.
3. Bailes JE, Cantu RC. Head injury in athletes. Neurosurgery 2001;48:26–46.
4. Cantu RC, Mueller FO. Fatalities and catastrophic injuries in high school and college sports, 1982–1997. Phys Sportsmed 1999;27:35–48.
5. Cantu RC. When to return to contact sports after a cerebral concussion. Sports Med Digest 1989;10:1–2.
6. Colorado Medical Society. Report of the Sports Medicine Committee: guidelines for the management of concussion in sports. Denver, Colorado, 1991.
7. Kelly JP, Rosenberg JH. The development of guidelines for the management of concussion in sports. J Head Trauma Rehabil 1998;13:53–65.
8. Practice parameter. The management of concussion in sports (summary statement). Report of the Quality Standards Subcommittee. Neurology 1997;48:581–585.
9. Kelly JP, Rosenberg JH. Diagnosis and management of concussion in sports. Neurology 1997;48:575–580.
10. Kelly JP, Nichols JS, Filley CM, et al. Concussion in sports. Guidelines for the prevention of catastrophic outcome. JAMA 1991;266:2867–2869.
11. McQuillen JB, McQuillen EN, Morrow P. Trauma, sport, and malignant cerebral edema. Am J Forensic Med Pathol 1988;9:12–15.
12. Cantu RC. Second-impact syndrome. Clin Sports Med 1998;17:37–44.
13. Cantu RC. Cerebral concussion in sport. Management and prevention. Sports Med 1992;14:64–74.
14. Cantu RC. Head and spine injuries in youth sports. Clin Sports Med 1995;14:517–532.
15. Gerberich SG, Priest JD, Boen JR, et al. Concussion incidences and severity in secondary school varsity football players. Am J Public Health 1983;73:1370–1375.
16. Macciocchi SN, Barth JT, Alves W, et al. Neuropsychological functioning and recovery after mild head injury in collegiate athletes. Neurosurgery 1996;39:510–514.
17. Levin HS, Mattis S, Ruff RM, et al. Neurobehavioral outcome following minor head injury: a three-center study. J Neurosurg 1987;66:234–243.
18. Cantu RC. Return to play guidelines after a head injury. Clin Sports Med 1998;17:45–60.
19. Beuls EA, Vandersteen MA, Vanormelingen LM, et al. Deformation of the cervicomedullary junction and spinal cord in a surgically treated adult Chiari I hindbrain hernia associated with syringomyelia: a magnetic resonance microscopic and neuropathological study: case report. J Neurosurg 1996;85:701–708.
20. Vigil DV, DiFiori JP, Puffer JC, et al. Arachnoid cyst and subdural hygroma in a high school football player. Clin J Sport Med 1998;8:234–237.
21. Raschka C, Weber R, Draf W. Frontal sinus impression fracture as a collision sequelae in football. Sportverletz Sportschaden 1994;8:46–49.
22. Broaddus WC, Holloway KL, Winters CJ, et al. Titanium miniplates or stainless steel wire for cranial fixation: a prospective randomized comparison. J Neurosurg 2002;96:244–247.

◆ 45 ◆

How Important Are Stingers?

Robert C. Cantu

Brief Answer

A stinger is an injury to a peripheral nerve, not to the spinal cord. Pain usually lasts for seconds to hours, but painless myotomal weakness may persist for days. Persistent or worsening weakness may be evaluated by electromyography (EMG) or magnetic resonance imaging (MRI). Recommendations for return to play range from almost immediate return to the same game after transient first-time occurrences to termination of the season if several prior episodes have occurred earlier in the same season.

Background

Stingers are also known as "burners." Both terms are descriptive of a specific type of upper limb sensory disturbance that may occur as a result of athletic injury. Stingers are peripheral nerve injuries, not spinal cord injuries, and are not directly related to the presence of central cervical spinal stenosis. Stingers are also distinct from the burning hands syndrome,[1] which is a separate clinical entity reflective of a central cervical spinal cord injury.

Literature Review

Both compressive and tensile (i.e., traction or stretch) overload have been implicated as the cause of stingers, although precise localization of this injury; that is, cervical spine versus brachial plexus, has been controversial. A variety of mechanisms have been described, including tensile injury to the upper trunk of the brachial plexus,[2–8] tensile injury to the cervical nerve root–dorsal root spinal ganglion complex,[4,9–12] compressive injury to the cervical nerve root–dorsal root spinal ganglion complex,[8,12–14] and compressive injury to the brachial plexus.[15,16] Compelling neuroanatomic features of the cervical nerve root–dorsal spinal root ganglion complex place it at greater risk than the brachial plexus for this injury.[17]

Pearl

Stingers are peripheral nerve injuries, not spinal cord injuries, and are not directly related to the presence of cervical spinal stenosis.

Assessment

The clinical assessment of a stinger requires an understanding of the sport and of the skill level of the athlete. For example, a tensile overload mechanism of injury occurs when the head and shoulder of the symptomatic limb are forcefully moved in opposite directions. A compressive overload mechanism occurs when the head and neck are forced into the extreme ipsilateral posterolateral quadrant, narrowing the cervical intervertebral foramen and compressing the cervical nerve root-dorsal root spinal ganglion complex. In football, tackling and blocking are the most common activities that cause stingers, with the tacklers or blockers usually sustaining the injuries.

The hallmark of a stinger is unilateral upper limb involvement following a traumatic event like those described above. The development of simultaneous bilateral cervical radiculopathy is very uncommon, and involvement of more than one limb should always prompt a consideration of spinal cord injury. The athlete typically experiences a lancinating, burning pain and dysesthesia, usually in a nerve root or dermatome pattern. A detailed assessment on the sidelines should include determination of the mechanism of injury; distribution and duration of symptoms; and evaluation of active range of motion of the neck only within pain tolerance to determine the presence of rigidity and/or pain provocation (to avoid the development of complications from a potentially unstable spine). Passive range of motion examination; that is, the patient remains passive while the examiner moves the patient's neck, is contraindicated if the player is symptomatic.

Pearl

Involvement of more than one limb should always prompt a consideration of spinal cord injury.

Neurologic examination emphasizing motor and sensory deficits in the distributions of the fifth, sixth, and seventh nerve roots is essential (Table 45-1). A quick neurologic assessment that measures only finger grip strength is inadequate.

Table 45-1 Innervation of Muscles Commonly Affected following a Stinger

Muscle	Myotome	Peripheral Nerve
Rhomboid	C5	Dorsal scapular
Supraspinatus	C5,6	Suprascapular
Infraspinatus	C5,6	Suprascapular
Deltoid	C5,6	Axillary
Biceps	C5,6	Musculoskeletal
Wrist flexors	C6,7	Median
Wrist extensors	C6,7	Radial
Triceps	C7,8	Radial

The duration of pain following a stinger varies from seconds to hours, rarely persisting for days or longer. However, specific myotomal weakness without pain may continue for days or longer, demanding frequent serial examination in the acute postinjury period. If weakness persists for more than 2 weeks, or worsens over the first few postinjury days, ancillary testing is reasonable and appropriate to determine precisely the site of injury and the degree of axonopathy.[18] EMG can be performed as early as 7 to 10 days following the onset of symptoms.[19] An EMG may be the most sensitive test for evaluating axonal loss in the presence of clinical weakness.

Pearl

Specific myotomal weakness without pain may continue for days.

Rehabilitation

Following a burner or stinger, the decision to return an athlete to competition is highly dependent on a well-designed treatment program. A conservative treatment plan, especially for a high-caliber or elite athlete, does not necessarily imply a wait-and-see approach. Rather, the plan should be proactive and aggressive. A comprehensive cervical spine rehabilitation program progresses over specific stages: protection of the injured structure, control of pain and inflammation, correction of flexibility and strength imbalances, correction of postural dysfunction, and emphasis on sports-specific exercise. Return-to-play decisions should be based on clinical, electrodiagnostic, and imaging findings, with additional consideration given to whether the injury is a first-time or recurrent problem. In each case, there must be a full recovery of strength in the affected muscles, and the patient must be asymptomatic with full pain-free range of cervical spine motion. Furthermore, the player must have completed a comprehensive rehabilitation program and exhibit balance, flexibility, and strength through the cervical and thoracic spine and shoulder girdle. If an EMG is done, absence of acute axonopathy in the shoulder girdle or extremity should be documented. If an MRI is done, absence of a substantial nerve root compressive lesion such as a disk herniation, large foraminal osteophyte, or marked stenosis should be documented.

Recommendations

Because the literature contains only class III data, only level III recommendations may be made. In terms of the timing of return to competition following a first stinger, if there is full clinical neurologic recovery within 15 minutes, the individual can return to the same game. If full clinical recovery occurs within 48 to 72 hours, return in 1 week is acceptable. Following a recurrent stinger in the same season, normally the individual is held from practice or competition for the number of weeks that corresponds to the number of that stinger. After three or more stingers, especially in the presence of acute EMG findings or imaging evidence of a neurocompressive lesion, the season should be terminated. These guidelines, however, do not necessarily apply to all scenarios. As with any other athletic injury, other medical and nonmedical factors may play a role in determining when an athlete can and should return to competition following a stinger.

References

1. Maroon JC. "Burning hands" in football spinal cord injuries. JAMA 1977;238:2049–2051.
2. Archambault JL. Brachial plexus stretch injury. J Am Coll Health 1983;31:256–260.
3. Clancy WG, Brand RL, Bergfeld JA. Upper trunk brachial plexus injuries in contact sports. Am J Sports Med 1977;5:209–215.
4. Funk FF, Wells RE. Injuries of the cervical spine in football. Clin Orthop 1975;109:50–58.
5. Hunter C. Injuries to the brachial plexus: experience of a private sports medicine clinic. J Am Osteopath Assoc 1982;91: 757–760.
6. Jackson DW, Lohr FT. Cervical spine injuries. Clin Sports Med 1986;5:373–386.
7. Robertson WC, Eichman PL, Clancy WG. Upper trunk brachial plexopathy in football players. JAMA 1979;241:1480–1482.
8. Wroble RR, Albright JP. Neck and low back injuries in wrestling. Clin Sports Med 1986;5:295–325.
9. Chrisman OD, Snook CA, Stanitis JM, et al. Lateral flexion neck injuries in athletic competition. JAMA 1965;192:613–615.
10. Marshall TM. Nerve pinch injuries in football. J Ky Med Assoc 1970;68:648–649.
11. Speer KP, Bassett FJ III. The prolonged burner syndrome. Am J Sports Med 1990;18:591–594.
12. Watkins RG. Nerve injuries in football players. Clin Sports Med 1986;5:215–246.
13. Poindexter DP, Johnson EW. Football shoulder and neck injury: a study of the "stinger." Arch Phys Med Rehabil 1984;65:601–602.
14. Rockett FX. Observations on the "burner." Traumatic cervical radiculopathy. Clin Orthop 1982;164:18–19.
15. DiBennedetto M, Markey K. Electrodiagnostic localization of traumatic upper trunk brachial plexopathy. Arch Phys Med Rehabil 1984;65:15–17.
16. Markey KL, DiBennedetto M, Curl WW. Upper trunk brachial plexopathy: the stinger syndrome. Am J Sports Med 1993;21: 650–655.
17. Sunderland S. The brachial plexus: normal anatomy. In: Nerves and Nerve Injuries, 2nd ed. New York: Churchill Livingstone; 1978:856.
18. Wilbourn A, Bergfeld J. Value of EMG examination with sports-related nerve injury. EEG Clin Neurophys 1983;55: 42P–54P.
19. Herring SA, Weinstein SM. Electrodiagnosis in sports medicine. Phys Med Rehabil State of the Art Rev 1989;3:809–822.

◆ 46 ◆

Do Return-to-Play Recommendations After Concussion Differ for High School, Collegiate, and Professional Athletes?

Henry Feuer

Brief Answer

The medical principles for treating concussions in athletes are essentially the same at the high school, college, and professional levels. Consensus exists about the broad concepts underlying the management of these head injuries, but no concussion grading system has been universally accepted. Furthermore, although some studies have begun to report prospectively collected observational data about the neuropsychological effects of sports-related concussion, no prospective studies have established criteria for return to play. Particularly at the college and professional levels, decisions may be influenced by extrinsic social and economic pressures and by an individual player's personal and career goals.

Literature Review

Medical management is fairly straightforward for sports-related head injuries at the ends of the spectrum of severity; that is, very mild concussions on the one hand and moderate to severe head injuries on the other. For the former, numerous sets of published guidelines for return to play are very similar (class III data)[1,2]; the choice of which set to use depends greatly on personal preference and experience. The latter are treated according to established principles familiar to every neurosurgeon.

For injuries between these two extremes of severity, such as more serious concussions and mild head injuries with seemingly good recovery despite abnormal imaging studies, management decisions require a great deal of personal judgment. Factors that must be considered include the individual's symptoms, signs, neuropathology, residual deficits, and social circumstances. There exists little useful evidence-based literature about differences in recommendations for high school, college, and professional athletes in terms of management protocols for concussions and other head injuries. The main principle agreed to by all is that before an athlete may resume participation, he or she must be completely asymptomatic (class III data).[1–3] Neurocognitive, neuropsychological, and neuroimaging studies that are currently in progress or already published may help define sound protocols based on outcomes and on comparative data for high school, college, and professional teams.[4–6]

Pearl

For injuries between the extremes of severity, that is, neither very mild nor obviously serious, management decisions call for a great deal of personal judgment.

Because of the paucity of evidence about whether recommendations differ for athletes at different levels of competition, the answer to this question must be based largely on personal experience and on expert opinion; that is, on class III data, as detailed below.

Background

The following reflections are from my personal experience as a neurosurgical consultant for head-injured athletes in most central Indiana high schools, for 10 universities and colleges in Indiana, and for the Indianapolis Colts football team. I am also a consultant to the National Football League (NFL) Combine (i.e., the centralized evaluation program in which all NFL teams and scout-selected college football players participate every year) and a member of the NFL Committee on Mild Traumatic Brain Injury, and I have stood on the sidelines during college and professional football games for many years. My colleagues and I also care for and evaluate head-injured race drivers in various auto-racing leagues, including IRL and NASCAR.

Screening Prior to Play

Indiana high schools are required to ask students only two relevant questions: "Have you ever had a head injury?" and "Have you ever been knocked out or been unconscious?" If the response to either question is yes, further information is obtained during a physician interview. If the player has no residual signs or symptoms from a remote brain injury that was not serious enough to cause prolonged loss of consciousness or hospitalization, he is ordinarily allowed to play without further testing. On the other hand, if the previous injury was considered serious, full details are obtained from the medical record. Depending on the nature of the injury, and if there is no clinical evidence of residual neurologic deficit, I usually recommend that he be allowed to participate in all sports. However, the parents and player are counseled regarding cumulative injury that could occur during collision or contact sports. In almost every instance, the family takes my advice to permit or restrict the child from playing. I express my opinion in a letter to the referring physician, with a copy to the high school athletic department (with the permission of the player and family), confirming that I have counseled that player and family. If the athlete is to practice with the team, I usually have to fill out a form for the school. In reality, it is rare that I have found it necessary to reject a player with a previous head injury who has recovered well enough, both mentally and physically, to be eligible for his high school team. On a few occasions, second opinions have been sought after I have rejected a player, and my decisions have always been upheld.

Most colleges usually require completion of a standard application form for all sports that is somewhat more specific than that used by high schools. For example, the Indiana University Athletic Department application form asks, "Have you been knocked out or experienced a concussion in the last three years, and if yes, were you hospitalized overnight?" If affirmative, medical records will be obtained by university staff prior to the time of my consultation. If the injury was remote and I can ascertain that there are no residual deficits, I usually grant permission to play. If the applicant played high school sports without a neurologic problem, my decision is easier. If the records suggest that a serious head injury occurred, I feel obligated to pursue a further workup, which may include magnetic resonance imaging (MRI) and a neurocognitive test battery by a neuropsychologist with experience in sports-related head injury. If an athlete is asymptomatic and the neurocognitive tests are normal, an abnormality on the MRI would not necessarily exclude the player. The imaging study also serves as a baseline in the event of further injury. Each case is considered individually, and the player is counseled. Sometimes, before rendering an opinion, I may run the case by some of my colleagues in sports neurosurgery. The university almost always accepts my advice. No waivers (a release of liability for an injury) are offered to recruits by college teams with whom I work. Occasionally a family will ask for a second opinion if I advise against play, particularly if a scholarship is at risk. My recommendation that a player not be accepted because of a previous head injury has never been reversed by a second consultant and has never resulted in legal action.

Pearl

The author's recommendation that a player not be allowed to participate in a sport because of a previous head injury has never been reversed by a second consultant and has never resulted in legal action.

Although "Have you had a head injury?" is the only question usually asked in the application, screening of professional athletes who have had a concussion is much more thorough. If the response is affirmative, the team physician gathers the medical history and does the initial screening. If he is unable to make a decision, he will seek my advice. Most situations can be resolved by phone. For example, if a candidate had two previous concussions with brief loss of consciousness and he played his last year of college with no injuries or symptoms, he usually is cleared. On the other hand, if a player has had more than two concussions or has had a severe head injury, I feel it is important for me to examine the player. I usually obtain an MRI and neurocognitive testing. After reviewing all of the studies, I make a recommendation to team management, and they weigh the situation according to their needs and the risks involved. If the player or the team has any concern about potential cumulative or additional injury, the player will usually be asked to sign a waiver after the risks have been thoroughly explained. A waiver would release the professional team from all liability should another concussion occur that renders the athlete unable to play. However, the athlete might still qualify for compensation based on the terms of his contract. Professional teams are extremely careful during the selection process because they are concerned about having to assume liability for a subsequent injury. Because of the teams' thoroughness in screening athletes, on only one occasion have I had to reject a player after I personally obtained a history that he had had numerous concussions.

Pearl

Professional teams are extremely careful about signing players with histories of head injuries because they are concerned about having to assume liability for a subsequent injury.

Concussion Requiring Removal from Play on Day of Injury

For high school players, I rarely deviate from the guidelines for return to play after a concussion. I usually abide by a combination of the recommendations of Cantu[7,8] and the American Academy of Neurology (Class III data).[9] The high school athletic trainers and team physicians in our area are usually familiar with these concussion guidelines. In most cases, either the trainer or team physician will do the routine sideline neurologic exam, administer a sideline cognitive test, and make the appropriate decisions during a game. I usually see those players with persistent symptoms that prohibit return to play.

For college players, the situation is usually similar, except a team physician is present during each game. He or she is usually a physician with some sports medicine expertise. Guidelines are generally followed, but return to play is sometimes based on "sound clinical judgment"; that is, the physician's experience with concussion management (J. P. Nevins, personal communication). During a college football game, even though the team physician or sports medicine expert is present on the sidelines, he or she does usually not go onto the playing field until called by the trainer, who traditionally is the first to evaluate the injured player.

In professional football, the team physician, who also has special expertise in sports medicine, always goes onto the field if a player appears to be injured. For professional athletes, concussion guidelines may be interpreted somewhat more liberally. For example, the American Academy of Neurology Guidelines[9] require that the injured athlete with a grade II concussion (transient confusion, no loss of consciousness, symptoms lasting more than 15 minutes) or grade III concussion (any loss of consciousness) have no symptoms for at least 7 days and have normal neurocognitive testing before being allowed to return to play. I usually adhere to these arbitrary time requirements for high school and college players. However, the professional player with no symptoms and normal tests may occasionally plead to return to competition sooner than 7 symptom-free days, particularly if pressured by coaches or an agent. Recent evidence supports the safety of this practice (class III data).[10] Concussion guidelines for athletes are essentially rules of thumb; they are not legal documents and are not based on prospective, evidence-based studies. Therefore, there is some leeway in dealing with mature professionals, provided all risks are outlined and all parties agree. In two decades of experience with the NFL, I cannot recall a single instance of a bad outcome when a concussed player returned to play when all symptoms had resolved, regardless of the duration of the symptom-free interval. I have never personally seen a second impact syndrome.

My policy for professionals is that the athlete who has had a Grade I concussion (no loss of consciousness, symptoms resolving within 15 minutes) must be completely asymptomatic before returning to the game, and I clearly and personally determine and document that he has no symptoms or abnormal signs. With Grade II or Grade III concussions, the athlete must undergo a neurocognitive test battery on which his performance must be back to his preseason baseline.

Pearl

Concussion guidelines for athletes are essentially rules of thumb; they are not legal documents and are not based on prospective, evidence-based studies.

When dealing with concussions in professional race-car drivers (a noncontact high-velocity sport), I never deviate from the strictest guidelines because an accident could result in a life-threatening injury to the driver and others. The extrinsic pressures in this sport are often tremendous. Team owners, who may have significant investments in their vehicles and who depend heavily on their drivers, may convince the driver to seek second opinions from selected specialists in various parts of the country. Fortunately, the strong medical community associated with professional racing understands the utmost importance of racing safety.

Pearl

The strictest guidelines are followed in sports like automobile racing, in which an accident could result in life-threatening injuries to spectators as well as to the driver.

External Factors

Pressure from the adolescent player, high school coach, and parents occurs commonly, especially when the young athlete is a starter, a star, or a scholarship candidate. I disregard these pressures and stick to generally accepted guidelines. The high school player is a minor and may not have the judgment or maturity to enter into a rational decision-making process. Also, one must be aware that the high school athlete is likely to minimize persistent symptoms in order to return to play sooner. Another issue that arises in high school is that a good athlete may play several sports. The guidelines need to be individualized for the sport. For example, I might not allow a football player who has suffered a serious concussion to return to football or other collision sports, but when that player becomes asymptomatic I may allow him to return to a contact sport like wrestling, which usually begins shortly after the end of football season.

Pearl

Although it may be difficult, the physician should remain objective and resist pressures from coaches, players, alumni, and others.

Because of pressures from alumni and media and because of the possibility of a professional contract, an ambitious college player may attempt to return to play too early after a head injury. I consider each player individually, and I may allow my professional judgment to supersede generally accepted guidelines if there is apparent full recovery. Is this dangerous? Although such a practice may be associated with some increase in risk which all parties involved must accept, the risk is still very low. Long before concussion guidelines for athletes were first published in the 1980s, I had learned to rely on my extensive experience with college teams and with managing head-injured patients. I am not aware of any asymptomatic player I permitted to return to play who subsequently had an adverse neurologic event.

In professional football, the injury is always captured on television. The physician on the field must be absolutely familiar with accepted immobilization procedures, especially with a suspected spinal injury, because it is likely that every action will be recorded and scrutinized. Often there is immense pressure from numerous sources, including the player, to grant permission to resume play, and permission to return to play usually generates a press release. It is important to remain objective and not to be influenced by these pressures. For example, a player may insist that he is ready to return because he has been allowed to practice (with a different-colored jersey that signifies no contact) and has experienced no problems. However, if his neurocognitive tests have not returned to baseline, I will refuse permission. In such a circumstance, the player may insist on a second opinion (from a specialist in neurologic disorders who has no connections with the team), usually at the urging of veteran teammates or his agent. The bottom line is the same as in high school and college: no return to action until symptom-free, with no signs of residual impairment.

In high school and college football, I adhere to the general rule that three concussions disqualifies an athlete for the rest of the season. However, when dealing with the pros, I take into consideration that the professional season lasts longer. For example, I recently treated a football player who had had two concussions in preseason games. He missed 6 weeks on my advice, and then he returned to play. Four months later he had a mild concussion in a playoff game. His sideline tests were normal, and I felt it was safe for him to resume play.

Conclusions

The decision-making process involved in allowing athletes to return to sports after a concussion varies somewhat among the high school, college, and professional levels. The medical issues are the same, and social, economic, and personal pressures are present at every level. However, the pressures are most obvious at the professional level. Generally accepted guidelines have been created, but these guidelines are rules of thumb and are not based on prospective, controlled trials; they are level III recommendations based on class III data. However, the guiding principle at all levels is that a player must not be allowed to return to the game until he is asymptomatic, without residual signs of neurologic deficit. In addition, formal neuropsychological testing is becoming an integral part of the athlete's neurologic evaluation.

Recommendations (Level III)

1. A general rule at all levels of competition is that an athlete must not be allowed to return to competition until he or she is asymptomatic.
2. Experienced physicians should be allowed to exercise their judgment in individual cases, even when their decisions seem to run counter to generally accepted (but arbitrarily constructed) guidelines.

Acknowledgments

Drs. Joseph Maroon and Robert Cantu have encouraged and supported me, and their efforts have promoted ongoing research in concussions in athletes for many years.

References

1. Cantu RC. Classification and clinical management of concussion. In: Bailes JE, Day AL, eds. Neurological Sports Medicine: A Guide for Physicians and Athletic Trainers. Rolling Meadows, IL: American Association of Neurological Surgeons; 2001:25–33.
2. Roos R. Guidelines for managing concussion in sports: a persistent headache. Phys Sportsmed 1996;24:67–74.
3. Kelly JP. Concussion in sports and recreation. Semin Neurol 2000;20:165–171.
4. Johnston KM, Lassonde M, Ptito A. A contemporary neurosurgical approach to sport-related head injury: the McGill concussion protocol. J Am Coll Surg 2001;192:515–524.
5. Lovell MR, Collins MW, Iverson GL, et al. Grade 1 or "ding" concussions in high school athletes. Am J Sports Med 2004;32: 47–54.
6. McCrea M, Guskiewicz KM, Marshall SW, et al. Acute effects and recovery time following concussion in collegiate football players: the NCAA Concussion Study. JAMA 2003;290:2556–2563.
7. Cantu RC. Guidelines for return to contact sports after a cerebral concussion. Phys Sportsmed 1986;14:75–83.
8. Cantu RC. Posttraumatic retrograde and anterograde amnesia: pathophysiology and implications in grading and safe return to play. J Athl Train 2001;36:244–248.
9. American Academy of Neurology, Quality Standards Subcommittee. Practice parameter: the management of concussion in sports (summary statement). Neurology 1997; 48:581–585.
10. Pellman EJ, Powell JW, Viano DC, et al. Concussion in professional football: epidemiological features of game injuries and review of the literature–part 3. Neurosurgery 2004;54:81–96.

♦ Part VII ♦

Trauma Systems

◆ 47 ◆

Which Specialty Should Be in Charge of Neurotrauma Patients? Do Patients with Head or Spinal Cord Injury Require a Specialized Neurosurgical Intensive Care Unit?

Jeffrey M. Lobosky

Brief Answer

This chapter reviews the available literature on whether designated neurotrauma intensive care units (NTICUs) improve outcome in neurotrauma patients and on whether neurosurgical expertise is important in the management of these complex patients. Unfortunately, evidence-based studies of these issues are scant and consist mainly of class III data. Although defensible conclusions cannot be drawn from the available literature, reason and experience suggest that caring for these patients in an NTICU with meaningful participation by neurosurgical specialists can optimize outcomes.

Background

A generation ago, little could be offered the neurotrauma patient beyond hematoma evacuation for head injury and spinal stabilization for traumatic spinal cord injury. As our understanding of the pathophysiology of neurologic injury progressed, new treatment protocols provided a variety of interventions, pharmacologic as well as surgical, to optimize recovery. The use of controlled ventilation and osmotic diuretics to reduce cerebral edema and the introduction of high-dose barbiturate therapy for the treatment of intractable increased intracranial pressure (ICP) necessitated that these patients be observed more closely than in the past. Sophisticated monitors, including ventriculostomy catheters, pulmonary artery and jugular venous bulb catheters, arterial and central venous pressure lines, and brain tissue oxygen probes, became available and continue to be added to the armamentarium of the neurosurgeon. The technical expertise needed to insert and use these tools became considerable. At the same time, the knowledge required to properly manage fluid and electrolyte balance, nutritional support, and ventilatory parameters began to increase in volume and complexity. Thus, the concept of an NTICU was born.

Pearl

Many anesthesiologists, trauma surgeons, pulmonologists, and other specialists have a strong interest in critical care medicine, including the management of neurosurgical patients.

The care of neurotrauma patients has historically fallen upon neurosurgeons. As technology and knowledge of neurophysiology advanced, training programs provided neurosurgical residents with intensive care experiences that prepared them to "captain" the team addressing neurologic injury. Simultaneously, other specialists, most notably anesthesiologists, trauma surgeons, and pulmonologists, developed an intense interest in critical care medicine, including the management of neurosurgical patients. This became most evident in the polytrauma patient, in whom the various specialties had overlapping interests. In many centers, a cooperative team approach emerged, encompassing several specialists providing expertise directed toward their particular organ systems.

The different trends summarized above have sometimes led to controversy about who should have primary responsibility for managing head-injured patients and where it should be done. It might seem that a neurosurgeon's training and experience would make him or her best prepared to provide optimal care for a patient with a neurologic injury. Furthermore, who could argue with such treatment being delivered in an intensive care setting that is specifically focused on the neurosurgical patient? Despite the inherent logic of these conclusions, however, there is no strong evidence to support these contentions, and, indeed, some studies can strongly argue the contrary.

Literature Review

The question as to whether a patient fares better when admitted to an NTICU as opposed to a general ICU or other setting is not easily answered. The question implies that all NTICUs are comparable in terms of available services and the expertise and interests of their staffs. Ghajar et al[1] surveyed the care of comatose, head-injured patients in a pool of over 600 trauma centers, 34% of which had designated NTICUs, and found disturbing variability in the management of these patients. Even in some NTICUs directed by neurosurgeons, there was a reluctance to utilize ICP monitoring routinely, as well as a reliance on such therapies as excessive hyperventilation and high-dose steroids, which have been shown to be detrimental or ineffective in the treatment of severely head-injured patients. Jeevaratnam and Menon[2] and McKeating et al[3] reported a similar experience in the United Kingdom and proposed the establishment of guidelines to be adopted by all ICUs caring for head-injured patients.

Pearl

Even in some NTICUs directed by neurosurgeons, there was reluctance to utilize ICP monitoring and reliance on hyperventilation and high-dose steroids, which have been shown to be detrimental or ineffective.

Evidence supporting improved outcomes from care in an NTICU has been offered by Warme et al,[4] who looked retrospectively at the outcomes of two groups of severely head-injured patients treated at the same institution before and after the establishment of an NTICU. The number of good outcomes increased dramatically in the latter group. A second study out of Sweden by Nordstrom et al[5] arrived at a similar conclusion. Hyman et al,[6] looking at the experience at Vanderbilt, suggested that treatment in a neurosurgical intensive care unit resulted in improved patient care as well as outcome. It must be remembered that these data are retrospective and anecdotal, but they do suggest that patients may indeed benefit from treatment in a specialized neurosurgical intensive care unit *if* that facility adheres to accepted standards of patient care. Simply calling a unit an "NTICU" offers little advantage to patients if they are not being appropriately monitored and treated.

Pearl

Many neurosurgeons have willingly abdicated their role to intensivists, trauma surgeons, and even nurse practitioners and physician assistants.

The role of neurosurgeons in the management of neurotrauma patients has been the subject of much recent debate.[7–10] During the last decade, neurosurgeons have, with disturbing frequency, willingly abdicated their role in neurotrauma care to intensivists, trauma surgeons, and in some instances to nurse practitioners and physician assistants. This has led to a sounding of alarms throughout organized neurosurgery and has prompted other specialists to question the necessity of neurosurgeons in the care of traumatic brain injury.[11–18] A recent survey of members of the American Association for the Surgery of Trauma highlighted the perception that neurosurgeons are providing inadequate care for victims of trauma.[17] Respondents emphasized the resistance of neurosurgeons to participate in the management of patients without "surgical" lesions and their reluctance to insert ICP monitors in comatose patients.

The reasons for neurosurgical "nonparticipation" are diverse. Invariably, surveys reveal a high degree of anxiety regarding exposure to malpractice actions by emergency room patients despite the fact that the few studies investigating this issue fail to substantiate this concern.[19,20] The frequency of less-than-perfect outcomes despite neurosurgeons' best efforts and the impact of the unpredictability and inconvenience of trauma on their schedules also contribute to neurosurgeons' reluctance. Most important, however, is the dismal reimbursement most surgeons realize for their many efforts. These factors have conspired to create a critical shortage of neurotrauma manpower in many communities, leading to the closure of many trauma centers and obligating trauma surgeons to identify alternative means of appropriately caring for neurologically injured patients.

Some reports suggest that general surgeons and trauma surgeons can be trained to perform emergency craniotomies and drill burr holes for intracranial hematomas.[12,15,16,18] Although the majority of these recommendations relate to practices in rural settings where neurosurgical expertise is geographically distant, the time is coming when trauma surgeons will seek similar privileges in more suburban and urban locales where neurosurgeons are practicing but are resistant to providing the necessary care to neurotrauma patients.

Havill and Sleigh[12] reported that the mortality rates of patients treated in their tertiary referral trauma center without neurosurgical specialists compared favorably with those of other adult series of TBI patients. Visvanathan[18] detailed the outcomes of head-injured patients, both surgical and nonsurgical, managed on a general surgery service and advocated more extensive neurosurgical training for the general surgical staff. The implications of these and other studies are that management of severe head injury is not beyond the realm of a general or trauma surgeon with additional training and that outcomes in such scenarios could be expected to approach those in the neurosurgical literature.[15,16]

Pearl

Brain surgery is best performed by brain surgeons.

However, there also exist class III data that completely refute the above notion and reiterate that brain surgery is best performed by brain surgeons. Wester[21] looked at outcomes of patients undergoing emergency surgery for acute epidural hematomas by nonneurosurgeons and concluded that it was more effective to transfer the patient to a facility with neurosurgical expertise even if such a transfer delayed the operation. In a subsequent paper, he went on to suggest that even with additional training, the number of craniotomies performed by general surgeons or orthopedists would be inadequate to maintain sufficient skills. He concluded that efforts would be best directed toward improving the speed and accuracy of diagnosing patients with significant neurosurgical lesions and toward effecting a more rapid transfer to designated neurosurgical centers.[22] Simpson et al[23] reported that emergency craniotomies performed by general surgeons in rural settings were often ineffective at removing a hematoma or were undertaken too late, resulting in adverse patient outcomes.

Even more provocative is the use of nonsurgeons, including medical intensivists, physician assistants, and other midlevel practitioners, to provide bedside care for the neurotrauma patient. The shortage of manpower at Hurley Medical Center in Flint, Michigan, for example, necessitated the use of physician assistants as house staff for its level II trauma center. Miller et al[14] reported that traditional parameters of quality care, such as transfer time to the operating room, ICU or floor, as well as length of stay, all compared favorably to parameters in the literature. Indeed, length of stay in the NTICU decreased 33%. Kaups et al[13] examined complication rates for ICP monitors inserted by neurosurgeons, general surgery residents, and midlevel practitioners. The results were almost identical in each group, leading to the conclusion that nonsurgeons could safely perform this invasive procedure. Bochicchio et al[11] reviewed similar data for ICP monitors inserted by intensivists and likewise discovered complication rates comparable to those in published neurosurgical series and lower than the rate for central venous catheterization.

Recommendations

Pearl

Evidence-based reports that answer these questions are simply nonexistent.

So what is the correct answer? Do victims of neurotrauma fare better in an NTICU with their treatment directed by neurosurgeons? Or can nonneurosurgeons provide a comparable level of care in a variety of alternative environments? The class III evidence that characterizes the available literature cannot support a definitive conclusion.

However, to many of us who remain actively involved in the care of victims of neurotrauma, the answers are apparent, even if they only have the strength of level III recommendations. No one has a better understanding of the intricate physiology of the central nervous system or is better trained to provide both surgical and nonsurgical interventions to ameliorate devastating insults to the brain and spinal cord than a neurosurgeon. Furthermore, delivery of that care in a setting where the latest technologic advances are readily available and where direct patient care is provided by nursing and support staffs with considerable neurosurgical expertise confers an immeasurable advantage. These points support the conclusion that neurotrauma patients are best managed by neurosurgeons in a designated NTICU.

The above conclusion, however, is not without qualifiers. The optimal management of these challenging patients requires that neurosurgeons remain abreast of current advances in the management of trauma patients. Furthermore, neurosurgeons' input is critical in creating and maintaining a high level of expertise in an NTICU. Their participation in establishing and revising treatment protocols, training nursing and ancillary service personnel, and assessing outcomes is invaluable. Neurosurgeons must ensure that the treatment provided in these specialized units complies with established guidelines. It is not coincidental that guidelines for management of traumatic brain injury were established by neurosurgeons, not trauma surgeons or intensivists. It is thus oxymoronic for an NTICU to function without a neurosurgeon.

Finally, the entire treatment staff, including neurosurgeons, must realize its limitations. Such limitations may be related to technical skills, knowledge, or time, and thus a "team" approach to the management of these complex patients may be optimal.[7,10,24] However, the success of such an approach requires ongoing communication among the trauma team members, a clear understanding of specific responsibilities, and a common objective of providing the highest quality of care for these patients.

It is erroneous to assume that any neurosurgical involvement is better than no neurosurgical involvement. If, as a member of the trauma team, the neurosurgeon is reluctant to insert appropriate monitors, is unavailable to respond to critical issues in a timely fashion, is unaware of current treatment guidelines to optimize outcomes, or is incapable of effective communication and cooperation with other members of the team, then his or her participation is both detrimental and counterproductive. In such instances, it would be far better for care to be directed by the intensivist or trauma surgeon. Outcomes are maximized when treatment is provided by those who are most interested and dedicated to delivering quality care. Neurosurgeons must understand that the growing trend of nonneurosurgeons managing neurotrauma is a direct response to neurosurgeons' failure to participate. With highly qualified, aggressive neurosurgical involvement, it is possible to reverse this trend and optimize neurotrauma care.

References

1. Ghajar J, Hariri RJ, Narayan RK, et al. Survey of critical care management of comatose, head-injured patients in the United States. Crit Care Med 1995;23:560–567.
2. Jeevaratnam DR, Menon DK. Survey of intensive care of severely head injured patients in the United Kingdom. BMJ 1996;312:944–947.
3. McKeating EG, Andrews PJ, Tocher JL, et al. The intensive care of severe head injury: a survey of non-neurosurgical centres in the United Kingdom. Br J Neurosurg 1998;12:7–14.
4. Warme PE, Bergstrom R, Persson L. Neurosurgical intensive care improves outcome after severe head injury. Acta Neurochir (Wien) 1991;110:57–64.
5. Nordstrom CH, Sundbarg G, Messeter K, et al. Severe traumatic brain lesions in Sweden, II: impact of aggressive neurosurgical intensive care. Brain Inj 1989;3:267–281.
6. Hyman SA, Williams V, Maciunas RJ. Neurosurgical intensive care unit organization and function: an American experience. J Neurosurg Anesthesiol 1993;5:71–80.
7. Belzberg H. The intensive care unit: who's in charge? Clin Neurosurg 1989;35:63–67.
8. Chesnut RM. Evolving models of neurotrauma critical care: an analysis and call to action. Clin Neurosurg 2000;46:185–195.
9. Meagher RJ, Narayan RK. The triage and acute management of severe head injury. Clin Neurosurg 2000;46:127–142.
10. Pitts LH. Neurosurgical critical care: who's in charge? Clin Neurosurg 1989;35:55–62.
11. Bochicchio M, Latronico N, Zappa S, et al. Bedside burr hole for intracranial pressure monitoring performed by intensive care physicians: a 5-year experience. Intensive Care Med 1996;22:1070–1074.
12. Havill JH, Sleigh J. Management and outcomes of patients with brain trauma in a tertiary referral trauma hospital without neurosurgeons on site. Anaesth Intensive Care 1998;26:642–647.
13. Kaups KL, Parks SN, Morris CL. Intracranial pressure monitor placement by midlevel practitioners. J Trauma 1998;45:884–886.
14. Miller W, Riehl E, Napier M, et al. Use of physician assistants as surgery/trauma housestaff at an American College of Surgeons-verified level II trauma center. J Trauma 1998;44:372–376.
15. Rinker C, McMurry FG, Groeneweg VR, et al. Emergency craniotomy in a rural level III trauma center. J Trauma 1998;44:984–990.
16. Schecter WP, Peper E, Tuatoo V. Can general surgery improve the outcome of the head-injury victim in rural America? A review of the experience in American Samoa. Arch Surg 1985;120:1163–1166.
17. Valadka AB, Andrews BT, Bullock MR. How well do neurosurgeons care for trauma patients? A survey of the membership of the American Association for the Surgery of Trauma. Neurosurgery 2001;48:17–25.
18. Visvanathan R. Severe head injury management in a general surgical department. Aust N Z J Surg 1994;64:527–529.
19. Burstin HR, Johnson WG, Lipsitz SR, et al. Do the poor sue more? A case-control study of malpractice claims and socioeconomic status. JAMA 1993;270:1697–1701.
20. Fink S, Chaudhuri TK. Medical characteristics of 61 unwarranted malpractice claims. South Med J 1995;88:1011–1019.
21. Wester K. Decompressive surgery for "pure" epidural hematomas: does neurosurgical expertise improve the outcome? Neurosurgery 1999;44:495–502.
22. Wester T, Fevang LT, Wester K. Decompressive surgery in acute head injuries: where should it be performed? J Trauma 1999;46:914–919.
23. Simpson DA, Heyworth JS, McLean AJ, et al. Extradural haemorrhage: strategies for management in remote places. Injury 1988;19:307–312.
24. Lobosky JM. Neurosurgical critical care: a perspective from private practice. Perspect Neurol Surg 1997;8:111–121.

Should Head-Injured Patients Be Taken to the Nearest Hospital or to a Hospital with Neurosurgical Capability That Is Farther Away?

Sandra M. Wanek and Donald D. Trunkey

Brief Answer

All patients with severe traumatic brain injury (TBI) [Glasgow Coma Scale (GCS) score ≤8] should be treated according to standard Advanced Trauma Life Support (ATLS) guidelines. Specific attention should be paid to avoiding and treating hypoxia and hypotension. Although no class I evidence exists, ample class II and III evidence supports a level II recommendation to transport patients with severe TBI to definitive care at a hospital with neurosurgical and neurocritical care capabilities.

Background

TBI continues to be the most significant cause of morbidity and mortality in the United States among persons 1 to 44 years of age. Data from 1991 reveal that ~1.5 million people in the United States suffer TBI annually, with over 1.1 million of these patients receiving outpatient care or no care at all and 393,000 being admitted to a hospital (class III data).[1] A population-based study from San Diego County revealed that over 40% of all trauma deaths resulted from acute head injury (class III data).[2] The loss in potential years of life, productivity, and potential income is enormous. In the U.S. alone, the cost to society was estimated to exceed $40 billion annually in 1966[3]; this figure has increased significantly in the intervening years. Worldwide, TBI is the leading cause of loss of productive years of life from either death or disability.

To reduce the morbidity and mortality associated with TBI, efforts have been made both to improve treatment and, more importantly, to reduce its incidence. In some parts of the United States, legislation to require helmets for motorcycle riders and programs to encourage helmet use among pediatric and adult bicycle riders has been associated with significant decreases in both the proportion of severe head injuries among victims of motorcycle and bicycle crashes and in the mortality associated with these types of accidents (class III data).[4]

Once TBI has occurred, treatment must focus on the prevention of secondary brain injury (SBI). Although long recognized, the concept of SBI has only recently been formally characterized. As a result of the initial traumatic event, an intracranial hematoma may rapidly enlarge and cause mass effect and midline shift. Hypoxia and hypotension may contribute to ischemia and subsequent edema. Increased intracranial pressure (ICP) from a mass lesion or brain swelling may compromise cerebral blood flow by decreasing cerebral perfusion pressure, placing a patient at risk for cerebral ischemia, subsequent cerebral edema, frank herniation, and death.

Literature Review

What can we learn from the past? Walter B. Cannon was a physiologist who studied the pathophysiology of traumatic shock in soldiers during World War I. Despite austere conditions on the front lines, he was able to make some remarkable observations that remain valid today. The first of these was that the body requires a minimal blood pressure to preserve delivery of oxygen and removal of metabolic waste products. He determined this threshold to be a systolic blood pressure of 80 mmHg. In conjunction with two pathologists, Gomez and Pike, he also analyzed the tolerance for hypoxia of various tissues of the body. He found the nervous system to be the tissue most sensitive to hypoxia and anemia, with as little as 8 minutes of anemia resulting in death of pyramidal cells in the cerebral cortex. Other areas of the nervous system tolerated progressively longer periods of anemia, with the spinal cord tolerating up to 45 to 60 minutes. He concluded, "Injured nerve cells require a better blood supply for their restoration than uninjured cells do for mere maintenance."[5]

To accomplish the goals of preserving perfusion pressure and preventing hypoxia, Cannon strongly advocated the use of blood as a resuscitation fluid. Crystalloids could help restore blood pressure only temporarily, and they obviously could not carry oxygen to the tissues. Moreover, salt solutions contributed significantly to third-space fluid losses from increased capillary permeability if treatment had been delayed. Colloids were found to have beneficial effects if used early in those soldiers with mild to moderate injures. For those with serious wounds or for whom treatment was delayed, early surgical intervention to prevent further blood loss prior to resuscitation correlated with a better outcome. Low blood pressure prevented further blood loss for a period of time, but its occurrence placed the patient at increased risk for end-organ damage from hypoperfusion. Therefore, he concluded that blood and salt solutions should be used as temporizing measures to maintain a minimal blood pressure of 80 mmHg to preserve viability of sensitive tissues until definitive surgical care became available.

Pearl

From his studies of hemorrhagic shock in wounded soldiers in World War I, Cannon concluded that blood and salt solutions should be used as temporizing measures to maintain a minimal blood pressure of 80 mmHg to preserve viability of sensitive tissues until definitive surgical care became available.

More recently, in a retrospective review of the database of the Traumatic Coma Data Bank (TCDB), hypoxia and hypotension were identified as powerful independent predictors of outcome for patients with severe TBI (GCS $\leq$ 8) (class II data).[6] Data from 717 patients in the TCDB revealed that single episodes of hypotension (systolic blood pressure <90 mmHg) or hypoxia (apnea or cyanosis in the field or PaO_2 <60 mmHg by arterial blood gas analysis) were strongly associated with significant increases in morbidity and mortality after TBI. In particular, hypotension was associated with a 150% increase in mortality. Several other studies have reported similar results. Although class I evidence is lacking, the strength of the class II evidence supports a level II recommendation to both avoid and rapidly treat hypoxia and hypotension to improve outcome in patients with severe TBI.

Establishing an airway to prevent hypoxemia in TBI patients and giving fluids to treat shock are critical to ensure the best possible outcome. Ideally, such measures are initiated at the scene of the accident. In addition to the skills of the personnel, however, the existence of an organized trauma system also contributes significantly to improved patient outcomes. Historically, patients were taken to the nearest available hospital for treatment regardless of the resources available at that hospital. With the development of trauma systems, patients were initially treated at the nearest facility and then triaged after stabilization to the level of care appropriate for their injuries. Some studies now suggest that outcomes may be improved when patients with severe TBI are triaged from the scene directly to tertiary trauma centers with resources necessary to optimally care for brain-injured patients.

Pearl

Some studies have suggested that outcomes may be improved when patients with severe TBI are triaged from the scene directly to tertiary trauma centers with resources necessary to optimally care for brain-injured patients.

In 1987, Baxt and Moody[7] demonstrated a decrease in mortality from severe TBI patients who were transported via helicopter by trained personnel who could obtain a secure airway and administer intravenous fluids, as opposed to a cohort treated by basic life support providers and transported by ground. The mortality in the aeromedically transported patients was 31%, versus 40% in the ground-transported patients. The majority of the helicoptered patients were injured in rural settings, and despite a longer transport time than the urban ground-transported group (57 versus 23 minutes), they had significantly less mortality *and* morbidity (class III data). Presumably, the trauma system worked for these patients by ameliorating hypoxia and hypotension early and by delivering them to definitive care without undue delay. Mullins et al[8] evaluated the association between implementation of a statewide trauma system and changes in distribution of admissions and risk of death. They found that of all trauma patients, those with TBI benefited the most from triage to level I trauma centers. The risk of death was decreased, with an odds ratio [95% confidence interval (CI)] of 0.8 (0.69–0.94) (class III data). This study included both direct admissions from the scene and patients who were initially treated at lower-designated trauma centers first. As with the Baxt study, a portion of the improvement in outcome was likely due to implementation of statewide ATLS guidelines for resuscitation of patients.

Pearl

Implementation of a statewide trauma system, with triage of severe TBI patients directly to level I trauma centers, has been associated with decreased mortality, especially in severe TBI patients.

A study from Quebec in 1997 sought to evaluate the morbidity and mortality of severely injured urban trauma patients who were triaged directly to a level I trauma center versus mortality of those who were transferred after being initially stabilized at a lower-designated hospital (class II data).[9] With regard to head injury, there was little difference between the groups if the injuries were stratified to low (Abbreviated Injury Score [AIS]$\leq$2) or high (AIS$\geq$4) severity. For those with moderate injuries (AIS = 3), the mortality among transferred patients was significantly higher than that in the directly triaged group ($p = .05$). The odds ratio (95% CI) was 2.69 (1.00– 7.93). Although the Canadian health care system is different from the U.S. model, this observational study still supports the recommendation of directly transporting severe TBI patients to definitive care and bypassing lower-designated hospitals.

Recommendations

For patients who sustain severe TBI in urban and suburban areas, treatment should be centered on ATLS guidelines and rapid transport to a level I trauma center with neurosurgical and critical care capabilities (level II). More controversy surrounds recommendations pertaining to patients injured in rural areas. Ideally, such patients should be treated according to standard ATLS guidelines and flown via helicopter to definitive neurotrauma care (level II). Clearly there are times when this will not be feasible due to lack of resources, the weather, or the presence of other life-threatening injuries that need immediate attention. In these cases, the best care of the brain injury is to maintain adequate blood pressure and oxygenation with fluids and inotropes as indicated. Transport should be arranged as soon as possible. An excellent document regarding the prehospital management of TBI is the Brain Trauma Foundation's "Guidelines for Prehospital Management of Traumatic Brain Injury,"[10] available at *www.braintrauma.org* under the *Guidelines* section. These should be read by all who participate in the care and transport of these patients.

References

1. Sosin DM, Sniezek JE, Thurman DJ. Incidence of mild and moderate brain injury in the United States, 1991. Brain Inj 1996;10:47–54.
2. Shackford SR, Mackerzie RC, Holbrook TL, et al. The epidemiology of traumatic death: a population-based analysis. Arch Surg 1993;128:571–575.
3. Committee on Trauma and Committee on Shock, Division of Medical Sciences. Accidental Death and Disability: The Neglected Disease of Modern Society. Washington, DC: National Academy of Sciences National Research Council; 1966.
4. Mock CN, Maier RV, Boyle E, et al. Injury prevention strategies to promote helmet use decrease severe head injury at a level I trauma center. J Trauma 1995;39:29–33.
5. Cannon WB. Traumatic shock. New York: Appleton; 1923.
6. Chesnut RM, Marshall LF, Klauber MR, et al. The role of secondary brain injury in determining outcome from severe head injury. J Trauma 1993;34:216–222.
7. Baxt WG, Moody P. The impact of advanced prehospital emergency care on the mortality of severely brain-injured patients. J Trauma 1987;27:365–369.
8. Mullins RJ, Veum-Stone J, Hedges JR, et al. Influence of a statewide trauma system on location of hospitalization and outcome of injured patients. J Trauma 1996;40:536–545.
9. Sampalis JS, Denis R, Frechette P, et al. Direct transport to tertiary trauma centers versus transfer from lower level facilities: impact on mortality and morbidity among patients with major trauma. J Trauma 1997;43:288–295.
10. Brain Trauma Foundation. Guidelines for Prehospital Management of Traumatic Brain Injury. Available at *http://www2.braintrauma.org/guidelines/btf_guidelines_ prehospital.pdf*

Index

Note: Page numbers followed by *f* or *t* refer to figures and tables, respectively.